The Development of American Physiology

THE HENRY E. SIGERIST SERIES
IN THE HISTORY OF MEDICINE

The Development of American Physiology

Scientific Medicine in the Nineteenth Century

W. BRUCE FYE

THE JOHNS HOPKINS UNIVERSITY PRESS
BALTIMORE AND LONDON

© 1987 The Johns Hopkins University Press
All rights reserved
Printed in the United States of America

The Johns Hopkins University Press
701 West 40th Street   Baltimore, Maryland 21211
The Johns Hopkins Press Ltd., London

Consulting Editor in the History of Medicine: Caroline Hannaway

The paper used in this publication meets the minimum requirements of American
National Standard for Information Sciences—Permanence of Paper for Printed
Library Materials, ANSI Z39.48-1984.

Library of Congress Cataloging-in-Publication Data

Fye, Bruce.
The development of American physiology.

(The Henry E. Sigerist series in the history of medicine)
Bibliography: p.
Includes index.
1. Physiology—United States—History. 2. Physiolo-
gists—United States—History. I. Title. II. Series.
[DNLM: 1. Physiology—history—United States.
QT 11 AA1 F997d]
QP21.F9 1987   612′.00973   86-33801
ISBN 0-8018-3459-7

To my parents, wife, and daughters

Contents

CONTENTS

Acknowledgments

THIS BOOK REPRESENTS the culmination of research that began in 1976 when I was a fellow in cardiology at the Johns Hopkins School of Medicine. With the encouragement and indulgence of Victor A. McKusick and Myron L. Weisfeldt I was able to combine a two-year master's program in medical history with activities as a fellow and junior faculty member of the cardiology division. This special course was made possible by a grant from the clinical scholars program of the Robert Wood Johnson Foundation, and William B. Greenough deserves my thanks for helping to arrange it. A. McGehee Harvey served as my adviser during my appointment as a clinical scholar at Hopkins. His consistent encouragement, advice, and friendship have been deeply appreciated.

My interest in American physiology and its implications for the development of modern medical education in America can be traced to a casual reading of Wilburt Davison's essay "Osler's Opposition to 'Whole-Time Clinical Professors,'" and to the suggestion of Richard A. Wolfe that "full-time started with Henry Bowditch—you should look at his papers at the Countway." This perceptive observation led me to select Henry Bowditch as the focus of my 1978 master's essay at Johns Hopkins.

From 1976 to 1978 the Institute of the History of Medicine of the Johns Hopkins University served as the institutional focus for my historical activities. Lloyd Stevenson accepted me as a postdoctoral fellow; his reading of my essay on Bowditch was helpful. Jerome Bylebyl, Caroline

Hannaway, and Owsei Temkin freely shared their ideas and responded to mine with useful suggestions; they continue to do so. Janet Koudelka merits my thanks for her encouragement during the formative stages of my historical "life."

From our days together in Baltimore, William Coleman has patiently listened to my ideas and has shared his valuable insight into the history of modern biology with me on many occasions. His careful reading of a draft of this manuscript was helpful and was deeply appreciated. Once I left Johns Hopkins to enter medical practice at the Marshfield Clinic in 1978, I had less time for (but no less interest in) historical research. Once in Wisconsin, I came to depend on my colleagues in the history of medicine department of the University of Wisconsin for encouragement and inspiration. Ronald Numbers challenged me to complete this book when my enthusiasm waned in the midst of too many commitments. He, too, read the entire manuscript and made perceptive observations and valuable comments. His insight into American science and social history has been particularly helpful.

Something must be said about the challenge of completing this project in the context of a life as a practicing physician. I empathize with the part-time physiologists of a century ago, such as S. Weir Mitchell, who sought to combine research with a busy medical practice. It is not easy. My colleagues at the Marshfield Clinic, particularly the other cardiologists, have generously supported my historical activities that take me away from practice. Without their indulgence this book would never have been completed. My medical assistants over the years, Bernie Soley Roggenbauer, Vicki Greenwald, and Sheila Dietel, and my secretary Marilynn Tesmer have helped in many ways. I am deeply grateful to Nancy Northup who has been my stenographer for nine years and has typed thousands of pages of notes as well as all of the drafts of this book.

Although my research has been facilitated by a personal medical history book collection of several thousand volumes, I have depended on many librarians over the years. They have obtained hundreds of articles and volumes on interlibrary loan and have assisted me in many ways. My sincere thanks to the staff of the Welch Medical Library during the Baltimore years and to the staff of the Marshfield Medical Library and the Middleton Health Sciences Library of the University of Wisconsin since 1978. I would particularly like to thank Albert Zimmerman, Alana Ziaya, and Dorothy Whitcomb for the extraordinary effort they have expended on behalf of my historical work.

Archivists and librarians at many institutions deserve my gratitude for their valuable assistance in uncovering and copying the many manuscripts that were used in the preparation of this book. Institutions that have granted permission for using excerpts from their archival and manuscript materials in this book include the Academy of Natural Sciences of Philadelphia, the American Philosophical Society, the American Physiological Society, the College of Physicians of Philadelphia, Columbia University, Duke University, the Francis A. Countway Library of Medicine, Harvard University, the Historical Society of Pennsylvania, the Jefferson Medical College, the Johns Hopkins University, the Johns Hopkins Medical Institutions, the Medical and Chirurgical Faculty of the State of Maryland, the National Library of Medicine, the New York Public Library, Northwestern University, the Osler Library at McGill University, the Smithsonian Institution, the University of Alabama in Birmingham, the University of Michigan, the University of Pennsylvania, Washington University, the Wellcome Institute for the History of Medicine, Williams College, and Yale University.

The editors of the *Bulletin of the History of Medicine* and the *Journal of the History of Medicine and Allied Sciences* have given permission to incorporate in this volume some previously published material.

Many individuals throughout the country contributed in various ways to my research into the professionalization of physiology and the origins of modern medical education in America. Among them are Toby Appel, Saul Benison, Gert Brieger, Gerald Geison, Judith Walzer Leavitt, John Parascandola, Guenter Risse, and Charles Rosenberg. Henry Tom of the Johns Hopkins University Press provided many helpful suggestions and valuable criticism. I am grateful to him and his staff for the effort they have expended on this project.

Finally, on a more personal note, my parents deserve my deep appreciation for their support and their example. I wish to thank my wife Lois for her encouragement and her willingness to share me with both medicine and history. I also thank my young daughters Katherine and Elizabeth for their patience.

Introduction

DURING THE SECOND HALF of the nineteenth century, American physiology emerged from the amorphous "institutes of medicine" to become, in Abraham Flexner's words, "the central discipline of the medical school."[1] The forces that led to this transformation and its impact on the development of American medical education form the substance of this book. Two fundamental characteristics of contemporary medical education—the full-time faculty system and the research ethic—emerged as a result of the efforts of a coalition of reformers who sought to make medicine more scientific. The full-time faculty concept is the belief that teachers of the scientific medical branches (e.g., anatomy, physiology, pathology) should refrain from medical practice and devote themselves exclusively to their duties as teachers and investigators. This scheme was eventually expanded to include clinical teachers as well. By "research ethic" I mean the conviction that medical teachers have an obligation to society to attempt to expand medical knowledge through research. America's first professional physiologists were central figures in a coalition of scientists, educators, medical editors, and scientifically oriented physicians who sought to make American medicine scientific a century ago.

Although Americans made some notable contributions to science and technology during the first half of the nineteenth century, the nation lagged perceptibly behind Europe in the development of the new laboratory-based sciences. Americans were particularly sensitive to the superiority of European science in an era of heightened nationalism following the Civil War. Some Americans argued that greater support for research and more opportunities for scientific careers were necessary if the United States was to compete with Europe in the discovery of knowledge. Individuals such as Joseph Henry of the Smithsonian Institution and Louis Agassiz of Harvard set the agenda: convince college and university trustees that their faculties must undertake research for the good of their institutions and the welfare of the nation. They argued that all Americans would benefit from technological developments made possible by scientific research and cited many examples to support this claim: the train, the steamship, the telegraph, and improved and more efficient weapons, to name but a few.

Scientific schools founded in the middle of the nineteenth century reflected recognition of the need for native institutions to train Americans in the newer techniques and ideas of science. The scope of this enterprise expanded during the final quarter of the century with the advent of a new generation of university presidents at some of America's most prestigious institutions of higher learning. Charles W. Eliot of Harvard, James B. Angell of the University of Michigan, Andrew D. White of Cornell, and Daniel Coit Gilman of Johns Hopkins were young and ambitious. They shared an interest in science, visited European universities and laboratories, and sought to redirect American higher education so the nation would no longer be subservient to Europe for new knowledge and advanced training in the arts and sciences.

These progressive university presidents encouraged, to the degree their institutions' finances permitted, the adoption of the research ethic at their schools. In their view, a university professor could no longer simply transmit knowledge derived from standard printed sources; he had an obligation to add to the information base of his chosen field. During the last quarter of the nineteenth century, this research ethic, already well established in German universities, gradually permeated the elite institutions of higher learning in the United States. By the end of the century, it had made inroads into the basic medical science programs in the nation's leading medical schools as well.

Eliot, Angell, and Gilman had reason to be particularly interested in medical education. Harvard and the University of Michigan had medical schools, and Johns Hopkins, a wealthy Quaker merchant, had endowed a hospital as well as a university in Baltimore. Physiologists joined the reform movement when it was already under way. Indeed, these university presidents made possible their participation in it. The physiologists adopted the goals of the educational reformers because university presidents and their supporters were addressing the needs of the medical scientists who sought jobs and facilities where they could perform research.

In principle, the physiologists' goals were based on a system that worked well in Europe. The full-time faculty concept and the research ethic originated abroad and were transmitted to medical schools in the United States as part of the movement to reform higher education in the postbellum era. The challenge was to stimulate adequate philosophical and financial support to adopt the sophisticated and expensive European approach to medical teaching and research. Until there were rewards, or at least salaries and job security, for performing medical research, the reformers' goals remained elusive. Physicians derived their incomes from seeing patients, and medical teachers were paid to lecture. These well-established patterns in the United States were not easily influenced by simple rhetoric.

Once a physician was in practice, he was unlikely to alter significantly his opinions or behavior. Attitudes toward medical science and practice were shaped during medical training. The reformers concluded that an appreciation of medical science and research could best be introduced into the medical profession through its new graduates. If medical teachers were to be the agents of change, however, they had to reorder their priorities. They had to be imbued with a spirit of inquiry, and be willing to give up medical practice for the cause of scientific medicine.

To accomplish their goal of making American medicine more scientific, the reformers sought to replace the part-time practitioner-professors of the basic medical sciences with full-time scientists whose value system differed from that of their predecessors. The reformers argued that medicine could be elevated from the level of an empirical craft to the stature of a science only through research. Moreover, this research had to be sponsored by the medical schools or special institutes committed to investigation, and society should be willing to pay for it.

Those who wanted to reform American medicine hoped to endow it with the authority of science. This is where physiology, the science dealing with the functions of living organisms, entered the picture. Claude Bernard, the leader of French physiology, set the agenda in 1865, when he claimed that "experimental physiology is the most scientific part of medicine, and . . . in studying it, young physicians will acquire scientific habits." Experimental medicine, synonymous with scientific medicine in Bernard's view, could only be fostered by "spreading the scientific spirit more and more among physicians." Thomas H. Huxley, the British champion of scientific education, had claimed a decade earlier that "physiology is *the* experimental science *par excellence* of all sciences." Although it took half a century, this philosophy was adopted in American medical schools. As historian Owsei Temkin observed two decades ago, "During the last hundred years, medicine has come to place an almost unprecedented reliance on physiology. This juncture was reached when experimental physiology became the foundation of experimental medicine."[2] Anatomy, the most traditional scientific course in the medical curriculum, did not serve Bernard's purpose; it was descriptive, not experimental, and experimentation was the only method by which medicine could advance.

Physiology provided the link between the larger educational reform movement championed by the university presidents and the previously ineffective efforts of physicians to elevate the standards of American medical education. The physiologists adapted the agenda of the educational reformers to suit their needs, and the needs of those who shared their interests, concerns, and ambitions. To show the central role the physiologists played in the movement to make American medicine more scientific, I explore two related themes. First, I describe the individual, institutional, and social factors that contributed to the emergence of physiology as a discipline in the United States. To accomplish this, I review the careers of four pioneering American physiologists: John C. Dalton, Jr., S. Weir Mitchell, Henry P. Bowditch, and H. Newell Martin. Their careers illustrate the critical stages of the professionalization of physiology in America. Second, I attempt to elucidate the relationship of the evolution of this discipline to the introduction of the full-time faculty system and the research ethic into medical education in the United States.

Although many fields, nonscientific as well as scientific, emerged as distinct disciplines during the closing years of the nineteenth century, the elevation of physiology to the status of a profession had major implications for medical education and practice. Even though physiology remained dependent on medicine for its manpower, funding, and many of its research themes throughout the nineteenth century, it also gained in stature. Experimental approaches championed by leaders of science in Europe resulted in discoveries that had practical implications for physicians and their patients. Description was gradually giving way to laboratory-based experimentation, the approach best understood by a younger generation who had been exposed to it in the European universities. With success came authority. Physiologists and their full-time colleagues in the other basic medical sciences ultimately became the spokesmen for the new scientific medicine. Moreover, they played a major role in reshaping the philosophy and structure of American medical education.

To be sure, physicians had long attempted to add to their prestige and influence by claiming their practice was based on science. American physicians could not credibly make this assertion in the mid-1800s. Aside from a few notable successes like the highly regarded experiments of William Beaumont and the discovery of anesthesia, Americans made relatively few contributions to medical knowledge during most of the nineteenth century.[3] American physicians were too busy earning a living from medical practice to devote time to research, and the United States had almost no full-time medical scientists in this era. Most of America's medical professors cared little for science; their goal was to train "practical" physicians.

In 1846, there were only two hundred medical school professors to instruct more than four thousand pupils in the nation's thirty-three regular medical schools. Each school had an average of six professors, virtually all of whom were active practitioners who devoted a few hours a week to didactic instruction.[4] Currently, there are about fifteen times as many medical students, but nearly three hundred times as many medical faculty members—and these are full-time, not part-time, medical teachers. A century ago there were fewer than a dozen full-time physiology professors in America's medical schools. Today, there are seven hundred full-time professors of physiology and a total of fifteen thousand paid positions in the basic medical sciences in America's medical schools.[5] Unlike their predecessors of a century ago, most present-day physiology "teachers" engage primarily in research, not instruction. This book seeks to explain the origins of this dramatic increase in the number of medical school teachers and the even more significant shift in the focus of their activities.

In the middle of the nineteenth century, traditional methods of pursuing scientific research were coming under increasing scrutiny. Virtually all individuals who viewed themselves as scientists in antebellum America were amateurs in the sense that they did not earn their living primarily from their scientific activities. Some held teaching positions in institutions of higher learning, but they were paid to teach, not to do research. Knowledge was generally advanced by men inspired by their own intellectual curiosity and motivated by their own determination. There was no institutional pressure to undertake research, and few rewards, either in prestige or money, to encourage it. Individuals without means found it necessary to develop elaborate and innovative arrangements to subsidize their research. They might teach at a school or college, go on the lecture circuit at the height of the lyceum movement, write textbooks, or have a paying job unrelated to their scientific interests. Johns Hopkins's first president, Daniel Gilman, claimed this situation still existed in the United States in the 1880s.[6]

The second half of the nineteenth century was a time of rapid and dramatic change in many aspects of American society. Developments with special relevance to the professionalization of physiology included the university movement, the endowment-of-research crusade, the trend toward specialization in many fields of endeavor, and the persistent efforts of a few scientists to establish career opportunities for themselves, their protégés, and their colleagues. Americans' expectations for their health and their society grew as discoveries and new techniques were reported from the European laboratories and clinics. The call to reform American medical education became more impassioned and unrelenting. Traditionalists argued, however, that the American context demanded nominal entrance requirements and a brief course that emphasized practical rather than theoretical knowledge. America's unique geographic and cultural characteristics had long been the scapegoat for the unwillingness of medical schools to elevate their standards. Eventually, this excuse seemed hopelessly inadequate to justify the widening gap between American and European contributions to medical science.

After several decades of frustration, the reformers finally triumphed—not as a result of a sudden coup orchestrated by America's handful of scientifically oriented medical teachers, educators, scientists, or their supporters, but by a prolonged campaign to change the medical profession's and society's attitude about the role of science in medicine. Eventually their plan worked. As older professors died, retired, or went into full-time medical practice, they were replaced by younger individuals, most of whom had received postgraduate training abroad. There, they witnessed the elaborate German system of medical education that supported full-time scientists to do research and train others to carry out investigations. When they returned to the United States, some young medical graduates sought, and won, scientific posts in America's leading medical schools. Gradually, the practitioner-teachers were relegated to a secondary role in teaching the scientific courses, and ultimately they were limited to teaching the clinical branches.

To illustrate the maturation of American physiology I have chosen four important individuals. Dalton was his generation's leading champion of vivisection, the fundamental technique of experimental physiology. He was ill and occupied with administrative duties in 1887 when Mitchell, Bowditch, and Martin suggested the formation of a national society for physiology to their scientific colleagues. A combination of individual, institutional, and regional factors shaped the careers of these four physiologists. The larger social context also influenced their roles in the professionalization of American physiology and the reform of medical education.

Following their contact with European physiology, the four wanted to reform the teaching of this subject in America. Each was deeply interested in research and sought access to laboratory facilities in which to carry on his experiments. Experimental physiology now necessitated a stable institutional focus and a source of financial support. The expectations of the earliest physiologists I consider, Dalton and Mitchell, were modest; their model was French physiology. Their mentor, Claude Bernard, worked under humble, almost primitive conditions when they studied with him in 1850. When they returned to antebellum America from Europe the United States had no physiological laboratories. Their ambitions for themselves and for physiology were moderated by the contemporary state of science and medical education in the United States. Dalton and Mitchell did not require elaborate facilities for their research, and neither established advanced training programs in physiology. They did transfer the philosophy and the techniques of French physiology to America, however. Both taught the subject using vivisections and demonstrations and tried to imbue their pupils with a respect for medicine as a science based on experimentation rather than speculation.

Two decades after Dalton and Mitchell studied with Bernard, another American, Henry P. Bowditch, found circumstances in the French physiologist's laboratory intolerable. Aware of the superiority of the new German physiological institutes, Bowditch left Paris to study with the new leaders of medical science including Carl Ludwig. The agenda and the facilities of the German physiologists exceeded those of the French, and it was the German model of science and medical education that Bowditch sought to introduce into America in the early 1870s. After spending nearly two years in Carl Ludwig's physiological institute at Leipzig, Bowditch returned to the Harvard Medical School, where he established the first physiological laboratory in America in which advanced workers were taught firsthand the new techniques of experimental medicine. Moreover, Bowditch introduced (on a rather modest scale) a program of European-style biomedical research at Harvard. He wanted a laboratory based on the German model, one large enough and sufficiently well equipped that several individuals could use it for their investigations. Bowditch confronted significant opposition but succeeded in achieving his goals because of family ties, independent wealth, and the influence of Harvard's new president, Charles W. Eliot.

Another ambitious scientist brought the hybrid British-German style of physiology to America in the 1870s under circumstances even more favorable than Bowditch's. H. Newell Martin, a native of Ireland, received his scientific training from Michael Foster and Thomas Huxley and viewed physiology as the fundamental component of the larger science of biology. When Martin came to the well-endowed Johns Hopkins University, with Daniel Gilman's help, he successfully introduced a sophisticated program of physiological research and advanced training into the United States. At the new Johns Hopkins University, Martin found unprecedented philosophical and financial support for his program. Committed to establishing physiology as a discipline in America, he eagerly sought advanced students for his program at Johns Hopkins.

The physiologists were not always successful in their efforts to promote scientific medicine. Mitchell remained in full-time practice after he was unable to win a physiology chair early in his career. He failed in his attempts to convince the trustees at Philadelphia's two prestigious medical schools that by 1860 physiology was an experimental, not a descriptive science. Mitchell also found them unresponsive to the assertion that a medical teacher who performed research was preferable to one who simply transmitted facts discovered by others. Mitchell's failure to win a physiology chair shows how local circumstances had the potential to retard, as well as facilitate, the growth of experimental physiology. Although not a professional physiologist, Mitchell had a profound impact on America's second generation of medical scientists. After not winning a physiology chair he joined the ranks of the educational reformers. It was in this capacity, and as a founder of the American Physiological Society, that he contributed to the introduction of the research ethic into American medicine.

Dalton, Mitchell, Bowditch, and Martin appreciated the importance of developing a network of influential friends and colleagues to achieve their goals. As Mitchell's career illustrates, trustees often made institutional decisions on the basis of influence rather than substance in this era. The four were eager to proclaim the importance of all science, and in particular their science, physiology, to the medical profession and to society as a whole. They did so by writing popular treatises and articles and by delivering lectures to nonmedical as well as professional groups. The physiologists believed science would ultimately benefit if the nation's youth received better instruction in science and were taught to appreciate its value to society.

Although they are not emphasized in this book, the scientific contributions of these four physiologists should not be overlooked. Their credibility in the world of scientific medicine, and among the reformers, was

due to their publications, and those of their pupils, as well as their philosophy. The medical and scientific communities of America and Europe held each of the four in high esteem. They were widely acknowledged as among the most productive American medical scientists during
their active careers. Bowditch and Martin produced men as well as
knowledge. Their pupils, and individuals influenced by Dalton and
Mitchell, swelled the ranks of the reformers during the closing years of
the century.

These four pioneers of experimental medicine trained or strongly
influenced most of the second generation of professional American physiologists. It is no coincidence that Harvard and Johns Hopkins were the
sites of the first successful programs in experimental physiology in America. To a significant degree, Charles Eliot and Daniel Gilman were responsible for shaping the local circumstances that made it possible to
introduce European-style experimental physiology into their institutions. Physiologists and other basic medical scientists trained in, or affiliated with, these two institutions played a significant role in the reform
of medical education during the closing years of the century.

The discipline of physiology grew slowly during the first two decades following the establishment of America's first physiological laboratory for students at the Harvard Medical School in 1871. Economic
and other social factors retarded the acceptance of the full-time faculty
model and the research ethic by America's medical schools. A century
ago most American medical practitioners were unconcerned with medical education beyond the financial threat the steady outpouring of new
physicians posed to their practices. They confronted intense competition
from a surplus of regular physicians and aggressive homeopaths and
other sectarian practitioners, and they had to deal with the harsh reali-
ties of country practice, or, if they practiced in a city, the threat of losing
their patients to specialists. When they became convinced that the reform of medical education along the European scientific model would
benefit them individually and collectively in the eyes of their patients,
America's practitioners began to join the scientists in their efforts to elevate the standards of medical education and encourage research by medical teachers.

The development of bacteriology was a critical event for the reform
movement that sought to make medicine scientific. Bacteriology lent
substance to the reformers' claims that research could benefit mankind.
The identification of bacteria helped prove the germ theory of disease
and held out the promise of a reduction in morbidity and mortality as
more was learned about the life history, spread, and effect of these organisms. The physiologists used the development of this collateral sci-

ence, which some initially claimed was part of physiology, to encourage the further development of their own discipline. As enthusiasm for bacteriology and its implications for public health reform grew, the physiologists and their allies had a practical reason for the scientific training of medical students; few contested this point.

The microscope joined the stethoscope as a symbol of the scientific physician. The value of the microscope in research lent credibility to the claim that medicine was scientific. Vivisection, not microscopy, was the fundamental method of experimental physiology, however. The new enthusiasm for the use of the microscope in medicine served the purposes of the reformers: its successful employment required specialized training by scientific teachers. Scientific practice, even the appearance of scientific practice, could enhance the image of physicians and increase their chances of financial success. In a popular guide addressing the social and economic aspects of medical practice, Baltimore physician Webster Cathell declared in 1882: "If, at your office and elsewhere, you make use of instruments of precision—the stethoscope, ophthalmoscope, laryngoscope, the clinical thermometer, magnifying glass and microscope, make urinary analyses, etc., they will not only assist you in diagnosis, but will aid you greatly in curing people by heightening their confidence in you and eliciting their co-operation."[7]

Economics was an important determinant of the philosophy and structure of medical education as well as medical practice. The fundamental reason for the repeated failures of earlier efforts to reform American medical education was the cost of the proposed curricular and staffing changes. Medical schools with short terms and a course confined to didactic lectures were at least marginally profitable. Any change to a longer or more sophisticated curriculum was financially risky. Students' fees were insufficient to support the new medical education. The scientific reformers of the progressive era were optimistic, however. They believed they could succeed if their cause was joined by enlightened medical practitioners, educators, medical editors, and influential members of American society. Endowment was becoming fashionable, and if attracted to medical education, it could be used to introduce the full-time faculty system, the research ethic, and other reforms in America's medical schools.

The physiologists became active spokesmen on behalf of the endowment of medical schools. Dalton, Mitchell, and Bowditch were responsible for attracting substantial endowments to their institutions. Alumni were told of the practical advances that resulted from the European system of medical education and research. Moreover, they were warned that competing medical schools would gain prestige through the construction of laboratories. Only a small percentage of alumni were willing to invest in their alma maters, however. The most promising source of money to supplement the students' fees was from philanthropists. But they too had limitations on the amount of money they would spend. The reformers persuaded philanthropists to support only those institutions willing to adopt or expand the new philosophy of scientific medical education.

To fulfill the promise of the full-time system, fundamental changes in the requirements for medical students were also necessary. The medical matriculants must be better prepared and have some knowledge of physics and chemistry, the foundations upon which the new experimental medical sciences were built. In addition to a new cadre of scientific teachers, laboratories were necessary—not just a small chamber or two for the private use of the professor, but large rooms amply supplied with modern instruments of precision and apparatus for experimentation. Practical training demanded additional staff to aid the professor in elementary teaching and in the laboratory. As the new philosophy of scientific medical education evolved, changes occurred at many levels. The new orientation toward practical laboratory training and bedside teaching affected everyone involved in learning, teaching, and practicing medicine. The physiologists and their scientific colleagues successfully lobbied for more time in the curriculum, laboratories for practical training, and additional staff in the basic medical sciences. Enthusiastic new scientific teachers worked hard to create an atmosphere that encouraged interest in science and a respect for research among their pupils.

The training, methods, and aspirations of basic science teachers in the nation's medical schools was gradually, but perceptibly changing. By the 1880s, the methods of investigation used to study the functions of the animal organism had become complex. Physiological research now depended on vivisection that required elaborate apparatus, sophisticated instruments of precision, and trained assistants. Medical practitioners could no longer perform significant physiological research during a few sporadic hours snatched from medical practice. It was claimed, and events confirmed, that it was now unlikely that a lone physician, however well intentioned, could be a successful and productive investigator in physiology. When physiology was redefined by Claude Bernard, Carl Ludwig, and other Europeans as an experimental rather than a descriptive science, the requirements for its pursuit changed. Only in the context of an institution, and a well-endowed one at that, could one hope to undertake successful physiological research.

The growing complexity of physiological research and the demands for more than simple lectures in physiology had major implications for those who taught or wished to teach this subject during the closing years of the nineteenth century. Previously, little more than a casual interest in physiology or comparative anatomy was required. The essence of the subject was simply transmitted to the unsophisticated student body in the form of didactic lectures; expectations of both teacher and student were minimal. Once a commitment to experimentation and research credentials were required of the professor of physiology, its traditional teachers found themselves in an increasingly untenable position. Instructors who had sought the chair of physiology to gain prestige and attract referrals to their medical practices now had to make a palpable commitment to science. By the 1890s, postgraduate training in an institution with a formal program in experimental physiology became a requirement for those hoping to teach physiology in one of America's leading medical schools.

The scientists who came to occupy the chairs of physiology and their full-time colleagues in the other basic medical sciences were obvious beneficiaries of the movement to reform medical education. They were now paid for doing science; their careers were subsidized by endowed medical institutions. There were trade-offs, however. The new standard demanded that teachers of the scientific branches devote all their time to academic duties. However tempting a medical practice might have been for financial, intellectual, or social reasons, it precluded success as a physiologist, or so the professionals claimed, and influential educators, scientists, and elite physicians came to believe. Amateurs were eventually excluded from teaching physiology as more and more institutions adopted the full-time faculty structure and the research ethic.

The professional physiologists were competitive for another reason: they were more mobile than the practitioner-teachers who were dependent on medical practice for most of their income. Consequently physiologists could switch institutions in order to find the most desirable full-time position. In 1868, when Mitchell failed a second time to win a physiology chair in Philadelphia, he gave up hope of ever getting an academic position in this subject. He did not consider moving to another city; his ties were to Philadelphia, and his practice was successful and growing. Full-time paid positions for physiologists were virtually nonexistent in this era, and it would have been risky for Mitchell to give up the security of friends, family, and a successful practice to relocate. A generation later, however, a few full-time positions in physiology made it possible for individuals to devote themselves exclusively to this science. William Howell, one of Martin's first pupils, moved from Baltimore to Ann

Arbor to Boston and back to Baltimore between 1887 and 1893 in an attempt to improve his lot as a full-time physiologist. Had he been a practitioner, these frequent moves would have been impossible.

The professional physiologists and their scientific colleagues in the developing fields of physiological chemistry, bacteriology, experimental pathology, and pharmacology grew in number and influence in the closing years of the nineteenth century. This group of basic medical scientists came to be viewed as the leaders of the new scientific medicine. University presidents, philanthropists, and many Americans were persuaded that medicine was a science and that the progress of medicine depended, in large part, on the efforts of the physiologists and their scientific colleagues in related biomedical disciplines. The full-time basic scientists also gained power in their own institutions. Although they were not practitioners, and could be criticized for not appreciating the challenges faced by physicians, the full-time basic scientists who embodied the research ethic became role models for many of the next generation of physicians. Nearly all medical graduates still went into practice, but they held a different view of the relevance and importance of research.

Basic science faculty members came to know the pupils early in their schooling, spent more hours with them than the part-time clinical teachers, and were more readily available: they did not have a practice to draw them to the office, home, or hospital where patients required care. Henry Bowditch became dean of the Harvard Medical School; the individual first approached had declined to serve because of the demands of his practice. Other physiologists also gained positions of influence within their institutions. Dalton became president of the College of Physicians and Surgeons of New York, and Mitchell became a member of the board of trustees of the University of Pennsylvania. In these positions, they encouraged the support of medical science and contributed to the establishment of the full-time faculty system and the research ethic in their medical schools. Their influence was felt beyond their local institutions as they participated in specialty organizations.

The establishment of the American Physiological Society represented the formalization of a network of scientists who shared common interests and concerns. Mitchell, Bowditch, and Martin collaborated in the formation of this society which demonstrated to the world that physiology had come of age in America. It was now a full-time profession with a commitment to research and to making America's physicians more scientific.

The public, too, benefited from the related developments of the professionalization of physiology and the adoption of the research ethic by America's leading medical schools. As the reformers had predicted, the full-time, research-oriented medical faculty members made more scientific discoveries. The reformers had long argued that Americans possessed the intelligence necessary to make meaningful contributions to knowledge; they simply needed the time and means to achieve this goal. During the twentieth century, as unprecedented philanthropic (and, later, government) support permitted the elevation of the standards of medical education, the expansion of the full-time system, and the adoption of the research ethic by many American medical schools, the United States steadily gained prominence in the world of biomedical science.

Canadian-born William Osler, one of America's leading physicians, claimed in 1901 that "the most distinguishing factor of the scientific medicine of the century has been the phenomenal results which have followed *experimental investigations. . . .* The researches of the physiological laboratories have enlarged in every direction our knowledge of the great functions of life." He asserted that the study of physiology and pathology during the second half of the nineteenth century had done more to emancipate medicine from "the thraldom of authority" than all the efforts of physicians since the time of Hippocrates. Osler was optimistic about the future since specialization in science, a characteristic of the age, was "the most important single factor in the remarkable expansion of our knowledge" and would surely lead to further breakthroughs.[8] Sociologist Joseph Ben-David agreed, and showed that "the development of scientific research into a separate profession brought about a considerable acceleration in the process of discovery."[9]

The success of American medicine in the twentieth century can be traced to the introduction of the research ethic into America's medical schools and collateral developments in the preliminary and professional training of physicians in the United States. Consistent financial support, first by philanthropists, and later by the federal government, was necessary to import and customize the European model of scientific medical education. The goals of America's first professional physiologists and their scientific colleagues seemed ambitious a century ago. Today, the contribution they made to the development of modern medical education and the research establishment in the United States is little appreciated. It is my hope that this book demonstrates the critical role they and their scientific colleagues played in making American medicine scientific.

CHAPTER ONE

John Call Dalton, Jr.

Pioneer Vivisector and America's
"First Professional Physiologist"

S. WEIR MITCHELL CLAIMED that John Call Dalton, Jr., was "our first professional physiologist."[1] Dalton (1825–1889) earned his living by teaching physiology and by writing physiology texts. Giving up medical practice to become a full-time physiologist and medical teacher distinguished Dalton from physicians who made contributions to physiology but whose income was largely derived from medical practice or whose teaching responsibilities included other subjects in addition to physiology. William Beaumont, Samuel Jackson, and Robley Dunglison contributed to this science but none merits the distinction of being called America's first professional physiologist.

Dalton's significance to American science and medicine transcends his role as the nation's first professional physiologist. A pupil of Claude Bernard, he introduced the French style of physiology with its emphasis on vivisection into the United States. For the first time, American medical students were taught physiology by demonstrations including vivisection in addition to traditional didactic lectures. During a career at the College of Physicians and Surgeons of New York that spanned most of the second half of the nineteenth century, Dalton taught thousands of medical students and served as a role model for future physicians and physician-scientists. He possessed, in Mitchell's words, "the rare gift of making those who listened desire to become investigators."[2]

An avid experimentalist, Dalton made several discoveries in gastrointestinal physiology and neurophysiology. The scope of his research was broad, however, and included studies in embryology and microscopic anatomy as well as experimental physiology, subjects considered part of physiology in America in the mid-nineteenth century. Although Dalton introduced experimental demonstrations into his physiology course, he did not develop a physiological laboratory for students. His research was carried out in a small private laboratory at the college. A prolific author, Dalton wrote elementary textbooks for the lay public and secondary school students in addition to numerous scientific articles and a highly regarded physiology text for physicians and medical students.

Dalton's most important role in the development of American physiology was his sustained, articulate, and effective response to the American antivivisection movement, precipitated, in part, by his use of vivisection in New York. He realized, however, that any restriction imposed on experimentation because of the New York–based antivivisectionists would have national impact. For two decades, Dalton was the chief spokesman for the scientific community in their battle with the antivivisectionists. In this role, the New York physiologist outlined the benefits of research to mankind in a thoughtful and persuasive manner.

Throughout his life, Dalton participated in several local and national societies. This involvement enhanced his visibility and fostered his image as a leader of medical science in America. In his late fifties, Dalton became president of the College of Physicians and Surgeons of New York, one of the most prestigious medical schools in the United States. Recognizing the growing importance of restructuring both the philosophy and content of medical education in America, he worked hard to obtain endowments for laboratories and salaries in the closing years of his life. Dalton's long career at one of the nation's leading medical schools demonstrated the feasibility of a life devoted exclusively to physiology teaching and research.

Dalton was born in Chelmsford, Massachusetts, in 1825 and was the son of a prominent local medical practitioner. His father graduated from Harvard College and attended medical lectures at Harvard and the University of Pennsylvania before receiving his medical degree from Harvard in 1818. The elder Dalton then entered practice in the village of Chelmsford where he replaced Rufus Wyman who had been appointed superintendent of the asylum for the insane in Charlestown. The friendship of the Wyman and Dalton families had a significant effect on young Dalton.[3] Dr. Dalton relocated his practice to the growing community of Lowell in 1831 when his son was six. It was in this town of eight thousand people and fifteen physicians that John Jr. was introduced to the practice of medicine. Young Dalton's interest in the scientific side of medicine can be traced, in part, to his acquaintance with Jeffries Wyman, the physician-naturalist. Jeffries, Rufus Wyman's son, was also born in Chelmsford and served as apprentice to Dalton's father when John was eleven.

Following graduation from the Harvard Medical School in 1833 and completion of an apprenticeship in the elder Dalton's office in 1836, Jeffries Wyman entered practice in Boston. Dr. Dalton encouraged Jeffries to practice in Boston but cautioned, "To be sure, a young man must wait patiently for patronage, but when it does come, it is worth having."[4] Jeffries's older brother, Morrill, was a successful physician in Cambridge, but Jeffries's Boston practice grew slowly.[5] Jeffries, like many other aspiring American medical graduates of the era, had traveled abroad for postgraduate study. While in Europe he was exposed to many leaders of French medical science, including François Magendie, the great pioneer of vivisection and experimental physiology.

A career in medical science and teaching rather than practice appealed to Wyman as it would to his young friend and protégé Dalton. Upon his return from Europe, Wyman settled in Richmond, Virginia, where he had been appointed professor of anatomy and physiology in the medical department of Hampden-Sidney College. When asked by one of his colleagues in Richmond whether he anticipated opening an office to see patients, Wyman replied, "I told him that if I held the professorship I had no wish to practice, & if I did not, my residence here would soon terminate."[6] By the age of thirty, Wyman was already a productive naturalist and the author of more than a score of papers. He grew frustrated with the intellectual isolation of his Richmond post, however, and revealed to his brother Morrill his desire to obtain a teaching position in natural history at Harvard.

Wyman's opportunity to return to Boston resulted from the resignation of John Collins Warren as Hersey Professor of Anatomy and Surgery at Harvard. Warren's resignation led to a reorganization of the chair: surgery was separated from anatomy and two anatomy chairs were established. Oliver Wendell Holmes became the Parkman Professor of Anatomy and Physiology at the Harvard Medical School in Boston, and Wyman was appointed Hersey Professor of Anatomy at Cambridge. As would be the case with Dalton, Wyman believed that the basic medical sciences were an essential part of the medical curriculum.[7]

The elder Dalton acknowledged his former pupil's Harvard appointment, "I cannot resist sending you my congratulations on your appointment to a Professors chair in our honored Alma Mater. . . . I have watched with never flagging interest your own & Morrill's advancement to distinguished positions in your professions & I trust that health & long life wait upon you to enable you to attain its very first ranks."[8] Although the younger Dalton's education at Harvard College and Harvard Medical School coincided with the time Wyman spent most of the year in Richmond, there is no doubt that the physician turned naturalist was a role model for Dalton.

Another individual who influenced Dalton during his youth was Elisha Bartlett. Following his medical education in Providence, Rhode Island, Bartlett spent a year of postgraduate training in Europe and returned to become one of the chief American proponents of the French school of medicine. Bartlett practiced in Lowell but was a peripatetic professor who taught pathological anatomy, materia medica, and the theory and practice of medicine at several medical schools during the 1830s and 1840s. As two physicians in the small town of Lowell, Bartlett and Dalton's father probably came into frequent contact. Young Dalton was exposed to Bartlett's enthusiasm for the French school expressed in his volume of biographical sketches of the leading physicians and surgeons of Paris.[9]

In 1844, the year Dalton graduated from Harvard College and enrolled in the Harvard Medical School, Bartlett proclaimed the independence of pathology and physiology, writing, *"Pathology is not founded upon physiology. The latter is not the basis of the former. The one does not flow from the other. Our knowledge of the one does not presuppose our knowledge of the other."*[10] Bartlett's statement anticipated the specialization that would characterize the basic medical sciences during Dalton's career. Ultimately, Dalton sought a position where he could devote himself to physiology as a subject independent from either anatomy or pathology, sciences with which it had long been combined under the title "Institutes of Medicine."

Attempting to explain the variations in scientific output in France, Great Britain, and the United States, Bartlett argued that the means and facilities for original research were superior in France compared with the other two countries. He also suggested other factors that might explain the difference in scientific productivity among the three nations. Professional jealousy and concern for success in practice were less prominent in France, where a greater degree of interest in medical research was present than in Great Britain or America. Although Bartlett anticipated a gradual narrowing of the gap, he concluded that the social factors that accounted for the national differences in the nature and results of medical research in the three countries would persist for a considerable period of time. Although the discovery of anesthesia two years later drew the world's attention to American medicine, Bartlett's prediction was essentially correct. Americans made few significant contributions to medical science until the structure and philosophy of medical education in the United States evolved to encourage research and to subsidize individuals who wanted to undertake it. It was in this movement that Dalton played a significant role.

When he matriculated at the Harvard Medical School in 1844, Dalton came into contact with several other scientifically oriented physicians who had studied in Paris and shared the interests and concerns of Wyman and Bartlett. Among Dalton's teachers were Oliver Wendell Holmes, Henry Ingersoll Bowditch, and John Collins Warren. While supplementing his Harvard education in Paris in 1833, Holmes wrote to his parents, "Merely to have breathed a concentrated scientific atmosphere like that of Paris must have an effect on anyone who has lived where stupidity is tolerated, where mediocrity is applauded, and where excellence is deified."[11] Like Wyman, Holmes was a full-time teacher of medical science and served as a role model for Dalton.

Although he practiced in Boston for a few years, Holmes relinquished practice altogether when he accepted the chair of anatomy and physiology at Harvard Medical School in 1847. Dalton's interest in experimental physiology cannot be traced to Holmes, however. Holmes focused his Paris training on pathological anatomy under Pierre Louis and Gabriel Andral, and at Harvard he emphasized anatomy over physiology in his combined course. Like his teacher Louis, Holmes disliked vivisection, and he taught his brief physiology course by lectures alone. All other American teachers of physiology in this era also used the lecture approach. Shortly, however, Dalton became one of the most vigorous proponents of vivisection as a teaching method in physiology. While a medical student in Boston, he had witnessed the first operation performed using anesthesia and realized, as did others who employed vivisection, that anesthesia would facilitate many of their animal experiments.[12]

While a medical student, Dalton was elected house apothecary at the Massachusetts General Hospital, where he also served as house surgeon following his graduation. Dalton gained practical experience in pathology during the cholera epidemic of 1849, when he performed post-mortem examinations on the majority of the patients who died in the Cholera Hospital. At this early stage of his career, Dalton's scientific leanings were already apparent. He became an active participant in the Boston Society for Medical Observation, founded in 1846 by Henry I. Bowditch. The society met bimonthly at the Boylston Medical School where members presented papers based on carefully documented clinical or pathological observations. Dalton's presentations before the society reflected his familiarity with the contemporary medical literature, dedication to detail, and interest in medical chemistry.

Emulating his Harvard teachers and his mentors Wyman and Bartlett, Dalton traveled to Europe for postgraduate training. This experience was of great significance in shaping Dalton's career. When the Harvard graduate arrived in Paris in 1850, Claude Bernard had recently assumed many of François Magendie's teaching responsibilities. When Dalton took courses from Bernard, the French physiologist's activities were undertaken in the context of limited funding, marginal equipment, a small and damp laboratory, and minimal encouragement from the government or the medical profession. Although his laboratory was cramped and inadequate for pupils, Bernard's demonstrations utilizing vivisection were enthusiastically received by students, who came in increasing numbers from Europe, Great Britain, and America. One of Bernard's main goals was to establish physiology as an autonomous discipline. Although he had completed medical studies and an internship in Paris, Bernard never practiced medicine and was ambivalent toward practitioners.

Bernard was Dalton's most important role model: he was a scientist who devoted himself to teaching and research in physiology. Although Bartlett proclaimed physiology's independence from pathology, he held many positions and practiced medicine. Wyman and Holmes did not practice, but their scientific leanings were not toward experimental physiology. Dalton's interest in medical science had been kindled by his childhood models and medical school teachers, but his career was shaped by his exposure to, and admiration for, Claude Bernard. As noted by historian Bruce Sinclair, other American scientists' professional lives were shaped by European study. For Franklin Bache, Asa Gray, and Joseph Henry, he proclaimed their first trip abroad "a crucial watershed in their scientific careers."[13]

Dalton returned from Paris imbued with a scientific spirit that led him to seek a position where he could teach physiology. Although he studied under Bernard at a time when the French physiologist's support was at its nadir, Dalton returned to America enthusiastic about experimental medicine and the potential role of vivisection in teaching. As Wyman and Holmes did, Dalton wanted to support himself by teaching and writing rather than by medical practice. There are several possible explanations for Dalton's decision not to engage in the practice of medicine: he saw his father confront the challenges of country practice; he was aware of Jeffries Wyman's difficulties in establishing a practice in Boston and his success in obtaining a scientific teaching position; and he was discouraged by the impotence of contemporary practitioners in combating disease. During the cholera epidemic of 1849, Dalton saw more than half of the patients die shortly after their admission to the Cholera Hospital in Boston.[14]

Dalton's first position as a physiology teacher was at the Boylston Medical School in Boston. Incorporated in 1847, it was the first New England medical institution to offer a three-year graded curriculum in which the scientific courses preceded the clinical lectures. Dalton's career at the Boylston School was brief, however. Responding to the competition the new school represented, the Harvard medical professors adopted a plan of a continuous whole-year session that resulted in the dissolution of the Boylston School. Uncertain about his future at the Boylston School, Dalton sought other opportunities to teach physiology.

In 1851 Dalton was appointed to the chair of physiology at the Buffalo Medical College where he used vivisections to complement his lectures. The brief medical term made it possible and his dependence upon students' fees made it necessary for Dalton to teach at more than one medical school. Lectures at Buffalo were delivered in the fall term, so some Buffalo teachers also held appointments at the Vermont Medical College in Woodstock, Vermont, where teaching began in early December.[15] Three years after he joined the Buffalo faculty, Dalton was elected professor of pathology and physiology at the Vermont Medical College. Dalton's appointment at Vermont was made possible by the resignation of Alonzo Clark who, with Elisha Bartlett, soon served as Dalton's link to New York City. Bartlett, who had known Dalton as a youth, taught at the Vermont School until 1853. During their final years on the Vermont faculty, Bartlett and Clark also taught at the College of Physicians and Surgeons of New York.

Dalton's physiology course at the Vermont Medical College was described by a contemporary reviewer:

> All the vivisections, which in the hands of Bernard have led to such splendid results, were repeated before the class. The action of all of the digesting fluids was examined in this manner, by means of fistulous openings. The various other phenomena, such as those referring to the nervous system, &c., which are more readily demonstrable to the eye, than understood from the study of books, were so presented that all had the opportunity of seeing for themselves.[16]

Dalton reported the results of his experiments on gastric juice in 1854, explaining he had "studied the gastric juice, at various times, by means of fistulae, artificially established in the stomach of the dog, after the method of Blondlot and Bernard."[17] While Dalton was studying with Bernard, the French physiologist was performing similar experiments.

In 1854, Dalton was invited to deliver lectures on physiology and microscopic anatomy at the College of Physicians and Surgeons in New York. The following year the professorships were restructured at the college, and Dalton was elected to fill the chair of physiology. By this time, the twenty-nine-year-old physiologist had already gained recognition as a popular lecturer whose students acknowledged his innovative use of vivisection. By the time he moved to New York, Dalton had published several papers that demonstrated his scientific talents, including an essay on the corpus luteum that won an American Medical Association prize.

The College of Physicians and Surgeons of New York was a direct descendant of the second medical school founded in America, King's College Medical School, chartered in 1767.[18] The college faculty acknowledged the increasing differentiation of the basic medical sciences in 1847 when they recommended the creation of a new chair of physiology and pathology, distinct from anatomy:

> The subject of physiology is now confided to the professor of anatomy. It has been found, however, that anatomy is required to be taught so minutely, to meet the wants of the students, that it is impossible for the same professor to do justice to the other branch. On the other hand, the recent application of improved microscopes to healthy and diseased structures, together with the great advances in the department of animal chemistry, and the light it has shed on the constitution of our bodies in health and disease, and upon healthy and disordered functions, leave an hiatus in these departments so great that, in the unanimous opinion of the Board, a new professorship is required.[19]

Alonzo Clark was selected to fill the chair of physiology and pathology created in 1847. Following the receipt of his medical degree from the College of Physicians and Surgeons in 1835, Clark studied in London and Paris where he was exposed to the leaders of the French school including Magendie, Andral, and Louis. Under the influence of these teachers, Clark began to shift his interest from chemistry to pathology. Clark's new course at the College of Physicians and Surgeons included demonstrations with the microscope as well as lectures on physiology and pathology. He did not employ vivisection, however, nor is there any evidence that he undertook research in either pathology or physiology.

The officers of the college were pleased with Clark's new course and applauded his innovations in medical teaching. Although Clark did not perform research, he recognized the growing importance of this activity. Indeed, he believed that physicians had an obligation to society to attempt to expand medical knowledge through research. In an 1853 address, Clark emphasized the interdependence of medical and scientific progress and explained that physiology had been "renovated" during the past two decades through experiment, the use of the microscope, and growing dependence on chemistry.[20]

A shift in Clark's interests during the 1840s made possible Dalton's appointment at the College of Physicians and Surgeons. Clark became increasingly involved in medical practice and was appointed attending physician at Bellevue Hospital in 1847. Reflecting the evolution of Clark's interests, the college restructured the chairs in 1854 so that pathology and practical medicine were united and physiology and microscopic anatomy became a separate appointment. This arrangement permitted physiology to assume, in Dalton's words, "a more independent position than before."[21]

Interest in science was increasing in New York when Dalton moved to the rapidly growing metropolis in 1855. The peripatetic European physiologist Charles-Edouard Brown-Séquard had recently visited America to lecture in several cities, including Philadelphia, Boston, and New York. Writing to Jeffries Wyman from New York in the fall of 1852 Brown-Séquard explained, "I am now lecturing . . . on Experimental Physiology and I am happy to say as a legitimate praise to the Medical Men of this country that in New York and in Philadelphia, I have met with much more Medical Men strongly interested in that Science than in Paris."[22]

Research, even the relatively simple research of the 1850s, cost money. The lack of financial support for experimentation discouraged many potential investigators. A motivated teacher in a tolerant institution could inaugurate a series of experiments, but without a source of income to subsidize the work, little could be accomplished. Dalton was aware of this problem, and it affected the goals he set for himself at the College of Physicians and Surgeons. Another medical scientist in New York, John W. Draper, explained the effect that limited funding had on his own research. Draper, professor of chemistry and physiology in the medical department of the University of New York, was a native of England who received his undergraduate education at University College,

London. He emigrated to America in 1832 hoping to find a teaching position in chemistry. After attending medical school at the University of Pennsylvania, where his interest in research was encouraged by Robert Hare and John K. Mitchell, Draper took a teaching position at the University of the City of New York where he hoped to continue his chemical investigations. He did not practice medicine but devoted himself exclusively to the teaching of chemistry and physiology when these chairs were united for him at the University of the City of New York in 1850.

In an 1853 address delivered to the alumni of the institution, Draper proclaimed that universities had an obligation to increase knowledge as well as to disseminate it. Draper denounced the common practice among American institutions of higher learning of measuring their success simply by the number of students they produced. Draper realized that research and laboratory training were expensive. Nevertheless, he was committed to practical laboratory training, even if his institution was not. He told the alumni:

> It will excite a smile among you to learn that the amount devoted to the support of the Laboratory, and intended also to meet the expenses of the course of lectures delivered to the Senior Class, was one hundred and twenty-five dollars a year; and, of late, even that has ceased. Yet, during the last fourteen years, the actual expenses incurred have been many thousand dollars; and it may, with perfect truth, be said, that the entire sum has come, not from the City, not from the University treasury, but from the private resources of a single individual.[23]

Draper, the "single individual" who subsidized the laboratory training, acknowledged that the purpose of his address was to stimulate endowment for his institution. Dalton, like Draper, became convinced of the importance of endowments for higher education in America. Gifts and endowments gradually came to institutions of higher learning, and later to medical schools. And medical scientists like Draper and Dalton catalyzed the endowment movement by emphasizing the utilitarian aspects of medical research. In the absence of endowments, extensive laboratory instruction and organized research were impossible in American medical schools.

Claude Bernard, Dalton's mentor, was becoming better known to American physicians during the 1850s. Americans learned of his remarkable discoveries in letters from recent medical graduates studying in Paris, and through his books and translations of his lectures. Some scientifically oriented American physicians were becoming impatient with the paucity of medical research on this side of the Atlantic. Francis

Donaldson, an American medical graduate who had recently studied in Europe, exclaimed in a review of Bernard's contributions to physiology: "That some of your readers will object to the conclusiveness of M. Bernard's doctrines, we doubt not; but we would remind them that it is scarcely fair to sit with folded arms, and reason about the probability of this or that physiological fact, without fortifying their opinions by experimental researches."[24]

Despite the pleas of Donaldson and others who shared his conviction that medical research deserved more encouragement in America, little could be accomplished without financial support. Research was neither expected nor rewarded. Dalton's appointment to the physiology chair at the College of Physicians and Surgeons was made not primarily on the basis of his commitment to, or accomplishments in, research. Students were not attracted to the New York institution simply because Dalton was a talented investigator. His popularity was due to his lecturing skills and his use of vivisection in classroom demonstrations. Nevertheless, his exposure to Claude Bernard and the techniques of modern experimental physiology made Dalton more desirable as a faculty member; he represented contemporary medical science at its best.

For most American medical graduates, the main purpose of study abroad was to increase their chances of success in the competitive world of medical practice. According to Benjamin Silliman, Jr., European training in modern scientific techniques could also enhance the competitiveness of a candidate for a medical school chair upon his return. The Yale chemist told one of his students in 1854:

> I think that there is a glorious field in Physiological Chemistry and
> my plan if I was of your age would be to go to Europe, perfect
> myself in general organic chemistry as a basis, study general and
> pathological anatomy at the same time and then turn in to the
> specialty of Physiological chemistry. . . . Such a preparation as I
> speak of would give a man great standing as a chemist and physi-
> ologist and open to him the best places in the country, which are
> in medical schools where such knowledge *made practical* and
> applied to the business of medicine, is most particularly wanted.[25]

Several Americans, writing in the middle of the nineteenth century, emphasized the growing practical utility of the basic medical sciences. William Cornell proclaimed the importance of comparative anatomy and physiology in 1854: "Almost all the knowledge we possess of the functions of the organs in our own species, has been derived from inspecting the organs and their uses in the lower animals. . . . Comparative anatomy and comparative physiology, then, are of great moment to every naturalist, and especially to every practising physician who wishes to employ the healing art *understandingly*."[26] Although this writer did not distinguish observation from experimentation, he did emphasize the importance of accurate observation. Two years earlier, Brown-Séquard wrote to Jeffries Wyman: "Fortunately the number of Speculative Physiologists is diminishing every year. I hope that, before long, under your influence and that of some other very intelligent young Anatomists existing now in the United States, theoretical physiology shall not be much longer taught in the best Medical Schools of this country."[27] Dalton had no intention of teaching theoretical physiology. Like his mentor Bernard, he sought to prove or disprove theory through experimentation.

The teaching of physiology was gradually assuming more importance in American medical schools as the country entered the second half of the century. In 1854, the committee on medical education of the American Medical Association resolved "that those medical colleges whose curriculum does not now include full courses of lectures on physiology and medical jurisprudence, be earnestly invited to make immediate provision for supplying the deficiency."[28] The authors of this report saw physiology as a science dependent on comparative anatomy, however. European experimental physiologists were rejecting this view, and Dalton's appointment in New York reflected the independence of physiology from both anatomy and pathology. In many people's minds, however, physiology remained a descriptive science more related to comparative anatomy than physics and chemistry.

When Dalton began teaching physiology at the College of Physicians and Surgeons, the population of New York was over one-half million people and the city had two other medical schools, the Medical College of the University of the City of New York and the New York Medical College. In his first introductory address as professor of physiology and microscopic anatomy, he outlined his philosophy of medical education. He advocated a graded curriculum in which the scientific courses preceded the clinical ones: "Instead of being homogeneous, the science of medicine is seen to be composed of several different departments,—the simpler of which must be thoroughly understood before we can approach the more complicated with any hope of success. A certain method, or order, in our studies therefore becomes necessary; for without it, progress is impossible." Dalton expanded on this theme:

> Anatomy is the description of the body in a state of rest. Physiology is the description of it in a state of activity. We see, then, that

the order in which these branches are arranged is not an arbitrary
one, but natural and necessary. One must precede,—the other
must follow. It is so with all the departments. But it is important
to bear in mind this fact:—that, *although the first is always a*
necessary preliminary to understanding the second, the facts of the
second cannot be, in the least degree, inferred from those of the
first, but must be studied by themselves.

Thus, in rhetoric reminiscent of Elisha Bartlett, Dalton declared, at
once, the interdependence, but independence, of the basic medical sciences. He rejected the traditional view of physiology as a speculative
science, or a science whose laws could be deduced from analogy, as comparative anatomists often claimed. Reflecting the influence of Bernard,
Dalton asserted that the "active phenomena" of the body must

be ascertained by direct observation and experiment. No knowledge of anatomy, however minute and thorough, could ever teach
us that the muscle fibre was contractile, or the nervous filament
sensitive. Those bodily phenomena, even, which are purely mechanical in their nature, require the same direct examination. The
structure of the heart may be learned by dissection; its rhythmical
and complicated movements baffle all a priori hypotheses and
must be actually *seen* to be understood.

Dalton also rejected the reductionist view of physiology promoted
by the German scientists Carl Ludwig, Ernst von Brücke, Hermann von
Helmholtz, and Emil Du Bois-Reymond: "I could name more than one
physiological writer, whose whole endeavor seems to be to reduce the
science, as it were, by force of arms, to a series of simple propositions,
which do not express its real character. They attempt to square physiology on the pattern of other sciences, instead of taking it as it really
presents itself, and studying it as chemistry and physics, they forget to
study it as physiology."[29] Although Bernard and these four German
physiologists all sought to expand understanding of the functions of the
living organism, their methods and philosophical approaches differed to
a significant degree. Du Bois-Reymond assessed the state of French
physiology during a visit to Paris in 1850 and informed his friend Carl
Ludwig, "The ignorance and limited view of even the best men here is
incredible. . . . Your textbook will be a couple of generations ahead of
the French conceptions."[30] Although nationalism played some role in
the mutual skepticism expressed by Bernard and the Germans, significant differences in their approach to physiology transcended national
boundaries.

Dalton was imbued with Bernard's philosophy of experimentation and shared his mentor's commitment to vivisection. For Dalton, the approach to the study of function and the method of teaching the facts derived from this study were equally important. He informed his pupils: "The *method* according to which scientific studies are to be pursued, far from being a matter of indifference, is of real and practical importance. A good method will do much to simplify and facilitate the student's labors; a bad one will certainly be the source of delay and perplexity."[31] Dalton's deep commitment to the experimental approach to physiology explains, in part, his willingness to confront the antivivisection movement when it arose a decade later.

His extensive 1857 review of two of Bernard's works provides further insight into the origin and nature of Dalton's interpretation of physiology. It opened with the claim that Bernard inaugurated a new epoch in experimental physiology. The New York physiologist declared, "He has first placed the science on its true footing, and has indicated the only course, that of experimenting upon living or recently killed animals, by which actual and satisfactory progress can be made. . . . He has shown us what the science really is, and how it is to be pursued."[32]

Dalton distinguished Bernard's course in experimental physiology from the systematic introductory courses delivered at most American medical colleges. Bernard sought to stimulate his audience by presenting them with the results of recent investigations as well as with questions that were inspiring new experiments. In this manner, Bernard attempted to teach the philosophy of research: a hypothesis suggests experiments that are varied until conclusions lead to a solution of the original problem. Dalton, like Bernard, tried to stimulate curiosity about life processes that could be satisfied only by experimentation. Although Dalton's students did not participate in actual experiments, he encouraged them to contemplate the intellectual process of experimental medicine and research. In his review, Dalton reiterated his commitment to the philosophical independence of, and practical distinction between, anatomy and physiology. It was not possible to deduce a physiological fact from an anatomical fact; function could not be predicted from structure.

The state of medical education in antebellum America mitigated Dalton's effort for experimental physiology. Few American medical students, including those at the College of Physicians and Surgeons, had more than a rudimentary high school education; many had less. Moreover, the brief four- or five-month curriculum precluded all but a cursory review of known physiological facts. There was no time for speculation about current controversies in medical science. In this era, the teaching of physiology was confined to the classroom; there were no physiological laboratories for students in any American medical school. Although constructed after Dalton's arrival, the new building erected at the college in 1856 did not include a physiological laboratory. Anatomy, the traditional medical science of student participation, fared better. The anatomical amphitheater in the new college building seated three hundred and the dissecting room had twenty-five tables. Dalton had a modest room in which he prepared his demonstrations and performed research.

A survey in 1858 of the medical institutions in New York City favorably reviewed Dalton's work at the college. In the opinion of the writer, New York's commercial character had led Americans to overlook its opportunities in the arts and sciences, but these were now being increasingly acknowledged. Discussing Dalton's course, the reviewer claimed:

> Probably a more full and perfect course of instruction in Physiology is here given than in any other institution in this country. Prof. DALTON devotes his whole course to this interesting branch. He demonstrates the structure and changes of such tissues as are necessary to his subject by microscopical illustrations, and illustrates questionable positions by vivisections on the lower animals. Prof. D. is a master of his subject, a fine speaker, and makes his hearers feel most forcibly the intimate and important relations of physiology to every other branch of medicine. Prof. D. is a young man; but if a good beginning, capacity, industry and high opportunities are any guarantee, it requires not a prophetic vision to see before him a brilliant future.[33]

Physiology was Dalton's future: it was his profession, not merely the sidelight of a busy practitioner who sought the prestige or extra income of a medical school chair. Unlike most contemporary American medical teachers, Dalton did not practice medicine. As a full-time physiologist, he devoted himself exclusively to instruction, investigation, and writing. His income from the sale of lecture tickets was supplemented by the proceeds from his textbook and primer, although the financial rewards from writing were not large in this era.[34] Dalton's lifestyle was a factor in his willingness to forgo the additional income a medical practice would have provided. A lifelong bachelor, he did not have to be concerned about supporting a wife and children. According to his friend and fellow physiologist S. Weir Mitchell, Dalton was not extravagant but "lived the simplest of lives—a bachelor, in a tiny suite of rooms, eating quietly at his club, unstirred by the venal ambitions of the roaring world of greedy trade around him in New York."[35]

It should not be presumed that medical practice guaranteed a stable, high income in the mid-nineteenth century. One writer claimed in 1858, "Physicians do not grow rich with rapidity—indeed, almost never . . . [although] if they choose the right places wherein to exercise their knowledge, and have the proper share of industry, together with even a moderate amount of ability, they will get 'a living.' "[36] Dalton's former Boston colleague Henry J. Bigelow pointed out the difficulty of being successful in science and practice at the same time. The prominent Boston surgeon denied that eminence in science predictably resulted in success in medical practice, or that a large medical practice implied that the physician was especially scientific.[37]

In 1859, Dalton published his textbook on human physiology, an octavo volume of 608 pages with 254 illustrations, nearly all of which were based on his own drawings.[38] In his preface, Dalton explained that the work was more than a textbook for students; it could also serve to update the practitioner on the dramatic new discoveries in physiology. He emphasized the practical value of these discoveries to the practicing physician, arguing they would aid in his understanding of the processes of disease and would ultimately lead to a more rational system of therapeutics. Dalton revealed that he had attempted to confirm many of the experimental results reported by others to justify the conclusions contained in his book. The work was, therefore, more than a simple reiteration of untested theories; it was based upon scientific observation and experimentation.

Dalton did more than simply edit foreign works. One reviewer, almost certainly Oliver Wendell Holmes, explained that even as a medical student Dalton "had a particular fancy for seeing and examining for himself." This reviewer claimed: "Dr. Dalton is one of the few native teachers of physiology who have made the discovery that an American has eyes, hands, organs, dimensions, senses, as well as a German or a Frenchman. He actually examines the phenomena he describes as they exist in Nature!"[39]

This claim is reminiscent of a criticism Holmes published in a review of another physiology textbook: "It is remarkable how few contributions have been made in this country to physiological science. . . . We accept the labors of such men as Professors Leidy, Wyman, Dalton, as evidence that American science is not necessarily to be an electrotype from that of the other hemisphere. . . . But still it is too true that our great want in physiological science is the spirit of observation."[40] Other reviewers of Dalton's *Physiology* shared Holmes's enthusiasm for the work. Commenting on the second edition that appeared in 1861, physiologist and army surgeon William Hammond proclaimed it "by far the most desirable text-book on physiology to place in the hands of the student which, so far as we are aware, exists in the English language, or perhaps in any other."[41]

During the first decade of his career as a physiologist, Dalton became widely known in America through his writings and his active participation in several medical and scientific societies. By 1860 he was a member of the New York Academy of Medicine, the New York Pathological Society, the American Academy of Arts and Sciences, and the Biological Department of the Academy of Natural Sciences of Philadelphia. Through these organizations, Dalton became personally acquainted with many of the leading scientifically oriented physicians of the day. This network of physicians and scientists would soon assume importance in Dalton's life. He turned to the members of these societies and others to gain support against the antivivisectionists who challenged him and other experimental physiologists before the decade was over.

In the spring of 1860, Dalton expanded his teaching activities and began lecturing on physiology at the Long Island College Hospital. His Long Island course, which began in March following the completion of his lectures at the College of Physicians and Surgeons, included vivisections and demonstrations on the use of the microscope.[42] Dalton's teaching and writing commitments limited the time available for research. Without consistent financial support for research, individuals were forced to emphasize income-producing activities. Medical practice, lecturing, and writing were financially rewarding, and research was often postponed or abandoned as demands on time grew. Research did not bring monetary rewards or prestige in antebellum America. Moreover, the nation's medical schools did not encourage their faculty members to do research. Ill-prepared students required elementary instruction, not sophisticated courses.

According to a committee of the American Medical Association, advanced courses, such as those taught by the leaders of European scientific medicine like Bernard, Brown-Séquard, and Virchow were inappropriate in the United States. American medical students lacked the extensive preliminary preparation of European physicians. The AMA committee also noted the lack of commitment to research among American medical teachers. This was not simply the fault of the individual, but was due to the relative emphasis placed on the various activities of a medical teacher. The committee noted a lack of any "official position" for an individual whose main responsibility was research; in America, research was seen as a distraction from the more important duties of simple instruction.

> This eminent physiologist [Dalton] is by mental constitution evidently qualified to hold the position in America which in Paris is occupied by M. Bernard. He should be exploring the dark and untravelled regions of physiology instead of leading undergraduates along its beaten track; his pen should be occupied in tracing new provinces of thought added by his genius to the ever-spreading map of discovered biological science, instead of writing text-books for students; and it is a curious illustration of the fact, that in his present academical position he is not the right man in the right place. . . . By natural bias this author is disposed to explore and demonstrate to physiologists new paths of biological research, while surrounding circumstances compel him to occupy his time in teaching the elements of his science to students. [43]

There was no alternative, however. No medical school paid its faculty to perform research. The AMA committee was addressing a national problem, not simply a problem at the College of Physicians and Surgeons of New York. The committee decried the utilitarianism of the American public and the medical profession; they felt this tendency was responsible for the lack of interest among physicians and medical publishers for articles or monographs based on research.

George Shrady, editor of the *Medical Record*, criticized the ambivalence of most American physicians toward science in an 1869 essay in which he claimed the American medical profession discouraged research. Shrady recognized that independent wealth was usually required to support a career in medical science, and that the overwhelming majority of physicians were attracted to the financial opportunities afforded by practice. [44] Elsewhere, Shrady explained that Claude Bernard had been enabled to pursue a research career by virtue of private economic support, "but to one Claude Bernard there are one thousand physicians who must make their profession pay their office rent and butcher's bills." Another obstacle, in Shrady's opinion, was the lack of interest among patients in medical research: "Patients, even the most intelligent of them, care little for abstract sciences." [45]

The conclusions of the AMA committee and the opinions of Shrady support the argument that individual, institutional, and local factors operated in a larger social context to retard the emergence of experimental physiology as a distinct discipline in the United States in the mid-nineteenth century. Only when there was a market for biomedical research in America, and a means to support it, would there be hope of establishing full-time careers for specialists in physiology who did more than teach the elements of the science and publish summaries of investigations undertaken abroad. Dalton only partially fulfilled his promise despite his status as a full-time teacher of physiology.

Dalton's career as a physiologist was shaped by the relative value of elementary teaching, writing textbooks, pursuing research, publishing original observations, and training advanced workers for careers in research and teaching. In America, medical students were admitted without regard for their prior educational experience, and medical teachers sought large classes. During his lifetime, however, forces within American medicine, science, and society would set the stage for a new definition of the responsibilities of the medical teacher and of the goals of a medical education. Dalton was an active participant in this reform movement during the final quarter century of his life, although it had little effect on his career.

In the spring of 1861, American society was disrupted by the outbreak of the Civil War. Responding to Lincoln's call for troops to protect the capital, Dalton applied for the position of assistant surgeon in the Seventh Regiment from New York. He spent two months in Washington in the early summer of 1861 and returned there in October to spend the winter in the service of the army. The disruption of his physiology work in New York became a source of concern to him, and he appealed to his fellow physiologist, William Hammond, then surgeon-general of the United States Army, to facilitate his release from service. By the fall of 1863, Dalton was back in New York and could once again devote himself to his career in physiology.[46] In 1864, Dalton gave up teaching at the Long Island College Hospital and confined his professional activities to the College of Physicians and Surgeons. He was succeeded at the Long Island College Hospital by Austin Flint, Jr., the son of a prominent New York physician. Like Dalton, the younger Flint studied under Claude Bernard and was a proponent of the use of vivisection in teaching and research. An active investigator and prolific writer, Flint had briefly served as Dalton's assistant at the Vermont Medical College. He was a founder of the Bellevue Hospital Medical College in 1868 and spent most of his professional career at that institution.[47]

Vivisection was a standard feature in physiology teaching in the New York medical schools by the mid-1860s. Not all American physiologists viewed this as a desirable trend, however. Robley Dunglison warned that the students might not learn the facts of physiology because the dramatic vivisections would distract them. He argued, "Vivisections have sufficiently established the reality of numerous phenomena, which do not require, therefore, hecatombs to ratify them. The great object, during the medical session, should be to teach 'physiology applied'; and it would, assuredly, be a step backward to restrict the expositions of the biological instructor to experiments and their results, or to 'operative physiology.' "[48] Dalton was soon confronted by more than philosophical discussions regarding the place of vivisection in physiology teaching; he bore the brunt of the antivivisection movement as it developed in New York.

Dalton's use of vivisection was confined to his classroom demonstrations and his private research. Although New York physicians or pupils occasionally witnessed his experiments, there is no evidence that Dalton sought to train advanced workers in the techniques of experimental physiology in the hope that they would become full-time physiologists. There was virtually no job market for full-time experimental physiologists in America in this era. The demand was for medical practitioners rather than for medical teachers or investigators. Those graduates who hoped to advance their standing in the profession by obtaining postgraduate training traveled abroad. American medical schools did not seek to compete with European institutions in the areas of laboratory or specialty training.[49] It is not surprising, therefore, that Dalton did not attempt to develop a program of advanced instruction or research in physiology at the College of Physicians and Surgeons. His limited facilities were undoubtedly a factor, but larger issues in American medicine and society led him to emphasize elementary teaching and writing.

Although Claude Bernard was successful in stimulating scientifically oriented physicians to perform research and use vivisections in teaching even though he was forced to tolerate primitive laboratory conditions during the early decades of his scientific career, he acknowledged the importance of adequate facilities, apparatus, and assistance. In 1867, the French physiologist made a plea for the public endowment of laboratories in which he attributed the growing disparity between the productivity of French and German physiologists to the superior facilities, apparatus, and support staff of the German scientists.[50] Nevertheless, Bernard was proud of his accomplishments. Three years later he claimed, "Despite the scanty means I had at my disposal, I took in numbers of students who today are professors of physiology or of medicine in various universities in Europe or in the New World."[51] Louis Pasteur expressed similar frustrations about the support for science in France and declared in 1868, "To be a scientist these days [one] needs private income or an invincible dedication."[52]

Dalton's mentor, Claude Bernard, proclaimed the crucial role of the laboratory in the training of scientific physicians in a comprehensive monograph on experimental medicine published in 1865. Bernard hoped this treatise would encourage investigation and the development of scientific medicine. Didactic courses, in Bernard's opinion, could arouse an interest in science among students and physicians, but scientists could only be created by exposure to laboratories: "The laboratory is the real nursery of true experimental scientists, i.e., those who create the science that others afterwards popularize. Now if we want much fruit, we must take care of our nurseries of fruit trees."[53]

Dalton may have wanted to enlarge the scope of his physiological activities at the college as he saw the growing emphasis on laboratory training in European universities. Whatever Dalton's goals in the immediate postbellum period, however, they were moderated by the local and national social context. Joseph Henry, writing to Louis Agassiz regarding Alexander Baird's election as president of the National Academy of Sciences, claimed, "In this Democratic country we must do what we can, when we cannot do what we would. . . . Why trouble yourself so much about the character of American science which can only be improved with the social and political conditions which tend to encourage and develop it."[54]

Shortly after the Civil War, the antivivisection movement spread to America and has affected experimental medicine to the present day. Objections to the use of animals for experimentation had been raised decades earlier in Great Britain and Europe. As early as 1828, a law had been passed in New York prohibiting cruelty to horses, sheep, and cattle. Until Dalton introduced vivisection into medical teaching, the humane movement in America focused on the treatment of domestic animals. The American antivivisection movement can be traced to Henry Bergh, the son of a wealthy New York shipbuilder who witnessed examples of cruel treatment of animals on the streets of Russia in 1864.[55] On his way home to America, Bergh visited London and learned of the activities of the Royal Society for the Prevention of Cruelty to Animals. In February 1866, Bergh delivered a public lecture on animal protection in New York City, and in April of that year, he organized the American Society for the Prevention of Cruelty to Animals. Similar regional societies were soon formed in Massachusetts, New Jersey, and Pennsylvania.

Bergh did not have to look beyond the limits of New York City to learn about vivisection. Dalton was neither discreet nor apologetic in using this technique in his demonstrations. Moreover, descriptions of vivisection were not confined to medical or scientific publications. The

New York weekly, the *Nation*, included an article in its first volume on the value of chemistry and physiology in the detection of poisons. The author declared:

> The frog is one of the most useful animals to man. . . . He has contributed more to the advancement of physiology than any other creature that inhabits the earth—allowing his abdomen to be ripped open, his brain exposed, and his nerves excised, without uttering a croak or moving a muscle; and, after all these things, he will live on in a state of quiescent beatitude as long as you please, whilst hour by hour the scientific physiologist watches him, and records the observed phenomena.[56]

The article was designed to point out the value of science to society rather than provoke an attack on animal experimentation.

Another of Bernard's American pupils, Francis Donaldson, professor of physiology, hygiene, and general pathology at the University of Maryland, responded to the early rumblings of the American antivivisection movement. In an 1866 introductory address, Donaldson emphasized the practical importance of physiology to physicians and argued that vivisection was an indispensable technique for advancing physiological knowledge. He acknowledged that the practice might seem cruel to individuals who failed to appreciate the benefits to mankind derived from animal experimentation. After listing several prominent European medical scientists who extensively employed vivisection, Donaldson credited America's pioneer experimental physiologists John C. Dalton, Jr., Austin Flint, Jr., S. Weir Mitchell, and William Hammond with making valuable contributions to medical science through their experiments.[57]

Dalton became the champion of vivisection on behalf of the medical and scientific community. George Shrady, the editor of the *Medical Record* and an 1858 graduate of the College of Physicians and Surgeons, encouraged Dalton to respond to Bergh's attack. Shrady characterized Bergh as a member of the class of zealous reformers sometimes called "world betterers," who were not discouraged by ridicule or failure.[58] In a letter to Edward Delafield, president of the College of Physicians and Surgeons, Dalton explained that the single object of vivisection was to discover knowledge to cure diseases and to reduce human suffering. He emphasized the critical importance of animal experimentation in physiological research and reminded Delafield that advances in medical practice were largely dependent on physiological discoveries. The New York physiologist declared that the greatest medical discoveries had been derived from vivisection and warned that the abandonment of the technique would have dire consequences for the well-being of mankind. Dalton stressed that anesthetics were used when a potentially painful procedure was undertaken on an animal and rejected Bergh's claim that vivisections were repeated at lectures simply to gratify "juvenile curiosity." He also denied that students and practitioners performed operations on living animals to acquire manual dexterity. Dalton explained that his response to Bergh's attack was "important to the cause of medical education, in which we, as well as the whole community, are interested."[59]

Shrady announced that Dalton would present a formal rebuttal of Bergh's claims at the New York Academy of Medicine on 12 December 1866. Dalton's articulate defense of vivisection before the New York Academy received wide circulation following its publication in the academy's *Bulletin* and as a separate pamphlet. In rhetoric reminiscent of his mentor Bernard he sought to impress his audience with the improvements in the medical art that could be attributed to animal experimentation. Dalton claimed, "It is not too much to say that *every important discovery in physiology has been directly due to experiments on living animals;* and that we owe many of those in practical medicine, surgery, and hygiene, either directly or indirectly to the same source."[60] His emphasis on the ultimate practical value of animal experimentation to mankind set the tone for the American response to the antivivisectionists. The balance of the address was a historical summary of contributions to practical medicine derived from experimental physiology utilizing vivisection. Among the advances Dalton traced to vivisection were the discovery of the circulation of the blood, the development of techniques for artificial respiration and blood transfusion, and the introduction of antidotes for venom.

The medical press was generally sympathetic to Dalton's views on vivisection. In response to the publication of his letter to Delafield, one correspondent claimed:

In this country, until quite recently, very little of this method of pursuing physiological study has been done. Professor Dalton, of the College of Physicians and Surgeons in New York, has probably made more researches in this way than any other American physiologist. The value of the results which he has obtained has been universally acknowledged by the medical profession; and as it is every day becoming more and more evident that the true practice of medicine must be based on the most accurate physiological knowledge, the value of the information gained in this way is becoming more and more demonstrated.[61]

Not only was there support for animal experimentation as the fundamental technique of physiological research, there was also enthusiasm for the value of demonstrations employing vivisection in the training of physicians. A Philadelphia writer who had both heard and read Dalton's address on vivisection expressed the hope that the medical schools faculties as well as the profession at large would soon acknowledge the necessity of teaching physiology through experiments.[62]

In February 1867, Dalton spoke on the subject to members of the Medical Society of the State of New York at their annual meeting in Albany. He informed his audience that Bergh was responsible for a bill before the New York state legislature that might restrict or prohibit vivisection. Offended, he claimed it contained "the most extravagant misrepresentations, calculated to mislead the members of the Legislature, and to injure in a serious manner the interests of medical science, and the cause of medical education."[63] Dalton read excerpts from Bergh's address:

> Of all the horrible sufferings inflicted upon the animal creation, those which are done in the name of anatomical science are at once the most fearful and revolting, and the most plausibly and tenaciously, though falsely advocated. Even for the monsters in human shape who nail, under this pretence, living dogs to a table, and then dissect them alive; and those who, fastening a horse so that he cannot stir a limb, begin, some to open his chest, some to saw into his skull, and others to probe the interior of his eyes— even for these are found apologists.[64]

Dalton drew an analogy between Bergh's efforts to suppress animal experimentation and the attempts to restrict human dissection a generation earlier. Opponents of these practices shared the same "ignorant and groundless prejudice," and Dalton argued that their success would significantly retard the advance of medical science and practice. The New York legislature had previously legalized anatomical dissection over the objections of some citizens, and Dalton hoped they would not now be persuaded to restrict animal experimentation because of the impassioned pleas of the antivivisectionists. In response to Dalton's presentation, a committee of the medical society was appointed to prepare a statement for the legislature on the implications of a bill restricting vivisection. Dalton forwarded his remarks on vivisection to his friend Jeffries Wyman and informed the Harvard scientist that the society

adopted "unanimously a Remonstrance to the Legislature against inter-
fering with physiological experiments."[65]

Bergh's campaign against vivisection was carried on primarily in
the daily newspapers of New York. Although he was successful in getting
his bill prohibiting cruelty to animals passed by the New York state legislature, vivisection was protected by an amendment proposed in response
to the New York State Medical Society's objection to any restriction of
animal experimentation. The bill, as passed, included the clause "nothing in this act shall be construed to prohibit or interfere with any properly conducted scientific experiments or investigations, which shall be
performed under the authority of the faculty of some regularly incorporated medical school or the university of the State of New York."[66]
Dalton was relieved that the legislature acknowledged the role vivisection played in medical teaching and research. Nevertheless, he would be
forced throughout his career to confront the antivivisectionists, led by
the "indefatigable" Bergh.

Dalton was not deterred from using vivisection in his lectures or in
his research. In 1871, he reported experiments performed on twenty
dogs in which he sought to prove the glycogenic function of the liver. He
explained that the nature of the investigation precluded the use of anesthetics and went on to describe the experiments in graphic terms. Three
assistants were necessary to hold the animal while Dalton excised the
liver through a large abdominal incision made with a single stroke of a
sharp knife. On the basis of these experiments, Dalton concluded that
sugar was a normal constituent of hepatic tissue.[67] Medical students at
the College of Physicians and Surgeons had no exposure to these experiments, however. Recalling his education there in the early 1870s, pathologist and medical educator William H. Welch remarked that there
was no laboratory training, although he viewed Dalton as "the embodi-
ment of scientific spirit and method, a direct, clear, and most attractive
teacher."[68]

Welch was stimulated by his experience at the college and at Bellevue Hospital to seek postgraduate training abroad that emphasized
physiology and pathology. He was unusually well prepared to take advantage of this European training having graduated from Yale College
and studied at the Sheffield Scientific School before his matriculation at
the College of Physicians and Surgeons. The lack of preliminary education contributed to the minimal interest of most American physicians in
experimental medicine. There was cautious optimism, however. Shrady
observed in 1871, "There seems to be a growing disposition on the part
of the students of our literary institutions to prefer scientific to classical

courses of study. This is certainly an indication of better things to come, and augurs well for the elevation of the standard of qualifications for medical students, for it is from such classes that we recruit our best men."[69]

Cornelius Agnew, a New York surgeon and ophthalmologist, expressed similar sentiments before the Medical Society of the State of New York two years later. A representative of the new generation of American specialists, Agnew had established an ophthalmological clinic at the College of Physicians and Surgeons of New York in 1866. He declared:

> We need in our profession in this country the influence of a
> learned class. We cannot, if we would, deny that such a class
> exists, but we need an enlargement of it. We need a class of men
> engaged in original researches; of men who can work more, and
> write more with less reference to the effect upon their
> practice. . . . We must attach to our colleges young men who
> have displayed a love of original research, an aptitude for teach-
> ing, or other qualities enabling them to advance the cause of med-
> ical education.[70]

Although contemporary introductory addresses, editorials, and correspondence reveal a growing interest in scientific medicine among American physicians, the United States offered virtually no opportunities for full-time careers in the basic medical sciences. William Welch informed his friend Frederic Dennis in 1877:

> I am anxious to stay in New York but must be in a position to
> support myself and am therefore ready to seize hold of any honor-
> able means of making a livelihood. . . . You know that my ambi-
> tion is less for acquiring a practice than it is for obtaining opportu-
> nities to follow up pathological investigations, and if I could
> support myself without practicing, I should be willing to relin-
> quish practice, but inasmuch as that seems to be out of the ques-
> tion in America, I still can not afford to throw away any opportu-
> nities for picking up a case here and there.[71]

Endowments were required for the support of scientific careers, but Americans had to be convinced that research was important and worthy of financial support.

The problem of public apathy toward research was not limited to the medical or natural sciences. John Tyndall, the prominent British scientist and advocate of scientific education and research, arrived in the United States in the fall of 1872. A lecture tour took him to several cities, where he was warmly received by individuals interested in science. At

Tyndall's farewell speech in New York Dalton heard the British scientist encourage his audience to work to obtain endowments for institutions of higher learning in America. Acknowledging the American tendency toward utilitarianism, Tyndall nevertheless urged the pursuit of pure science. He implored those considering a scientific career to "increase their fidelity to original research, prizing far more than the possession of wealth an honorable standing in science."[72]

Speaking of the physical sciences, astronomer Simon Newcomb complained in 1874, that the American people did not appreciate the value of scientific research. The public had to be educated so that prestige, if not money, would accrue to those who undertook scientific investigation.[73] Educating the public would be the approach used by the physiologists and their reform-minded scientific colleagues during the closing years of the nineteenth century.

Increasing prosperity in America was accompanied by a growing sentiment that wealthy individuals could be persuaded to support research in science and medicine.[74] Endowment could also change the character of medical education. Medical schools first turned to their alumni with little success. Daniel St. John Roosa urged the medical alumni of the University of the City of New York to donate to their alma mater in 1872:

> What we do need most, and first of all . . . are endowments for professorships. The teachers should be free from any taint of desire of large classes, merely that their salaries may be increased. We need more opportunities for special studies and investigations in chemical and physiological laboratories, in the dissecting-rooms, and the clinical wards. We also need libraries and scholarships, in short, what money will bring—money not to be spent on the outside of the cup and the platter, the college building and the lecture-room, but for the support of men who are willing to labor for science, if science can give them their bread-and-butter.[75]

The alumni of the College of Physicians and Surgeons, animated by the talk of endowments at rival New York institutions, established a committee to confer with the faculty to identify ways that their association might aid the school. Dalton was involved in the discussions in April 1873 to raise an endowment of $100,000. They proposed that this fund be used to endow a chair of pathological anatomy and establish "laboratories in chemistry, physiology and pathological anatomy, where original researches may be carried out under the guidance of proper instructors."[76] The alumni committee concluded that there was "no more certain way of advancing the standard of medical education than by furnishing the most ample facilities for the prosecution of studies and investigations in the purely scientific departments of medicine," and that the college urgently needed them.[77]

Pathology rather than physiology was the main beneficiary of the college's movement to enhance scientific teaching and research. Local circumstances determined the emphasis on pathology. Alonzo Clark, an influential faculty member who would soon be elected dean and president of the college, was interested in pathology. Moreover, Francis Delafield, the son of Edward Delafield who preceded Clark as president, hoped to devote himself to a career in pathology. The younger Delafield, following graduation from the college, traveled to Europe where he studied under Rudolf Virchow and other leaders of pathology. A demand for practical instruction in microscopical and pathological anatomy appeared in response to the growing acceptance of the cell theory and germ theory. In 1874, Charles Heitzman opened a private microscopical laboratory for training students and physicians in New York that "proved successful beyond all expectation."[78]

America's medical schools and hospitals gradually recognized the need to encourage the development of pathology. Although the limited resources available for the support of laboratory teaching were directed primarily at pathology at the College of Physicians and Surgeons, the growing interest among physicians in microscopy and bacteriology led to a heightened awareness of the importance of the basic medical sciences in general. As was the case with physiology, few American institutions provided opportunities for individuals interested in devoting themselves to pathology. Francis Delafield was appointed to the chair of pathological anatomy in 1877 and soon prepared a plan for the establishment of a pathological laboratory at the college.

Dalton was one of the main proponents of endowment to raise the quality of teaching and permit the introduction of laboratory methods at the college. He drafted a report on the goals of an endowment campaign in 1876 that emphasized the changes during his quarter-century career in medical education and the practical advances to society from research in the physical sciences. He predicted analogous gains from the growing emphasis on research in the life sciences. Medical practice was changing because of the discoveries attributable to the laboratory method and the introduction of clinical microscopy. Medical education had to change as well.

> Students of medicine cannot be properly instructed by lectures
> alone. In order to convey the requisite information in the best

manner, the lectures must be accompanied, in many cases, by illustrations and experiments, requiring special appliances suited for
the purpose. . . . For these reasons, the material requirements of a
Medical School at the present day are vastly increased over those
of a quarter of a century ago. More space is needed, and a greater
number of apartments, adapted for different uses. Well
appointed laboratories, for both investigation and practical
research and instruction, in chemistry, physiology and pathology,
are becoming indispensable for first-class institutions, and require
a corresponding outlay of money.[79]

Dalton did not explicitly outline his plans for laboratory instruction
in physiology, and he did not advocate practical laboratory exercises for
all students. The expense would have been prohibitive, and there was no
precedent among America's medical schools in the mid-1870s. The College of Physicians and Surgeons did not have sufficient endowment to
erect, equip, and staff a student physiological laboratory. Moreover,
Dalton would have had to make a major new commitment after teaching the subject for a quarter century. He had achieved great distinction
in his chosen field without extending his duties to include the instruction
of nearly one hundred students in the laboratory. Perhaps most important, he realized that student participation in repetitive laboratory exercises using animals would elicit harsh criticism from the antivivisectionists. He received widespread support for the use of vivisection in the
context of research, some support for its use as an educational tool in the
form of demonstrations, but essentially no support for its routine employment in elementary laboratory teaching. Although Dalton had been
successful in his attempts to block the aggressive verbal and legal attacks
of the antivivisectionists, the likelihood of future triumphs against Bergh
and his associates would be reduced if vivisection became part of a routine laboratory training program for medical students.

Bergh followed events at the college closely. John G. Curtis, a graduate of Harvard College and a recent graduate of the College of Physicians and Surgeons, became Dalton's assistant in the early 1870s. Although an active practitioner, Curtis shared the physiology teaching
responsibilities with Dalton. Curtis did not undertake any independent
research, but he occasionally assisted Dalton in experiments and frequently gave demonstrations before the medical students. In 1875,
Bergh attacked Curtis for using an unanesthetized animal in demonstrations before a class at the college. This charge signaled Curtis's entry
into the antivivisection debate, a fight to occupy him for nearly four
decades.[80]

Dalton remained the spokesman on behalf of animal experimentation and published a refined and enlarged justification for vivisection in 1875. In his introduction, he portrayed the protagonists as ignorant of the objectives of physiological experiments, the techniques themselves, and the history of medical progress.[81] Dalton expressed dismay at the persistence of the movement and warned that it threatened the advance of medicine. He claimed that the criticism of vivisection came from "nonprofessional sources" and, in order to demonstrate the support of the medical profession, Dalton published a series of resolutions condoning the practice. Letters on behalf of animal experimentation came from the Medical Society of the State of New York, the Medical Society of the County of New York, the New York Pathological Society, the Society of Neurology and Electrology, the New York Neurological Society, and various county medical societies in the New York area.

Testimonials from American and foreign physicians emphasized the practical benefits to humanity of animal experimentation. Edward H. Clarke of Harvard wrote, "The progress which has been made in therapeutics for the last quarter of a century . . . is largely due to experiments upon animals by physiologists. It would be difficult to estimate the amount of human suffering that will remain unrelieved if these studies cannot be carried on."[82] Austin Flint, Sr., one of America's most respected medical authorities, and the father of a prodigious vivisector, asserted, "Any one who is conversant with the great advances in knowledge of physiology, during the last half century, must be aware that they have been made chiefly through the agency of vivisections and other methods of experimentation on living animals. Our knowledge of diseases is always enlarged by advances in physiology."[83]

Organized medicine was now coming to the aid of the few individuals who practiced vivisection. The alliance between medical practitioners and medical scientists ultimately led to widespread reforms in the structure and philosophy of American medical education. The supporters of animal experimentation claimed that limiting vivisection had implications far beyond the effect it would have on the handful of American physiologists employing the technique in teaching and research: the entire profession and society would suffer from an injunction on the practice. The members of the Putnam County Medical Society of New York resolved "that the suppression of physiological and pathological research by means of vivisection would interfere materially with our progress in medical science, and thus prove a great detriment to the medical profession, and to the welfare of mankind."[84]

Representatives of organized medicine in New York extended their support of vivisection to include its use in teaching. They argued that demonstrations employing vivisection had great instructional value.[85] Support for Dalton and vivisection was not limited to the medical community of New York. Editorials also appeared in Boston and Philadelphia medical journals. Bergh and his associates could not be taken lightly after the success of the British antivivisection movement. By obtaining legal sanctions against vivisection, the British group had severely restricted its use in teaching and research.

Dalton continued to organize the medical response to the antivivisectionists and was active in the formation of the Committee on Experimental Medicine of the Medical Society of the State of New York in 1880. As chairman, he encouraged other influential physicians to join the committee, among them John Shaw Billings.[86] In the early 1880s, Dalton's former pupil and associate John Curtis became increasingly active in this organization and associated activities designed to frustrate Bergh's annual attempts to bring legislation prohibiting or severely restricting vivisection before the New York state legislature.

Concern about the quality and content of American medical education grew as more physicians returned from postgraduate work in Europe where they had seen the well-equipped medical laboratories at the continental universities. The growing contrast between American and European medical facilities and training threatened their national pride. Whereas Americans found the French laboratories of the 1870s vastly inferior to those at the German universities, the Parisian facilities had improved. One American warned in 1883 that individuals hoping to perform research in the laboratories of the College of France had better be familiar with the basic principles and techniques of scientific investigation. Only qualified individuals were admitted to the research laboratories, and "it is not pleasant to hear Americans spoken of as superficial or ignorant because some have made this mistake in regard to the object of these institutions."[87]

Not all physicians supported the trend toward student participation in laboratory activities, however. Albert Leffingwell graduated from the Long Island College Hospital in 1874 where he had been a pupil of Austin Flint, Jr. Leffingwell later served as a physiology instructor and was impressed by the enthusiastic response of medical students to vivisections.[88] By 1880, Leffingwell had become a spokesman for the antivivisectionists and proposed an intermediate position between Bergh's demand that all vivisection be stopped and Dalton's posture that any limitation was undesirable. Leffingwell condoned vivisection performed on animals that were completely anesthetized but encouraged the prohibition of any repetitive experiment performed simply for demonstrational purposes that resulted in pain to a warmblooded animal. Increasingly active in the American antivivisection movement, Leffingwell replaced Bergh as the leader of that cause upon Bergh's death in 1888. The demands of the antivivisectionists moderated somewhat under Leffingwell's influence. Nevertheless, the movement gained some credibility among the public by having a physician involved in its cause.

In view of the sustained antivivisection agitation, Dalton chose the subject of the experimental method in medical science for his Cartwright Lecture delivered at the College of Physicians and Surgeons in 1882. In this articulate review of important medical discoveries that had resulted from animal experimentation, he argued that research should be "followed and cultivated for its own results, whatever they may be, without demanding immediate returns of a kind that can be designated beforehand, and with entire confidence in the substantial value of this method, which has always been, and will always be, the only source of permanent improvement in medical science."[89] Dalton continued to emphasize the role of vivisection in research in his speeches and publications and avoided the controversial issue of repetitive exercises.

Once again seeking to gain supporters for research and vivisection, Dalton urged the American Medical Association in 1884 to form a committee on experimental medicine. This committee was charged with the duty of coordinating the opposition to any legislation that might retard medical research by restricting animal experimentation. In addition to Dalton, it included Horatio C. Wood, Jr., William Pepper, and James Tyson of Philadelphia; Christopher Johnston of Baltimore; John Shaw Billings of the United States Army; and Austin Flint, Jr., of New York.

Although Dalton devoted much time and energy as the spokesman on behalf of vivisection and experimental medicine, the focus of his investigations shifted from animal experimentation during the 1870s. He recognized the practical implications of the new germ theory of disease, and became interested in bacteriology. His interest in the germ theory derived, in part, from his experience in microscopy. It is also likely that it was encouraged by his brother Edward B. Dalton, an 1858 graduate of the College of Physicians and Surgeons who was appointed sanitary superintendent of the New York Metropolitan Board of Health in 1866.[90] John Dalton's writings revealed a sophisticated understanding of the contemporary interpretation of the relationship of bacteria to disease. The germ theory of disease and its practical extension, antiseptic surgery, provided Dalton with a potent new example of the growing interdependence of scientific research and practical medicine.[91] Although several years passed before Joseph Lister's formulation of the antiseptic approach to surgery gained universal acceptance, this development represented a dramatic illustration of the practical benefits of basic research to mankind. In his earliest papers, Lister acknowledged his debt to the experiments on fermentation of Louis Pasteur.[92]

Other subjects attracted Dalton's attention during the 1880s. Recent advances in cerebral localization and a longstanding interest in neurophysiology led him to investigate the location of the vision centers in the cerebral hemispheres. He had followed the development of photographic technology, and used new techniques to advantage in producing a massive atlas of the gross anatomy of the human brain in 1885. This handsome work included forty-eight heliotype plates with a detailed description of the cerebral cortex. Unlike many of his other publications, this atlas did not pose the threat of stimulating renewed attacks by the antivivisectionists.[93] He revised his popular textbook of physiology throughout his career as well. Dalton was, without question, one of America's most prolific medical authors during the second half of the nineteenth century.

In 1883, Dalton resigned as professor of physiology, and the following year succeeded Alonzo Clark as president of the College of Physicians and Surgeons. His assistant John Curtis was appointed professor and withdrew from medical practice to devote his entire time to his activities at the college. Curtis never cared for medical practice and gladly gave it up. Facilities for physiology and pathology teaching at the college had expanded in 1878 when the alumni association made funds available for the construction of a modest laboratory in a former storefront on the ground floor of the college building. Five years later a $10,000 gift for the purchase and maintenance of physiological apparatus in memory of Foster Swift, an 1857 graduate of the college, made it possible for Curtis to acquire sophisticated physiological instruments. Because the new ground floor laboratory did not provide adequate space for the installation of much apparatus, Curtis decided not to spend the entire gift until a more suitable laboratory was constructed at the college.

By 1880, some American physicians and their families had made gifts to various institutions on behalf of medical education and research. But these bequests were few in number and small in amount. The profession was encouraged to do more to support the advance of medical science and the elevation of the standards of medical teaching. In 1882, one writer urged physicians to set an example for wealthy citizens to endow American medical education:

What professor in a medical college, dying rich, has left any considerable portion of his fortune to the college in connection with which he has accumulated his wealth? We have never learned of one such. A few days since the news came to us that the late Professor Pancoast died very wealthy, estimated one million dollars, but it was added he left all his money to his family. To Jefferson Medical College he gave neither hundreds or thousands of his money. Is such an example likely to encourage the rich men of Philadelphia to leave portions of their wealth to Jefferson Medical College? Its own professors who have the means will not endow it, and why should strangers do better?[94]

The activities of the Alumni Association of the College of Physicians and Surgeons of New York demonstrated the willingness of some graduates to support the school's development. More was needed, however, and the college, located in America's wealthiest city, soon benefited from the growing philanthropic spirit of some of America's wealthiest citizens. During Dalton's presidency, the college received a gift of more than one-half million dollars from William H. Vanderbilt for the construction of elaborate laboratory and clinical facilities. In his letter announcing this gift, the financier and railroad operator explained:

> I have been for some time examining the question of the facilities
> for medical education which New York possesses. The doctors
> have claimed that with proper encouragement this city might
> become one of the most important centres of medical instruction
> in the world. The health, comfort and lives of the whole commu-
> nity are so dependent upon skilled physicians that no profession
> requires more care in the preparation of its practitioners. Medicine
> needs a permanent home where the largest opportunities can be
> afforded for both theory and practice. In making up my mind to
> give substantial aid to the effort to create in New York City one of
> the finest medical schools in the world . . . it seems wiser and
> more practical to enlarge an existing institution which has already
> great facilities, experience and reputation than to form a new one.
> I have therefore selected the College of Physicians and Surgeons
> because it is the oldest medical school in the state, and of equal
> rank with any in the world.[95]

There was precedent for endowing medical institutions in America. The most notable example was Johns Hopkins's bequest of three and one-half million dollars to found the Johns Hopkins Hospital. Indeed, it is likely that Vanderbilt was referring to Johns Hopkins when he mentioned his decision to endow an existing institution rather than encourage the formation of a new one. Dalton played a role in attracting Vanderbilt's huge gift, although the philanthropist's personal physician James W. McLane, a professor at the college, was largely responsible for securing it.

The College of Physicians and Surgeons was only one of many American institutions to benefit from philanthropy in the closing years of the nineteenth century. The unique economic and social circumstances of the age precipitated this movement with its major implications for higher education. Michael Mulhall, an Irish statistician and historian, declared in 1885, "When some future historian describes the progress of the nineteenth century, he will doubtless be struck by the enormous increase of wealth, especially in the interval between 1850 and the present date."[96] The reform of American medical education and the endowment of medical science ultimately resulted from the sustained financial support of a few philanthropists.

By the mid-1880s the leaders of the movement to reform American medical education were unanimous in their belief that adequate endowments were the only means to achieve their goals. One of Dalton's pupils, William G. Thompson, who had studied in London and at the University of Berlin following his graduation from the college in 1881, reviewed the status of American medical education four years later and concluded, "So long as a medical college is dependent entirely upon the fees of its students for support, the highest educational good can not be attained. The question concerns endowment." After describing the typical abbreviated curriculum of American medical schools, Thompson claimed:

> No wonder that our students, immediately after graduating, go by the hundred to Paris, Berlin, Vienna, etc., where the Government encourages professional schools, laboratories, and scientific bureaus by substantial support and thorough system. They go abroad, partially because it is the fashion, and gives them a sort of advertisement as having done the proper thing, and partly to learn a new and useful language, and study foreign methods of life. But the fundamental reason of their going is that, instead of sitting in a huge lecture-hall with two or three hundred other men, to take notes *verbatim* of a lecture which often might be read in a text-book at home, they can join small classes in which they practically demonstrate every fact for themselves, under the guidance of an instructor.[97]

Thompson recognized that the laboratory approach was far more costly than teaching by lectures and classroom demonstrations. Nevertheless, he advocated the construction of well-equipped and adequately staffed laboratories for teaching and research in chemistry, anatomy, physiology, and pathology. He believed this approach would signal a sharp rise in the standards of medical education in the United States that would ultimately result in foreign students coming to America for medical training.

Henry Noyes, another graduate of the college, shared Thompson's enthusiasm for the laboratory approach to medical teaching and research. Following a visit to Europe in 1885, Noyes expressed his awe at the modern research laboratories in several continental medical schools. Contrasting the European situation with that in the United States, he acknowledged the contributions made by American physicians despite meager facilities: "I pay willing tribute to men who sacrifice ease and health to pursuits of pure science; who must snatch time from bread-getting, who give public instruction . . . that they may contribute to the advance of scientific medicine. . . . But the advance of scientific study demands proper facilities in addition to the possession of talents."[98] To encourage American physicians to pursue scientific research, Noyes advocated providing them with financial support so they would have time for research as well as the necessary apparatus and assistance.

Wealthy citizens of New York responded to the calls for the endowment of medical science and medical education in their city. In 1884, Andrew Carnegie gave the Bellevue Hospital Medical College $50,000 for the erection of a laboratory building that provided opportunities for practical work in physiology, pathology, and therapeutics as well as private rooms for research. Cornelius Hoagland, a medical graduate of Western Reserve University, who became a millionaire through the manufacture and sale of baking powder, had a longstanding interest in microscopy. The developing field of bacteriology attracted his attention and his money when his grandson died of diphtheria in 1884. Hoagland donated nearly $200,000 to found a laboratory devoted to the basic medical sciences with emphasis on bacteriology at the Long Island College Hospital. The Hoagland Laboratory opened in 1888, the same year that the Loomis Laboratory at the University of the City of New York was established through a gift of $100,000 from Oliver H. Payne, a wealthy entrepreneur. These facilities, devoted to the basic medical sciences, included rooms for research as well as laboratories for the practical training of medical students.[99]

Each institution courted its patrons, and a certain degree of competition developed among the philanthropists as they contributed ever greater sums to their chosen charities. The medical schools of New York

City benefited disproportionately since they were located in the commercial and mercantile capital of the United States. Nevertheless, a new precedent with national implications had been established: the endowment of medical schools. Cornell University, Stanford University, and the Johns Hopkins University were examples of how endowed institutions could establish productive programs of scholarship and research. Growing recognition among American citizens, and particularly the wealthy entrepreneurs, that the endowment of medical research could yield palpable dividends through advances in public health, greater understanding about the pathophysiology and transmission of disease, and the discovery of specific cures served as a strong stimulus for the support of medical science. Dalton played a significant role in this movement.

Although as America's first full-time physiologist, Dalton was a pioneer, his agenda for physiology was quite modest. His emphasis was on classroom demonstrations and his own research. When funds became available to expand the scope of teaching and research at the college, Dalton had already relinquished the physiology chair. His successor John Curtis had the opportunity and responsibility of establishing a more comprehensive physiology program. Medical schools that received gifts from their alumni and philanthropists had to decide how to spend the money. One editor cautioned the officers of the College of Physicians and Surgeons not to commit the "too common error of spending the whole sum in new buildings and grounds, and having nothing left to sustain efficient laboratories and workers in the more purely scientific departments of medical instruction."[100]

Recognizing an opportunity to inaugurate a new era of laboratory training and research at the college through Vanderbilt's large gift, John Curtis traveled to Europe in 1886 to gain insight into the modern techniques of physiological teaching and research and to acquire apparatus. Curtis decided to go to Europe, in part, because of the recent exposure of his assistant Warren P. Lombard to European laboratories. Lombard had spent three years of postgraduate study in Europe following his graduation from Harvard Medical School where he had worked in Henry Bowditch's physiological laboratory.[101] Following his return from Carl Ludwig's Physiological Institute in Leipzig, Lombard, unable to find a paid teaching position in physiology elsewhere, became Curtis's assistant in New York in spite of the meager facilities. Lombard later recalled:

I had to do my first piece of research in the old building in the College of Physicians and Surgeons on Fourth Avenue, in a little

room that Professor John G. Curtis had used as a carpenter shop
to make models to illustrate his lectures. No janitors in those days.
I bought a broom and pail and removed the shavings and spiders.
Fortunately, I had bought a kymograph and induction coil before
I left Leipsig, and there was a firm bench, light, gas, and water.
What more could one want?[102]

This tongue-in-cheek assessment of the opportunities for physiological research at the college in the mid-1880s emphasizes the disparity between
what scientifically oriented physicians desired and what they had.

The first serious attempt to inaugurate an ambitious program of
laboratory training and research at the college occurred nearly thirty-
five years after Dalton had first introduced vivisection into the teaching
of physiology. Using college funds, Curtis purchased several major
pieces of physiological apparatus in Leipzig during his European visit. It
was Curtis's aim "to develop for the first time in the City of New York an
adequate and well-equipped physiological laboratory, which should
serve for teaching purposes and to which any properly trained person
could come with abundant opportunities for research."[103]

Dalton died in 1889. Upon hearing of his death, William H. Draper
expressed his sadness. The prominent New York dermatologist claimed
that Dalton had played a crucial role in the advance of the College of
Physicians and Surgeons by his "wonderful administrative ability . . .
lofty intelligence and thoroughly unselfish spirit."[104]

Dalton's major contribution to American physiology was his enthusiastic introduction of vivisection into teaching and, more important, his sustained and effective defense of the practice. He could have
been describing his own role in America when he elaborated François
Magendie's contributions to physiology:

> Coming at a time when the profession was unconsciously ripe for
> a more exact method of study, he gave the impulse and direction
> to a new movement. His untiring industry and the vigor and con-
> sistency of his ideas impressed themselves upon his associates and
> opened a fresh chapter in the history of physiological medicine.
> Notwithstanding the number and value of his own investigations,
> and of the new facts which he added to our knowledge, his influ-
> ence was still greater in the stimulus which he imparted to his
> contemporaries.[105]

Dalton did not establish a "school" of physiology as did Henry P.
Bowditch at Harvard and H. Newell Martin at Johns Hopkins. Nevertheless, as did his mentor Bernard, Dalton inspired many physicians to

acknowledge the central role of experimentation in the advance of medical science. Pupils who acknowledged their intellectual debt to Dalton included William H. Welch and William Halsted. Their enthusiasm for medicine as a science was inspired, in part, by Dalton when they were pupils at the college. When they became faculty members at the Johns Hopkins Medical School, Welch and Halsted were active participants in the reform movement to make American medicine scientific. Welch was a leading advocate of the full-time system of medical education; Dalton as a full-time medical educator was an early example. S. Weir Mitchell observed in his memorial address on Dalton, that he "was the first among us to give a life to the single pursuit of experimental physiology . . . [and] out of this singleness of pursuit and out of the fact that he was the first to content himself with physiology as a laboratory life-work there came to him a reputation above and beyond that which his discoveries justified."[106]

CHAPTER TWO

S. Weir Mitchell

Philadelphia's Frustrated Physiologist
and Triumphant Reformer

UNLIKE DALTON, WHO WAS successful in his quest for a scientific chair in a major American medical school, S. Weir Mitchell (1829–1914) of Philadelphia was unable to win an academic position in physiology.[1] Dalton and Mitchell were contemporaries whose early lives were subject to similar influences: both were sons of prominent physicians who respected medical science; both were graduated from prestigious medical schools; and, most important, both were devoted pupils of Claude Bernard. Although he made important contributions to physiology throughout his long career, Mitchell was an amateur physiologist who earned his living through medical practice. He understood the growing distinction between professional and amateur medical scientists. Mitchell, perhaps inadvertently, described his own circumstances in a comparison of Dalton's activities as a professional physiologist with individuals who made contributions to physiology when "they stepped aside from their other pursuits to follow experimental study for a brief season, and who went back again to the ordinary routine of their profession."[2]

Mitchell was not by choice an amateur physiologist. Local and institutional factors in Philadelphia prevented him from winning the chairs of physiology at the University of Pennsylvania and the Jefferson Medical College in the 1860s. These defeats did not diminish Mitchell's love of physiology, however. Indeed, they led him to work to improve opportunities for other Americans to pursue scientific careers. Despite his amateur status, Mitchell was one of the primary figures in the establishment of physiology as a discipline in America. Mitchell's defeats in the 1860s illustrate the importance of social and political factors in determining career opportunities and outcomes. It is impossible to know how the course of American physiology might have been altered had Mitchell been successful in his quest for an academic chair. It is clear, however, that the development of physiology in Philadelphia suffered. Philadelphia, long a leader in American science, lagged perceptibly in the movement to establish full-time chairs in the basic medical sciences, to introduce the research ethic into medical school teaching, and to initiate meaningful participation of medical students in laboratory exercises in physiology.

From the colonial period through the mid-nineteenth century, Philadelphia was widely acknowledged as the nation's leading intellectual center. Philadelphia societies with major commitments to scientific or medical research included the American Philosophical Society (1743), the Academy of Natural Sciences of Philadelphia (1812), and the Franklin Institute (1824). Physicians were prominent participants in these societies throughout the nineteenth century. A tradition of research by physicians of this city can be traced to John Morgan, one of the founders of America's first medical school (1765) at the College of Philadelphia. In his well-known address on medical education that year, Morgan emphasized the intellectual and practical benefits of research and experimentation. Anatomist and historian George Corner once claimed, "Had a program such as he presented to his trustees in 1765 been followed wherever medical schools grew up in the new country, American medicine need not have taken a century and a half to catch up with Europe."[3] Several physicians or scientists with medical training contributed to the recognition of Philadelphia as America's leading medical and scientific center in the late eighteenth and early nineteenth centuries. "Physiology first took root at the University of Pennsylvania," according to physiologist and historian John Fulton, when a professorship of the institutes of medicine was established in 1789; it represented "the first American physiological chair."[4]

The University of Pennsylvania was also one of the earliest medical schools in the United States to create a full-time position in a basic medical science. Joseph Leidy was appointed to the chair of anatomy at the university in 1853 and served as a role model for Mitchell.[5] As a youth, Leidy became interested in natural history, and while studying medicine he came under the influence of a number of scientifically oriented physicians including Paul Goddard and William Horner. Inspired by his exposure to continental scientists during a European journey in 1848,

Leidy gave up the practice of medicine after two years to devote himself to anatomical teaching and research. The concept of the full-time basic medical scientist was alien to American physicians in this era, however, and opponents to Leidy's 1853 candidacy for the Pennsylvania chair criticized him for devoting too much time to research and for not being an active medical practitioner.

Samuel Jackson, professor of the institutes of medicine at the University of Pennsylvania, addressed the ambivalence of medical practitioners and medical teachers toward research in antebellum America in an introductory lecture delivered in 1840, the year before Leidy matriculated at the university. Jackson encouraged his pupils to attempt to add to medical knowledge: "Whatever may be the particular bent of your genius, or the kind of talent you possess, there is, in medical researches, some one pursuit adapted to it. You have no excuse for negligence. The qualifications for these objects are industry, perseverance, application. These are in the power of each of you. They alone may enable you to establish important truths to be embodied in the science." Jackson was aware of the impediments to Americans pursuing scientific studies, however:

> It is unhappily true, that the active commercial spirit prevailing in
> this country and England, gives to the possessor of wealth, an un-
> due power and influence. It represses an intellectual class; it
> places the moneyed interest at the head of society. A scientific and
> literary class, possessing a weight and power in society, is yet to be
> formed in this country. Our literature and science are cultivated
> in subserviency to the advancement of fortune. We work for
> money; not for truth or fame. Combat against this feeling.[6]

A French observer of American culture, Alexis de Tocqueville, had reached a similar conclusion five years earlier. He applauded Americans for their contributions to practical science, but complained that they essentially ignored abstract or theoretical science. He attributed this shortcoming to the democratic nature of American society which did not permit the development of an aristocratic class with leisure for speculation and contemplation. Moreover, Americans sought money and power, and had little time left for purely intellectual activity.[7]

S. Weir Mitchell was born into the world of science and medicine in Philadelphia in 1829. He was the son of John K. Mitchell, a prominent physician, medical author, and scientist who taught chemistry and physiology at the Jefferson Medical College.[8] Weir Mitchell's grandfather was a Scottish physician who emigrated to America in the eighteenth century, and his father graduated from the medical department of the University of Pennsylvania in 1819. In 1841, a time of major reorganization at the Jefferson Medical College, Mitchell's father was elected to the chair of theory and practice of medicine. His scientific colleagues at Jefferson included Robley Dunglison, professor of the institutes of medicine and medical jurisprudence, and Franklin Bache, professor of chemistry. Weir Mitchell emulated his father who combined a career as a successful medical practitioner with his scientific and literary interests. His father's modest private chemistry laboratory in the Philadelphia Medical Institute made a strong impression on Mitchell as a boy. Mitchell believed that his father was best suited for a scientific career, but claimed that financial necessity forced him to devote most of his energy to medical practice.

At the age of nineteen, Mitchell enrolled in the Jefferson Medical College as one of more than two hundred students. There, he heard Robley Dunglison lecture on physiology. Although the lectures were didactic, without experiments or illustrations, they further stimulated young Mitchell's interest in the scientific side of medicine. He gained practical training in James Booth's chemistry laboratory. Booth, having recently returned from study abroad, was familiar with the newer chemical techniques. While medical students, Mitchell and his classmate Thomas Bache were invited to participate in research under Dunglison's direction. The probable reason the two young medical students were given this unusual opportunity is that both were sons of Jefferson faculty members. Mitchell and his friend studied the effect of the exposure of excised frog hearts to a vacuum. These experiments, performed when Mitchell was twenty-one, represent his first documented physiological research.[9]

Following his graduation in 1850, Mitchell traveled to Europe for additional medical study. Dunglison helped him plan his trip and provided a letter of introduction to the prominent British physiologist William Carpenter, well known to American medical students through his popular physiology text. Mitchell also studied in Paris, the leading city for medical training in this era. As Dalton had, he studied under Claude Bernard whose stature as a physiologist was rapidly growing. While studying in Paris, Mitchell contracted smallpox. The ambitious Philadelphian revealed his frustration to his sister in February 1851: "The little I have done here is child's play. I have learned next to nothing. I feel unsettled, and instead of a year of fair work which could show results, what do I have to exhibit?"[10]

Mitchell's plan to remain in Europe another year was thwarted by his father's declining health. The burden of a large medical practice led the elder Mitchell to urge his son to return home to join him. Upon his return to Philadelphia, Mitchell first confronted the role politics and personality disputes could play in an individual's career. He failed to win a position as intern at Pennsylvania Hospital because of persistent hard feelings from an earlier conflict between his father and members of the board of that institution.[11]

Within a year after returning home from Paris, Mitchell began delivering physiology lectures at the Philadelphia Association for Medical Instruction, also known as the "Summer Association." Brown-Séquard delivered a series of lectures at the Summer Association in 1852. Although not illustrated with vivisections, Brown-Séquard's course included extensive descriptions of research he had undertaken using this method.[12] Soon after inaugurating his physiology course, Mitchell established a modest laboratory in the Philadelphia School of Anatomy building used by teachers of the Summer Association. Mitchell's longtime friend and colleague William Keen claimed that here Mitchell taught "the first purely experimental course on Physiology in the city," beginning in 1856.[13]

Inspired by his exposure to Bernard and Brown-Séquard's Philadelphia visit, and despite a busy medical practice and his summer lecture course, Mitchell found time to initiate a series of experiments in 1853. He used microscopical and chemical analysis as well as vivisection in his research. The subject of Mitchell's first independent research project on uric acid crystals reflected the interests of his father, his chemistry teacher James Booth, and the French scientists Pierre Robin and Claude Bernard.

His third published paper, on the relationship of the pulse to respiration, provides valuable insight into Mitchell as a scientist at this early stage of his career. During his training abroad, financial support from a wealthy British relative enabled Mitchell to buy books and instruments. He employed one of these instruments, a haemadynometer, in his experiments. Mitchell was not working in isolation, but had the cooperation and encouragement of several scientifically oriented physicians who also taught at the Summer Association. He was assisted in his vivisections by other recent Jefferson graduates including Jacob Da Costa, George Morehouse, and John Brinton as well as their "private pupils."[14] Nevertheless, Mitchell's circumstances were not entirely conducive to research. He undertook his experiments in the evening, following the completion of his duties as a medical practitioner.

The low productivity of Americans compared with European medical scientists troubled Mitchell. He hinted at this concern in a review of a paper by Joseph Jones, a recent graduate of the University of Pennsylvania Medical School, and forcefully stated his view in an extensive survey of anatomical and physiological research in America he published in 1858.[15] The survey included an annotated list of recent American publications in anatomy and physiology and revealed Mitchell's familiarity with the medical literature. He harshly concluded:

> At best, it is a melancholy catalogue; and considering the adventurous ingenuity of the national mind, as well as the solid character of its achievements in other lines of scientific research, it is not easy to see why a science so eminently experimental as physiology, should be able to boast so few active laborers and so small a number of conspicuous results. Still, even the last year shows a remarkable improvement, and we may hope, at least, that he who ten years hence reviews the earnings of our physiological workers, may have a larger sum of original results to cast into the lap of the great Mother Truth.[16]

Mitchell's assessment was similar to that of Joseph Leidy, who had claimed five years earlier: "In our own country, but little yet has been done for the advancement of Anatomy and Physiology; nevertheless we have had some excellent observers and teachers."[17] Mitchell wanted to see research more widely undertaken in America. But few of Mitchell's or Leidy's contemporaries appreciated the distinction between teaching and research, and between sciences based on observation and those based on experimentation. This lack of appreciation became apparent when the young Philadelphia physiologist attempted to find a stable institutional base for teaching physiology and pursuing research in this promising science.

Although Mitchell sought to emulate his father's career in many respects, he received little encouragement from the senior Mitchell. Despite his profound interest in chemistry, his father did not encourage specialization in this or any other scientific field. Just as his son was completing his medical training, the elder Mitchell told his pupils:

> Among the errors into which many students fall in the pursuit of a medical education, none is more common than undue admiration of one branch and dangerous neglect of another. . . . One, enamored of the beautiful theories and admirable processes taught by the physiologist, abandons himself too exclusively to the cultivation of physiology. Devoting to it an undue proportion of time, and bestowing on the hours given to less favored branches less of

pleasurable excitement, he becomes insensibly little more than a physiologist.[18]

Although few American medical practitioners concerned themselves with the issue of medical research, a small but increasingly vocal segment of the medical and scientific communities argued that Americans must make greater efforts to expand man's knowledge of his body, his environment, and the universe. Mitchell's lineage, his European training, his publications, and his participation in a number of societies facilitated his entry into a network of American scientists who wanted to introduce the research ethic into American higher education. The Academy of Natural Sciences of Philadelphia, to which he was elected in 1853, served as his intellectual focus. Together with a score of scientifically oriented Philadelphia physicians, Mitchell participated in the founding of two local societies in 1857 that encouraged medical research: the Philadelphia Pathological Society and the short-lived Philadelphia Biological Society. These organizations were founded, in part, to fill a void in America. As historian Bonnie Blustein has claimed, "There was no place . . . for the physician-investigator comparable to that offered by the Continental universities and institutes."[19]

In 1858, Mitchell began a series of studies on the toxicology of snake venoms and arrow poisons with William Hammond, an army surgeon with a deep interest in physiological research. Mitchell may have met Hammond as early as 1848 when he came to Philadelphia for further training after his graduation from the Medical College of the City of New York. Following his enlistment in the army as assistant surgeon in 1849, Hammond held a variety of posts around America, although he viewed the Academy of Natural Sciences of Philadelphia as his scientific home.[20] Hammond and Mitchell were present at the founding meeting of the Philadelphia Biological Society, and it was mainly from Hammond that Mitchell derived his interest in the toxicology of snake venoms. As an army surgeon stationed in New Mexico and Kansas during the 1850s, Hammond became interested in the medical management of snake bites and investigated a purported antidote attributed to the French herpetologist Gabriel Bibron.[21]

Although Hammond had not studied abroad, he was familiar with the recent publications of the French and German physiologists. He observed that physiology was now based on chemistry and physics, and, for this reason, the tendency to explain function on the basis of vital force had greatly diminished.[22] Dalton, a disciple of the philosophy of Bernard had criticized the attempts of the German physiologists to reduce physiology to nothing more than physics and chemistry. Hammond, who had not been personally exposed to either group, was familiar with both, and consequently held a somewhat more balanced view.

Mitchell became interested in curare, a substance Bernard was actively studying when he was his pupil in 1850. Mitchell and Hammond's extensive study of curare published in 1859 reveals their experimental techniques.[23] They used pigeons, owls, mice, frogs, rabbits, alligators, and cats in their experiments. Their studies included microscopical examinations as well as detailed observations on the response of the pulse, respiratory rate, and temperature of animals administered curare by a variety of routes. In concluding their essay, they reaffirmed the central role experimentation must play in advancing medical knowledge.

Mitchell's collaboration with Hammond ended when the army surgeon left Philadelphia in the fall of 1859.[24] Aided by Joseph Henry of the Smithsonian Institution, Mitchell obtained snakes and continued his studies on venom. Mitchell reported his extensive experiments on the physiology and pharmacology of venom in an impressive monograph published by the Smithsonian in 1860. It contained little information of direct relevance to the practicing physician, but Mitchell informed his readers that a subsequent paper would deal with the medical aspects of serpent bites. In his clinical paper, published the following year, Mitchell emphasized the value of experimentation as a means to elucidate the pathophysiology of snake bites and identify possible antidotes.[25]

Hammond and Mitchell received national and international recognition for their studies on curare and venom. Claude Bernard, Mitchell's former teacher, and Brown-Séquard were among the Europeans who took notice of their publications. Oliver Wendell Holmes, who admired Mitchell's father's scientific and literary talents, wrote the young Philadelphia physiologist upon receipt of the venom monograph that he was "delighted with your numerous and well conducted observations and experiments. . . . I don't know that I have spoken strongly enough of the great excellence of your observations. They form a most original and important addition, as I think to physiological science."[26] Mitchell appreciated Holmes's encouragement and a quarter century later remarked, "The first letter that I ever received in recognition of any scientific work I had done, came to me when I was a young fellow from Oliver Wendell Holmes. He will never know how much good it did me."[27] Dalton was among those who acknowledged the significance of Mitchell's venom monograph: "The paper, in which the account of these experiments is given, has no superior in medical literature for the clearness and elegance of its style, the abundance of its material, and the precision of its results."[28]

Not all of Mitchell's teachers and colleagues encouraged his research efforts, however. He later recalled that Samuel Jackson "said to me most earnestly, 'If you want to practise medicine, do not venture to be an experimental physiologist. It will ruin you.'"[29] The experience of Robley Dunglison supported Jackson's claim that medical practice was incompatible with a significant commitment to science:

> In this country, the so called "practical" predominates, and it is constantly contrasted with the "scientific." . . . To be considered highly scientific and to have published largely on his own profession and more especially to be eminent in general literature is positively detrimental, by encouraging the idea, that the physician may be very learned and very scientific and literary but, for that very reason, probably not practical, and I am sorry to say, that this popular feeling has been occasionally taken advantage of by the members of his own profession, when an eminent member has come amongst them and it has been insidiously remarked, when his qualifications have been inquired into by the laity, that "he is undoubtedly a man of *science* and *learning* in his profession, but they do not know, whether he is a *practical* man." This, I know, has been repeatedly said of me, both in Baltimore and Philadelphia and even by one or more of my personal friends![30]

Yet Mitchell pursued his scientific studies with great vigor while conscientiously attending to his growing medical practice. By the early 1860s, Mitchell was widely acclaimed as America's leading experimental physiologist; his fame as an investigator even surpassed Dalton's. Brown-Séquard acknowledged Mitchell's contributions, writing in 1861, "I am very happy to see that you do so much for Physiology, and I congratulate you very sincerely for the advances this noble science owes to you already. You and your friend and scientific partner, Dr. Hammond, are the most original Physiologists of the United States."[31]

When the Summer Association disbanded in 1860, Mitchell lost his teaching position in physiology. In 1861, he was elected a member of the Boston Society of Natural History, and the following year a member of the American Philosophical Society. These new affiliations brought Mitchell into contact with other Americans who shared his commitment to original research. But his frustration grew as he found that he had less time to devote to his experiments. Mitchell complained to Jeffries Wyman: "My former work, such as it is, has been done in the face of extreme obstacles, arising from the fact, that I rely upon my practice to keep the pot boiling for myself & others. People wonder that men in Europe who have a *whole* life to give to science shd. do so much—I marvel that they effect so little. I can only work from June to October & that time I hope always to keep, in part at least, for science."[32]

The morbidity and mortality of the Civil War set the stage for an abrupt shift in Mitchell's career. Nearly all American physicians' practices were affected to some degree by this great conflict.[33] Hammond resigned from the chair of anatomy and physiology at the University of Maryland, which he had held for a year, to rejoin the army medical department as assistant surgeon at the beginning of the Rebellion. Concern for the care of sick and wounded soldiers led to the formation in 1861 of the Sanitary Commission, whose goals included the reorganization of the medical department of the army. Hammond came to the notice of the commission through his 1862 study of the military hospitals in Grafton, Virginia, and Cumberland, Maryland. His reputation as a medical scientist, the high quality of this report, and his early performance in the army led to Hammond's appointment as surgeon-general. This appointment placed Hammond in a position to change the career of his friend Mitchell.

The military hospitals in and around Philadelphia, which had more than twenty-five thousand beds for the sick and wounded, provided ample clinical material. Mitchell declined the position of brigade surgeon, preferring to stay in Philadelphia so that his medical practice would be less disrupted, and so that he could continue to care for his widowed mother. These responsibilities also prevented Mitchell from accepting Dalton's invitation to teach the physiology course at the College of Physicians and Surgeons of New York when Dalton was in the army in Washington. Shortly after his appointment as army surgeon in October 1862, Mitchell began to take an interest in cases of nervous disease. Soon, patients with this type of problem were referred to him, and Hammond created a special neurology ward for him in the new military hospital on Turner's Lane in Philadelphia.[34] The intensity of wartime duties, together with his own medical practice, made it difficult for Mitchell to continue his physiological studies. Early in the war, he informed his sister, "No physiology this summer but splendid hospital work."[35]

Mitchell was not the only Philadelphia physician who found that clinical duties limited the time available for laboratory work. Harrison Allen, a recent graduate of the University of Pennsylvania and resident physician at Pennsylvania Hospital, complained to Joseph Leidy in 1862 that the duties of his position as resident physician made it impossible for him to devote more than every other night and Sundays to scientific work at the Academy of Natural Sciences of Philadelphia.[36] Although his scientific productivity declined, Mitchell's physiological research did not cease despite his new Civil War commitments. In addition to neurological papers, he collaborated with George Morehouse in a study on the physiology of respiration in Chelonia and an investigation of the antagonism of atropine and morphine.

An opportunity arose in 1863 that Mitchell believed would provide him with an institutional setting where he could once again teach and perform research in physiology. Samuel Jackson had been ill for some time and resigned as professor of the institutes of medicine from the University of Pennsylvania in the spring of 1863. Even before Jackson's official resignation, Mitchell rallied his scientific colleagues to lend their support to his attempt to win the chair. William Hammond regarded Mitchell as America's premier experimental physiologist and encouraged Joseph Leidy to support him. He pointed out that Mitchell's election would acknowledge the value of his research, as well as his education and talents as a lecturer, and "his success would be a recognition of the claims of scientific labor which would gratify me."[37] Mitchell wrote Leidy, optimistically declaring: "I send a list of my papers. In the statement DaC[osta] gave you will find the essence of what I want you to add—please to send it to my house *tomorrow*. We have no time to lose. Dr. Jackson today gave me leave to canvass & authority to refer to him any trustees who want to know what he thinks. He will indorse me as a candidate as full as we could wish or ask—the track is clear."[38]

Mitchell spared no effort in eliciting testimonials from several prominent scientists who were familiar with his work. From Boston, he received letters from Jeffries Wyman, Louis Agassiz, and Oliver Wendell Holmes. He also sought the assistance of Joseph Henry, secretary of the Smithsonian Institution, who was deeply committed to the advance of experimental science in America. In requesting testimonials from these leading American scientists, Mitchell emphasized his personal interpretation of physiology as an independent science. Moreover, he reminded them of his dedication to research in contrast to the typical medical faculty member's disdain of experimentation and reliance upon didactic instruction. To Wyman, Mitchell confided:

I have been to Washington & secured warm letters from my friend Hammond & Prof. Henry. I am now awaiting yours & Agassiz to place all before the Trustees at once. What I want is this—That you should say with energy enough to reach Trustee brains what you think is my position as a man of science—as a physiologist— whether I am likely to illustrate the chair etc. . . . Of my opponent I have nothing to say but that he is a gentleman & that we are both *said* to teach well—But I shall feel it just a little hard if it should happen that I am beaten by one who has never added a leaf to the crown of the mistress in whose service I have spent so many hours of welcome labour. You will know *how* I feel & why the heaviness of the stake makes me so unscrupulous a beggar."[39]

Mitchell's supporters corresponded among themselves regarding his ambition for the Pennsylvania chair. Writing to Joseph Leidy in March 1863, Joseph Henry revealed that he had received a letter from Wyman emphasizing the value of Mitchell's scientific contributions. Henry also explained that he had written the trustees of the University of Pennsylvania urging Mitchell's appointment:

> I have advocated the proposition that, other things being equal, a position in one of our larger Institutions of learning ought to be given in preference to the candidate who has done most by original research to advance the branch of knowledge to which the vacant chair pertains. The adoption of this rule would not only stimulate original investigations, but also ensure a higher class of teachers. The man of original research as a rule must possess enthusiasm, in pursuit of his favourite subject, which cannot fail to be communicated to the pupils.[40]

Henry found little understanding of, or sympathy for, this distinction that he (and Mitchell) believed was so important. Nearly a decade later, Henry informed John Tyndall, "It is only after nearly twenty-five years of struggle . . . that I have begun to make the country appreciate the difference between the discovery of new truths, and the teaching of old ones."[41]

Although Mitchell initially believed "the coast was clear," other candidates were nominated to fill Jackson's vacant chair. The most formidable candidate, who ultimately won the contest, was Francis Gurney Smith, Jr.[42] Smith was the son of a prominent Boston merchant and held undergraduate and medical degrees from the University of Pennsylvania. He entered medical practice in 1842 and was appointed lecturer on physiology at the Summer Association the same year. Smith was attracted to physiology by Robley Dunglison, whose lectures he attended regularly. Following the custom of contemporary medical teachers, Smith edited a variety of British and European works, among them William Carpenter's popular physiology text.[43] A prolific editor, Smith gained widespread recognition when he brought out the second volume of Daniel Drake's classic work on endemic diseases of America and served as the editor of the *Philadelphia Medical Examiner* from 1844 to 1854. Although a common way for medical teachers to supplement their incomes, the editing and abstracting of the British and European literature, elicited harsh criticism from a number of Americans including Oliver Wendell Holmes.[44]

Smith was a popular and well-known teacher of physiology in Philadelphia. He had lectured on this subject for a decade at the Summer Association before becoming professor of the institutes of medicine in the Medical Department of Pennsylvania College. This school suffered financial difficulties, however, and closed because of declining enrollments as a result of the Civil War. Although Smith was interested in the scientific side of medicine and participated with Mitchell and others in the formation of the Biological Department of the Academy of Natural Sciences in 1858, he held the traditional view of the responsibilities of medical teachers. In contrast to Mitchell, Smith undertook little research in physiology. His only notable contribution was a study of human gastric juice inspired by Brown-Séquard's visit to Philadelphia and his access to Beaumont's experimental subject, Alexis St. Martin, in 1853.[45] Smith derived the majority of his income from a busy medical practice and supplemented it with student's fees and royalties from textbooks he edited.

Mitchell and Smith provided the trustees of the University of Pennsylvania with a distinct choice. Superficially, both were prominent Philadelphia practitioners who had taught physiology and were frequent contributors to the medical literature. Mitchell's publications, however, were based on extensive original research that employed vivisection. Smith's literary efforts, comprised almost entirely of editing or supplementing the writings of others, did not represent new contributions to knowledge. This distinction between the candidates did not determine the outcome of the contest, however. The university board selected Smith to succeed Samuel Jackson. This selection provides valuable insight into the priorities of institutional boards of trustees in an era when little or no distinction was made between teachers who simply transmitted known facts and those who attempted to expand knowledge through research.

Social, not scientific, factors influenced the trustees. Smith was an active member of the Protestant Episcopal Church and was one of the first staff members appointed to the Protestant Episcopal Hospital founded in 1852. Several Pennsylvania board members belonged to this church, and one of the most influential members of the board was Alonzo Potter, a prominent Episcopal minister and the founder of the Episcopal Hospital. Moreover, the board's twenty-four members included only three physicians, so there is little reason to believe the board members possessed any great insight into the special needs of medical education in America at this time. The election took place on 5 May 1863 with eleven board members present, of whom only one, George Norris, was a physician.[46]

"I have lost my election," Mitchell told Joseph Henry. "It ought to satisfy me as it did not turn upon the question of science or ability to teach but on such outside influences as age—church connections—& social pressure."[47] Mitchell's analysis is supported by the complaints of George Shrady regarding medical appointments. The New York medical editor observed in 1866, "As the case now stands, when a vacancy occurs . . . at the proper time, the requisite pressure, social, political, and even religious, is brought to bear upon the laymen who are primarily the power in this matter, and the thing is done."[48] The trustees, virtually all laymen, failed to appreciate the claims of Mitchell and his supporters regarding the importance of the candidate's commitment to scientific research. Even most contemporary American physicians did not value research or encourage interest in medical science. Speaking to a Philadelphia medical audience the same year as Mitchell's defeat, Alfred Stillé complained of their apathy toward science.[49]

Joseph Henry consoled Mitchell and asserted that the decision was not in the best interest of American science. He encouraged him to carry on his investigations and assured him that his contributions would ultimately be acknowledged and rewarded.[50] Holmes expressed similar sentiments and urged Mitchell to be patient, noting, "It is hardly desirable that an active man of science should obtain a chair too early—for I have noticed as you, doubtless, have that the wood of which academic *fauteuils* are made has a narcotic quality which occasionally renders their occupants somnolent, lethargic or even comatose."[51]

Had Mitchell won the Pennsylvania chair he almost certainly would have established a physiological laboratory in which to continue the work he had started in the Summer Association. There, aided by students and colleagues, he had performed many experiments and had served as a role model for Philadelphia students and young physicians interested in medical science. Now, without an institutional base, and with growing commitments to practice and wartime obligations, Mitchell's opportunities for physiology dwindled. The successful candidate, Smith, did not establish a physiological laboratory at the University of Pennsylvania until 1875. By that time, Mitchell was a member of the board of trustees at the university and encouraged this improvement. It was for his eloquence and the thoroughness of his didactic lectures, rather than for research, that Smith would be remembered.

After his defeat Mitchell continued to investigate the toxicology of rattlesnake venom. His intellectual energies became increasingly focused on diseases of the nervous system, however. He acknowledged the importance of the specialty hospitals founded by Hammond in facilitating his study of the nervous effects of wounds.[52] Mitchell's rich Civil War experience led him to publish several important papers with his surgical colleagues William Keen and George Morehouse. Medical historian William Norwood considered them one of the few significant contributions to medical science derived from the enormous medical experience of the Civil War.[53]

Despite his growing interest in clinical neurology, Mitchell still wanted a physiology chair—an institutional base for his scientific interests. He later claimed, "It is never very well to be absolutely isolated in your pursuits. I, myself, can well recall how little interest I found in this city in physiology when I first began to work at it practically. It was a real and serious discouragement. The reverse of this condition of intellectual loneliness has its use. All men do more and better work amidst the competitions of other workers."[54]

Another opportunity for a chair in physiology presented itself to Mitchell in April 1868 when Robley Dunglison resigned from the Jefferson Medical College. Dunglison, Mitchell's physiology teacher, had held the Jefferson chair for more than three decades. Requesting a letter of recommendation from Wyman, Mitchell exclaimed, "I have again to undergo the awful horrors of a canvass."[55] Wyman responded, "In truth I do not understand why the Trustees wish my testimonials, if they are in any way acquainted with the status of Physiology in this country. But after the result in the former canvass, I suppose we are not to presume that they know anything about it."[56] The Jefferson trustees received strong letters on Mitchell's behalf from Wyman, Joseph Henry, William Hammond, Louis Agassiz, John Dalton, Austin Flint, Jr., and Brown-Séquard.[57]

Louis Agassiz was a spokesman for the research ethic and appreciated the growing differentiation of science. Speaking of Mitchell's contest, he informed the Philadelphia physiologist, "You know as well as I do what deep struggle is going on in scientific circles among us, and how deeply the future prospect of science in the U.S. is involved in the contest, though the community at large knows nothing about it." Agassiz contrasted the typical candidate for a scientific chair who performed no research, but was a popular lecturer who simply recited the discoveries made by others, with the original investigator "upon whose effort in reality rests the progress of knowledge." The Harvard scientist explained:

Your friends feel happy to know that you belong to the small band which by original independent research contribute to the advancement of science and may before long place our country on a level with the most progressive nations. . . . I hope in the present case the selection of a professor of physiology in the most important medical school of the U.S. will be influenced chiefly by the opinion of the most competent men of the country, as I am satisfied that in that case your selection would be secure and that being placed in a position in which you can devote your abilities to the further advance of your science, there shall be another centre of real progress in one of our institutions of learning.[58]

Mitchell's opponent for the Jefferson chair was James Aitken Meigs, the son of a Philadelphia shoe merchant and 1851 graduate of the Jefferson Medical College.[59] An active medical practitioner, Meigs held a number of hospital positions. He also served as demonstrator to Francis Gurney Smith, Jr., whom he eventually succeeded as professor of the institutes of medicine in the short-lived Medical Department of Pennsylvania College. Meigs illustrated his physiology lectures with vivisections, a practice that was becoming increasingly popular in Philadelphia in the 1860s. With Mitchell and Smith, Meigs participated in the formation of the Biological Department of the Academy of Natural Sciences of Philadelphia. His scientific interests related primarily to ethnology and physical anthropology, however, fields to which he was attracted by Samuel George Morton and Joseph Leidy.

As Mitchell found, Meigs's medical practice limited the time he could devote to his scientific interests. He claimed in 1856, "A considerable amount of sickness is prevailing in my neighborhood, and my practice, therefore shortens my time for such [scientific] labors very much."[60] A frequent reviewer of new works in physiology for the *American Journal of Medical Sciences* and the *North American Medico-Chirurgical Review* in the late 1850s and 1860s, Meigs proclaimed the growing practical importance of physiology to the medical profession. He was convinced that "practical medicine can never become a rational, philosophical system, unless it is based upon a strictly scientific physiology."[61] Meigs had not studied abroad, but his reviews reveal his familiarity with the European literature of physiology and related sciences. In contrast to Smith, Meigs appreciated the research ethic; in an 1859 address he stressed the dichotomy between the professor who simply teaches known facts and the "experimental biologist" who investigates and seeks new knowledge.[62]

Meigs was qualified to hold the Jefferson chair: he was familiar with the contemporary literature of physiology; used vivisection in his physiology course; and proclaimed the importance of the basic sciences to the practicing physician. Moreover, he was one of very few medical teachers to acknowledge the research ethic. Nevertheless, Meigs was not truly an experimental physiologist as the term was coming to be defined in Europe, or would soon be defined in America. His scientific specialty was ethnology. It was not an impediment to his winning the Jefferson chair, however. As a result of the withdrawal of southern students at the outset of the Civil War, Jefferson had suffered a decline in enrollment greater than that of most other northern medical schools. In an attempt to attract more students, and to compete with the University of Pennsylvania, a special "summer course" was inaugurated at Jefferson in 1866. Meigs was selected to teach physiology in this summer course.[63] Already an adjunct member of the Jefferson faculty, he sought to succeed Dunglison upon his resignation in 1868.

As Mitchell did, Meigs eagerly elicited support from his professional and scientific colleagues, and the board received letters from individuals whose scientific interests reflected his own. Josiah Nott, Richard Owen, Daniel Wilson, and Paul Broca wrote the Jefferson trustees on Meigs's behalf. Ironically, Joseph Henry wrote letters of support for both Meigs and Mitchell. The Smithsonian Institution had long been interested in anthropology and ethnology, and Henry was aware of Meigs's contributions to these fields.[64] Few American physicians, let alone lay boards of trustees, recognized the growing differentiation of the basic medical sciences in this era. Writing in support of Mitchell, three weeks after he had written on behalf of Meigs, Henry informed the Jefferson trustees that he supported Mitchell because he had "an earnest desire to see our more important scientific positions filled by men of powers of original investigation, who have enlarged by their own labors the bounds of science, and added to the reputation of the country."[65]

Although an alumnus of Jefferson, the son of one of its most illustrious former teachers, and the recipient of strong letters of support from America's leading scientists, Mitchell was by no means confident of success. His experience in the 1863 Pennsylvania election demonstrated the unpredictability of trustees. Aware of the intense political feelings in America in this era, he appealed to Henry to exert his personal influence with George Woodward, a Democratic member of Congress who also sat on the Jefferson board.[66] Writing to one of the Jefferson trustees, possibly George Woodward, Mitchell explained:

> I am now able to say to you that I have the voice of every professor now at home as well as the expressed desire of Dr. Dunglison

that I should succeed him. Nevertheless, I run as I am told the
utmost risk owing chiefly to the possible absence of two trustees.
As for myself it is of course no light matter to see the just reward
of years of labour slip away for no fault of mine. You can understand therefore why I urge you to oblige me by returning for this
occasion.[67]

Lawrence Turnbull, Meigs's biographer, described the 1868 contest as "a most exciting canvass, in which the whole profession of the city
and county was interested." Meigs was "supported by a large number of
the medical men of Philadelphia, many of them using their utmost personal efforts on his behalf. They were attracted to him by his urbanity of
manner, willingness to assist them in any emergency, which with his
pleasant smile won their regard, and also their respect for his qualities of
head and heart."[68] A former student of Meigs, writing at the time of his
election, characterized him as

one of the most fluent & able lecturers I have ever heard. He has
had a large experience as teacher & lecturer on Physiology. . . .
He is at present actively engaged in practice and enjoys to a large
extent the confidence and respect of the community. He is young,
active & energetic, a man of exemplary habits and . . . a good
democrat. Anything that you may be pleased to do to promote his
interest will be serving as a great personal favor to me. I am now
living in hopes that some day I will be able to remove to Phila. &
pursue the practice of my profession & if I can secure the good
will of such a man as Dr. Meigs it would be a very great benefit to
me.[69]

Thirteen of the fifteen members of the Jefferson board were present
on 2 June 1868 when eight voted for Meigs and five for Mitchell.[70] As
was the case at the University of Pennsylvania, the Jefferson trustees included only one physician. The others were lawyers, politicians, businessmen, and philanthropists. The Philadelphia medical press greeted
Meigs's appointment with approval: "It is one of those appointments
based on real and widely acknowledged merit. . . . Without in the least
questioning the deserts of the other candidates, we think that all must
acknowledge that the Trustees have made a most judicious choice for the
position."[71]

Members of Mitchell's scientific network saw things differently. Responding to news of his defeat, Wyman informed him that Meigs also
requested a letter of recommendation, which he did not write, "as I
could only offer him second best." The Harvard naturalist continued, "I
cannot understand the result of the election, living so far away from the

scene of action & knowing nothing of the currents & counter-currents which finally control the issues of all such matters. It did seem to me that the trustees of the college had a chance which rarely happens in this country for strengthening their faculty & that they would be wise enough to profit by it. Your friends here will I am sure deeply feel the disappointment."[72]

As was the case in 1863, Mitchell felt the need to explain the circumstances of his defeat. He wrote to Wyman:

> Dr. Meigs by whom I have been defeated is not as *you* know a physiologist so that as you infer the contest turned on other than relative claims as biologists. The board of trustees is made up of democrats most of whom have been politicians & lived by that trade. They are nearly all men of the people & have risen from the ranks & several who are connected by family & other ties have long been looking forward to using their positions to place in the faculty a member of their clique & family. Political, social & family reasons decided the matter against the wishes of the faculty & the desires of the late Professor. I ought to explain what I mean by social reasons—Dr. Meigs is the son of a shoemaker here & has fought his way up with courage & intelligence.[73]

Mitchell's frustration in losing this chair is revealed in his closing comments to Wyman:

> Of course I felt bitterly the defeat of certain intellectual ambitions, but most of all the fact that I must continue to work as hard as ever at practice & so see it year after year encroaching on the little time I can give to science. Had I gotten this chair I meant to organize a physiological laboratory with a paid assistant & to have spent on this scheme at least a thousand a year. I could thus have accomplished a great deal of systematic research which is out of my power so long as only the afternoons of summer can be given to work.[74]

Writing to Joseph Henry, Mitchell declared, "I am very sorry to tell you that owing chiefly to the Democratic character of the Board of the Trustees I have lost the election. . . . It is my last chance of such a position & I am never likely to claim a repetition of the kindly service you have twice rendered me."[75]

Henry chose not to tell Mitchell that he had also written a letter on Meigs's behalf, but he did express his "personal mortification" that Mitchell had not won the Jefferson chair. Henry decried the role that politics had played in the contest and expressed regret that Philadelphia had lost its position as the scientific center of America. He hoped that the medical schools of that city would come to recognize the folly of selecting as professors men who were "popular expounders of science" rather than "men of original thought and research."[76]

It is tempting to speculate what it might have meant for physiology in Philadelphia and America had Mitchell won a chair. There is no reason to question his claim to Wyman that he would have established a physiological laboratory at the Jefferson Medical College. A decade earlier, while a teacher at the Summer Association, he had involved students and colleagues in research in which vivisection was employed. An institutional base at the University of Pennsylvania or the Jefferson Medical College would have provided Mitchell with the opportunity to involve students in experimental work once again. Henry P. Bowditch, who departed for Europe for postgraduate study the same year as Mitchell's Jefferson defeat, founded a physiological laboratory at Harvard in 1871 that provided opportunities for research for advanced pupils. Mitchell remained rueful over his defeats despite an increasingly successful career as a neurologist. Acknowledging the publication of a recent paper based on research performed in Bowditch's physiological laboratory a few year after his Jefferson defeat, he declared to James J. Putnam, "It is very pleasant to see the gradual awakening in America of physiological research &—I have only the vain regret that I am not also one of the present workers."[77]

Mitchell and his network of scientific colleagues were not the only ones who sensed problems with the state of medical science in Philadelphia. In a discussion on national and regional differences in productivity in medical research, George Shrady acknowledged the growing interest in experimental medicine in Boston and New York. The provocative medical editor expressed the hope that Philadelphia would regain its stature by encouraging rather than "persecuting" leaders of scientific medicine.[78]

Unlike Dalton of the College of Physicians and Surgeons of New York, or Henry Bowditch, who became Harvard Medical School's first full-time physiologist in 1871, Meigs continued to practice medicine after his appointment to the Jefferson chair. Meigs's decision to continue practice had significant consequences for physiology at Jefferson. One of his biographers claimed, "In his thirty years' practice he was very successful, having devoted himself to it very closely. . . . The cause of science has suffered from these engrossing cares, which he never could be prevailed upon to resign."[79] Meigs believed the medical profession discouraged its members from pursuing scientific research. He attributed this attitude to the financial aspects of medical practice and to the "baser sort" of doctors who were obsessed with wealth. He rejected the notion that medical practice and research were incompatible. Although he argued that the powers of observation—so important to the medical practitioner—were enhanced by research, he did not encourage his pupils to pursue their scientific interests. In 1870 he told the Jefferson students, "I must warn you to commence your career by binding yourselves, Ulysses-like, to the mast of your profession, lest in your occasional incursions into the domain of science, the voice of the siren estrange you *wholly* from your first love, and ruin your prospects as medical men."[80]

Although Meigs had used vivisections in his physiology lectures and demonstrations at Pennsylvania College in the 1850s, he did not continue this practice when he assumed the Jefferson chair in 1868. It is possible that the growing antivivisection sentiment discouraged him from doing so. Moreover, Meigs's research in anthropology and ethnology did not require the use of vivisection, so he had no incentive for its inclusion in his Jefferson program. Meigs was, nevertheless, highly regarded as a teacher and was respected as a practitioner. Ironically, historians of anthropology, themselves seeking individuals who shaped that discipline, identify Meigs as one who failed to achieve the level of distinction to which he seemed destined. Aleš Hrdlička attributed this failure to his preoccupation with other interests, and concluded that Meigs's scientific impact was largely limited to his own generation—he left no disciples.[81]

Meigs left no mark on physiology in Philadelphia. He divided his loyalties between practice and science, ethnology and physiology. His commitments and activities were too diffuse for him to serve as a meaningful role model during a period when American medical science was evolving into distinct disciplines. Moreover, the descriptive sciences of ethnology and anthropology did not require the team approach and involvement of one or more assistants necessary for complex physiological experiments. Meigs could pursue his ethnological research in relative isolation in contrast to Dalton or Mitchell, who required assistants to perform their vivisection-based research. It is important not to lose sight of the context, however. There was essentially no job market for biomedical scientists in this era. Consequently, as was the case with Meigs, the overwhelming majority of physicians interested in science were forced to practice to subsidize their scientific activities. Indeed, it is unlikely that Mitchell would have completely given up his medical practice had he won the Jefferson chair. Unlike Dalton, Mitchell found medical practice rewarding. Although he realized it reduced the time he could devote to research, Mitchell, as did Meigs, viewed the activities as complementary. The fundamental difference between Meigs and Mitchell was their scientific focus. Mitchell was an experimental physiologist as the term was coming to be defined; Meigs was not.

Henry Chapman, a medical graduate of the University of Pennsylvania, succeeded Meigs, who died at the age of fifty in 1879.[82] Chapman saw the dilemma posed by attempting to combine medical practice with the physiology chair. Following two years as resident physician at the Pennsylvania Hospital, he had gone to Europe for three years of postgraduate study. His interest in scientific medicine had been stimulated primarily by Joseph Leidy who sponsored his membership in the Academy of Natural Sciences of Philadelphia in 1868. While in private practice, Chapman served as Leidy's assistant at the University of Pennsylvania from 1873 to 1876. By this time, he had written a monograph on evolution and more than twenty scientific papers. When he was selected to succeed Meigs, he was a lecturer in physiology at the University of Pennsylvania.

Chapman recognized the desirability of full-time positions in the basic medical sciences; he also understood why they were unlikely to occur in America:

> Everything in the long run is a question of finance, as a great philosopher once said. The reason why the anatomists, physiologists, and chemists in this country are not as distinguished as those in Germany is very evident; they do not make their studies the business of their lives. They do not live in their laboratories, but in their carriages going from patient to patient, or are engaged in occupations foreign to their specialties. Science is a jealous, unprofitable mistress in one sense. . . . It is impossible for any one to study these sciences, teach them properly and practise medicine; he must either neglect his lectures, or his patients.

Chapman was fully aware of the conflict between science and practice, but he failed to accept the solution that was increasingly being offered by the reformers of medical education: endowment. He rejected the claim that endowments would lead to a higher standard of American medical education, and asserted, "Patronage is always followed by intellectual apathy and degradation."[83] He challenged Dalton's emphasis on vivisection in physiology teaching and complained, "In many places the study of human physiology seems to have degenerated into little else than vivisections or experiments upon living animals."[84]

Horatio C. Wood, Jr., an 1862 medical graduate of the University of Pennsylvania, a pioneering pharmacologist, and Mitchell's close friend, was a staunch defender of animal experimentation. Wood believed, however, that the practice was costly to the physician who undertook it, both in terms of dollars and reputation. As one who practiced vivisection, he reported that it could result in "loss of character and good-will amongst an influential and estimable, though misled, portion of the laity. I have known ladies to canvass against a doctor because he was a vivisector, and have seen cultured women leave the room at a social gathering because they could not associate with a vivisector."[85] He argued that vivisection should be encouraged, not combated, because "the personal sacrifices are too great, the rewards too impalpable, to induce many Americans to do the work." He argued for aid to support research rather than laws to discourage experimentation and declared that only a dozen individuals in the United States consistently used vivisection in the course of experimentation. This activity was confined, in Wood's opinion, to Baltimore, Boston, New York, Philadelphia, and Easton, Pennsylvania.[86] His assessment of the small number of vivisectors appears to be accurate. It was estimated in 1883 that of Philadelphia's 1,500 doctors only 6 engaged in vivisection, "and they only occasionally, and not as a continuous occupation."[87]

Henry Chapman introduced laboratory training in physiology at the Jefferson Medical College in 1880. The physiological laboratory was equipped with an extensive collection of modern apparatus he had acquired in Paris.[88] He held the chair of physiology at Jefferson for nearly thirty years, retiring in 1909. Although he was a founding member of the American Physiological Society in 1887, and the members toured his laboratory during their meeting the following year, Chapman had little influence on the professionalization of the discipline. Jefferson graduates or faculty members gave none of the presentations at the Philadelphia meeting, and Chapman was the only individual with a scientific tie to the Jefferson Medical College among the twenty-eight original members of the American Physiological Society.[89] Moreover, the only new member of the society elected before 1900 with an affiliation to Jefferson was Chapman's demonstrator and assistant, Albert P. Brubaker. Although the physiology course at the college advanced under Chapman's guidance to include routine laboratory exercises, the institution did not become a center for physiological research, nor did it produce any professional physiologists, save for Brubaker, in the nineteenth century.

Mitchell's 1868 defeat for the Jefferson chair may have alienated him from the college. His earlier defeat at the University of Pennsylvania did not have this effect, however, and he came to play a major role in

that institution. Mitchell's prominence as a specialist in nervous disor-
ders grew during the 1870s with the publication of several papers and
monographs on neurological subjects. Acknowledging the receipt of his
book on injuries of nerves, Oliver Wendell Holmes exclaimed, "I have
heard that you have become a great doctor."[90] Ironically, Mitchell was
elected a trustee of the University of Pennsylvania in 1875, joining the
group that had selected Francis Gurney Smith, Jr., in preference to him
for the vacant physiology chair only twelve years earlier.

Mitchell's appointment to the board of trustees of the University of
Pennsylvania placed him in a position to participate in important educational reforms at the institution during the final quarter of the nineteenth century. There had been earlier attempts to reform the medical
curriculum. From the standpoint of the basic medical sciences, one of
the most important events occurred in 1865 when an auxiliary faculty
was established. This faculty consisted of five individuals who were paid
a fixed salary for teaching scientific courses in the spring following the
completion of the regular session. Taught by didactic lectures the sub-
jécts included zoology and comparative anatomy, botany, geology and
mineralogy, hygiene, and medical jurisprudence. The auxiliary faculty
was made possible by George B. Wood who contributed $50,000 to en-
dow the five professorships. He had received undergraduate and medical degrees from the University of Pennsylvania and had held a variety
of appointments in the medical school throughout his long life.[91]

Although the auxiliary courses consisted solely of lectures without
laboratory work, their establishment did acknowledge the growing importance of the biological sciences and other subjects not part of the traditional American medical curriculum. The Pennsylvania innovation
was applauded by a contemporary writer who claimed the auxiliary
courses afforded "the best chance which is available to the students of
any medical school in America, for becoming acquainted with the elementary branches of scientific study, and thus fitting themselves for the
performance of thorough reliable work and original scientific investigation."[92]

The curricular reforms at the Harvard Medical School that followed shortly after Charles W. Eliot's election as president of Harvard
in 1869 were watched with great interest by several members of the University of Pennsylvania faculty. One of the Harvard developments was
the establishment of a full-time, salaried chair of physiology in 1871.
Alfred Stillé, professor of medicine at the University of Pennsylvania,
wanted to see salaried professorships expanded to include the entire

medical faculty at his institution. He argued, "In every country of continental Europe professors have fixed salaries. It is these salaried teachers to whom the progress of medicine is mainly due. They are able to pursue their studies and experimental researches without being harassed by questions of finance. . . . And so it might still be in our own country."[93] He believed the University of Pennsylvania could play a leading role in advancing American medical education by adopting a system of fixed salaries.

Stillé's campaign for reform was joined by Horatio Wood, Jr., the nephew of the influential University of Pennsylvania faculty member and trustee George Wood. Young Wood shared several interests with Mitchell including toxicology and diseases of the nervous system. Wood learned of the inner workings of the Pennsylvania board of trustees from his uncle George Wood who had served as a member of that body from 1863 until his death in 1879. Wood's perspective on the reform movement at the University of Pennsylvania appeared in his letters to another reformer of medical education, army surgeon John Shaw Billings. He claimed that some members of the medical faculty viewed his uncle's creation of the auxiliary faculty with indifference or hostility. He explained, "The want of cultivation of his friendship and the personal jealousy shown to some of his young protégées aided very much in his perceiving the necessity of reform and the fact that the faculty of medicine are besottedly old fogeys and opposed to any raising of the medical department."[94]

Mitchell replaced George W. Norris, an eminent surgeon who died in March 1875, on the university board of trustees. Horatio Wood proposed that Mitchell should succeed Norris, but revealed to Billings that his uncle George Wood "did not like him at first but finally became very well satisfied to nominate & push him & in spite of the active & bitter opposition of the old faculty he was elected. We now felt that we had scored one—as Dr. M. was openly a reformer. This election of Mitchell, although so briefly described here required a weeks work of both Pepper & myself."[95] Henry Chapman informed Joseph Leidy that Mitchell's nomination "has made considerable talk. He is disposed from what he has said to me to take an active part in the Medical Department of the University and the Faculty are already wrathy about it, particularly Carson."[96]

Mitchell played an active role in restructuring the curriculum at the University of Pennsylvania beginning in 1875 as a member of the board's Committee of the Department of Medicine. Mitchell, Horatio Wood, and their reform-minded colleagues confronted a conservative medical faculty, however, whose dean, Robert E. Rogers, proclaimed medical instruction at the university unequaled in extent or comprehensiveness in America.[97] Rogers compared the university's curriculum with that of the Harvard Medical School and mentioned that Pennsylvania students now had the opportunity to work in the new physiological laboratory.

A new medical hall constructed at the university in 1874 included a modest laboratory where Francis Gurney Smith, Jr., taught physiology experimentally and by demonstrations. The laboratory was "under the charge of the Professor of Physiology, aided by the Demonstrator. Its main object is to afford the Student an opportunity to study Physiology by experiment and personal observation. The functions of the various organs, and the sources, constitution, and destination of the secretions and excretions, are studied in the living and dead subject by the student, either singly or in classes."[98] Despite this claim, and an announcement that opportunities were available for advanced students to participate in research in the physiological laboratory, Smith reluctantly used vivisection in his course, and avoided this technique if any other approach was feasible.[99] Moreover, it was not Smith who encouraged the expansion of physiology teaching at the university. Horatio Wood and William Pepper had served on a university committee of hospital professors that advocated a three-year medical curriculum that would include laboratory work in physiology during the first year.[100] Mitchell and the members of this committee were the active promoters of the expansion of the university's physiology program; Smith was a rather reluctant participant.

The changes in the medical curriculum at Harvard were a potent stimulus for the young reformers at the University of Pennsylvania. Among the reformers at Pennsylvania was James Tyson, an 1863 medical graduate of the institution who had a special interest in physiology and pathology. A former assistant to Smith, Tyson was appointed lecturer on pathological anatomy and histology upon the organization of the new university hospital medical faculty. Tyson wrote to Calvin Ellis, dean of the Harvard medical faculty in December 1874, "The young men here, as you know are a unit in approval of the Harvard plan as it is now called throughout the land, but those in authority still object to it. I have read your announcement carefully and it seems to me in the matter it contains throughout, the best argument I have yet seen in favor of the system, and I am anxious that all connected with our school should be possessed of it."[101]

On the eve of the nation's Centennial, Mitchell's friend Wood assessed the status of American medical education and advocated specific reforms. He compared the philosophy and structure of medical education in England, France, Germany, and the United States, and characterized the American system as "wretched." Although he acknowledged that facilities for medical education were improving in the nation, Wood complained that these facilities did not imply higher requirements for graduation. He applauded the Harvard reforms, and argued that the graded course of instruction and practical training in the laboratory and the clinic at that institution would inevitably result in better qualified medical graduates. The new Harvard program, modeled after European medical education, meant, in Wood's view, that "its medical diploma is the *only one* issued by any prominent American medical college which is a *guarantee* that its possessor has been well educated in the science and practice of medicine."[102]

The University of Pennsylvania could not allow the Harvard reforms to go unanswered. As was the case at the College of Physicians and Surgeons of New York, the alumni at Pennsylvania agitated for changes at the medical school. The proposed reforms at Pennsylvania were similar to those adopted at Harvard, and endowment was the means by which they were to be accomplished. As spokesman for the Pennsylvania reformers, Wood announced: "Laboratories must be provided, hospitals established and supported, a corps of competent instructors appointed and salaried. In no other way can medical education in the United States be placed on the same level as that of other civilized countries, and the public be efficiently protected against the disastrous activity of a multitude of untrained and reckless practitioners."[103] The reform movement at Pennsylvania gained momentum, and Wood, Mitchell, Pepper, and Tyson won concessions from the conservative faculty. Unwilling to accept the changes, Robert Rogers resigned as dean and was succeeded by Joseph Leidy. Mitchell welcomed Rogers's departure, and believed it would permit the introduction of a mandatory three-year curriculum and associated reforms at the university.

Never fully committed to physiology, Francis Smith resigned from his chair at the University of Pennsylvania in 1877. Mitchell, defeated by Smith for the chair nearly fifteen years earlier, was now in a position to influence the future development of physiology at the university. Smith informed the trustees, "The state of my health for the last few years makes it advisable for me to diminish my labours, & I have, therefore, decided to relinquish my professorship & devote myself to the practice of my profession."[104] Despite the creation of a physiological laboratory in 1874, Smith maintained his busy practice and had little interest in expanding his duties at the university. He was unwilling to spend either time or money on behalf of his chair. Smith's demonstrator Isaac Ott explained to Harvard's full-time physiologist Henry Bowditch: "It is not likely that Prof. S[mith] will add much to the laboratory as I have heard indirectly that he thought it expensive. . . . [He] still thinks of running up to Boston but I don't think he will take the time as he has a large obstetrical practice."[105]

Smith's resignation provided an opportunity for the University of Pennsylvania to appoint an individual committed to expanding the scope of the physiology course. In an editorial entitled "A Step Forward in Medical Education" one Philadelphia writer explained, "In the selection of a new professor of physiology, the trustees are searching for a tenant willing to devote all his time and study to the consideration of physiological questions."[106] Mitchell's goal of establishing a physiological laboratory for working scientists at the University of Pennsylvania might now be realized. Such laboratories already existed at Harvard Medical School and the recently opened Johns Hopkins University in Baltimore. Henry Bowditch's physiology program at Harvard was successful, and Newell Martin's biology department at Johns Hopkins, with its emphasis on advanced education and research in science, was attracting widespread attention.

Mitchell was impressed by the laboratories at Johns Hopkins, which he visited in 1877 while he was in Baltimore to deliver an address to members of the Medical and Chirurgical Faculty of Maryland. He congratulated the Johns Hopkins officials for providing the "young profession" with such sophisticated laboratory facilities. Nearly a decade after his defeat for the Jefferson physiology chair, he remarked, "As I walked through these laboratories and saw what splendid hospitality and to what opportunities you invite the young and eager investigator, I had but two regrets,—that I am not twenty-one, and that I was not born in Baltimore." The Baltimore audience heard him present themes about the importance of research that he had developed fifteen years earlier. These ideas were no longer abstract or ephemeral; there was growing support for research among the medical and lay populations. Mitchell added new arguments to old ones, and informed his audience that laboratory research was now "the true test by which we stand or fall in the eyes of the vast jury of other workers in science. The public are also beginning to comprehend this, and to feel that a doctor who has signalized himself by physiological and chemical studies is a man who has a double claim to respect." He invoked a persuasive argument regarding the role science might play in elevating the regular medical profession. Science, in Mitchell's opinion, was the major difference between the regular practitioners and the "organized quackeries." He invited anyone to point to a significant discovery in physiology or chemistry made by a homeopath. He rejected the view that science and practice were incompatible, and revealed that he now advised young and able physicians to devote time to laboratory work and research. "To spend a few years in such work is not only to give himself the best of intellectual training, but is also one of the best means of advancing himself and fortifying his position when by degrees he becomes absorbed in clinical pursuits and daily practice."[107] Experience in the laboratory and participation in research not only advanced science; it made better doctors. Simply to state that research was important had not been enough; other arguments were necessary, Mitchell and his reform-minded colleagues now realized.

Mitchell's claim that homeopathy was not based on science was echoed by others attempting to encourage intellectual and financial support for scientific investigation. This argument was particularly persuasive for contemporary regular practitioners confronting intense competition from homeopaths and other sectarians. Alonzo Palmer of the University of Michigan medical school explained how science could undermine the strength and credibility of the homeopaths. Commenting on the growing understanding of the bacterial origins of many diseases, he declared in 1882, "In view of the present state and drift of science . . . how absurd become the dreams of exclusive systems . . . [which] must recede more and more into the obscurity of past follies as science advances."[108]

Mitchell's enthusiasm for medical reform and his encouragement of research and laboratory training were shared by James Tyson, Horatio Wood, and William Pepper. Pepper, the son of a prominent Philadelphia physician and Pennsylvania faculty member, was an 1864 medical graduate of the university. Like Mitchell, Pepper gained from his father "an idea of the fascinating nature of medical investigations."[109] Early in his career, he became interested in pathology and, with Mitchell, was a member of the Pathological Society of Philadelphia and the Academy of Natural Sciences. In 1871, Pepper visited numerous European medical centers in preparation for his role in the planning of new hospital facilities at the University of Pennsylvania. Five years later Pepper was elected to the chair of clinical medicine and, with Mitchell, Wood, and Tyson, coordinated the curricular reforms initiated at the university in the 1870s.

In an 1877 address on higher medical education, Pepper expressed views similar to those articulated by his friend Wood two years earlier. After reviewing the status of medical education in Europe and the recent

Harvard reforms, he focused on the need for greater emphasis on preliminary education and practical training. He also advocated the establishment of "fixed salaries" for the medical faculty, thereby removing the financial incentive for large classes that encouraged a didactic rather than a personal and practical approach to instruction.[110]

Mitchell, Pepper, and their fellow reformers had a major impact on the structure and philosophy of medical education at the University of Pennsylvania. During the 1870s, the staff of the medical school expanded from seven to eleven professors, and from a single demonstrator of anatomy to more than twenty-five demonstrators and assistants.[111] This dramatic shift to practical laboratory education occurred suddenly, and had not been anticipated when the 1874 medical hall was planned. Only four years later, Leidy, the new dean, complained that the recently completed medical building was inadequate for the new laboratory-intense medical curriculum. A new laboratory building at the university was proposed as the solution. Mitchell and others on the board of trustees quickly acted on this suggestion and a building was promptly erected.

Mitchell was the primary speaker at the dedication of the new laboratory building at the University of Pennsylvania in 1878. His address reflected his continued commitment to experimental medicine and his interpretation of the growing interrelationship of science and medicine in American society:

> Fifty years ago the public concerned itself little as to any form of scientific progress. . . . [However] the profession of Medicine as such, no longer lives a life of intellectual seclusion. The increase in the number of scientific men, not physicians; the diffusion of knowledge as to Anatomy and Physiology; the ever-increasing interest in all forms of scientific activity; the growing value attached to Hygiene and to large measures of sanitary use; and what I might call the secularization of every addition to medical knowledge, by its instant record in newspapers, popular science journals, and reviews, have combined to give us, as a profession at least, what we once lacked,—a court, where we are heard with respect, and, for the most part, judged with fairness and interest.

Mitchell argued that scientific training using instruments of precision in the laboratory would contribute to the development of a higher caliber of medical practitioner with benefits for the individual patient and society.

Despite his defeats in the 1860s, Mitchell maintained his interest in physiology and his commitment to research. Having recently visited

Johns Hopkins, and aware of the activities in Bowditch's Harvard physiological laboratory, he told his audience that the University of Pennsylvania, with its new hospital and laboratories, must also emphasize research. Research had become more complex: "Nowadays every research involves the use of expensive apparatus such as only a great school can provide. To such scientific hospitalities this University invites all who can prove their ability to make the world of thought more rich by honest use of the means she offers." As did Dalton, Mitchell recognized the critical need for endowments if laboratory training and research were to become the responsibility of medical schools. "This Commonwealth, and the rich within it, can reach us with help which was never more needed than now. They can remember us in wills . . . by endowing medical and other professorships; they can give means to assist poor and able men to carry on original researches; they can enable us by larger salaries to secure the whole time of the highest talent." In his closing comments, Mitchell anticipated a trend that would evolve in American medical education during the next quarter century. He explicitly encouraged the establishment of the full-time system for basic medical scientists, whereby qualified individuals would be enabled by the provision of adequate institutional salaries and apparatus to devote their lives to teaching and research. If this plan was adopted, Mitchell argued, future generations of physiologists would not have to earn their living by practicing medicine.[112]

William Pepper expanded these themes in an address at McGill University in 1885. Acknowledging the recent gifts of Johns Hopkins, William H. Vanderbilt, and Andrew Carnegie to medical institutions, he declared, "No gifts promote more directly the best interests of the Community than do these in support of the new and higher medical education. . . . The amounts needed are large. There are several chairs in each Faculty, the incumbents of which should receive an ample fixed salary, since their time must be devoted to scientific work which brings no other remuneration. These professorships should all be fully endowed." Emphasizing recent developments in bacteriology, he exclaimed, "Happily the day has come when, even in this practical country, there is a growing recognition of the importance of pure science, and of the influence of abstract scientific investigations upon our material welfare & progress."[113]

As physicians and laymen alike came to acknowledge the relevance of science to practical medicine, increasing attention was focused on how to encourage scientific careers and medical research. The endowment of professorships, which would free medical teachers from their financial dependence on practice or students' fees, gained increasing attention in the 1880s. A Philadelphia writer put it quite simply in 1882, "If we desire deep investigation into the hidden truths of nature we must pay for it."[114] The growth of bacteriology made it easier for scientific physicians to prove that medical research could benefit mankind. The emergence of pharmacology had a similar although less dramatic effect. Commenting on the efficacious new remedy for angina pectoris, nitroglycerin, a Philadelphia writer observed, "One of the most important additions recently made to practical therapeutics is *Nitro-Glycerin*. . . . The applications of Nitro-Glycerin to the treatment of disease are directly deducible from the physiological study—another proof, if more were needed, of the value of the physiological method."[115]

Francis Smith's resignation from the physiology chair provided the University of Pennsylvania with an opportunity to hire a full-time physiologist with a commitment to research and practical laboratory training. Models for the full-time basic medical scientist existed in Europe and at the Harvard Medical School. Mitchell and his reform-minded colleagues at Pennsylvania knew what they wanted; the problem was to find a suitable individual for the physiology chair. Brown-Séquard briefly considered applying for the post, but when he was offered the chair of physiology at the College of France previously held by Magendie and Bernard he decided not to pursue the Philadelphia position.[116] Brown-Séquard then encouraged his assistant Eugene Dupuy to apply for the Pennsylvania physiology chair.

Dupuy had accompanied Brown-Séquard to the United States on several occasions and was known to many of the leaders of American medical science. Although he had an impressive bibliography and produced strong letters of recommendation from leading European scientists and Henry Bowditch, Dupuy was not awarded the chair. Despite the great success of Louis Agassiz at Harvard and the appointments at Johns Hopkins of Newell Martin and other foreign scientists, the University of Pennsylvania was more provincial, and sought an American for the position.[117]

The physiology chair stood vacant for more than a year, and anxiety grew among some members of the Pennsylvania faculty. Mitchell unsuccessfully tried to convince John Dalton to accept the position. D. Hayes Agnew, the influential professor of surgery, informed James Tyson, "The continued vacancy of this chair, I think, is prejudicial to the interests of the University, and should be filled at the earliest possible day. At present there seems to be no gentleman specially prominent in the Country who is available for the position, and there is no reason to believe that after the lapse of another year anyone can rise into such prominence as would make it longer desirable to delay the appointment."[118] Agnew concluded his letter by strongly recommending Harrison Allen for the position. The medical faculty supported this recommendation and the board of trustees unanimously chose Allen to fill the chair.

Horatio Wood noted the expediency of this appointment for both the institution and the individual:

> At a time when there was no available American physiologist the high esteem in which he was held as a scientific investigator and teacher led the Faculty of Medicine in the University of Pennsylvania to ask for his election to the Chair of Institutes, although everyone knew that his studies had hitherto been in different lines. His acceptance of the Chair was without doubt largely founded upon the absence of any anatomical prospects.[119]

Mitchell was frustrated that a true experimental physiologist could not be found for the position. The provincialism of the university, the scarcity of individuals willing to devote themselves exclusively to physiology, and the relative lack of mobility of most medical teachers who depended upon medical practice to supplement their salaries combined to determine the selection of Smith's successor.

When they selected Harrison Allen, Mitchell and the trustees chose an individual dedicated to science and research; they did not, however, select a physiologist. An 1861 medical graduate of the University of Pennsylvania, Allen had taught zoology and comparative anatomy in the auxiliary faculty a decade earlier and had been eager to obtain a regular post in anatomy for many years. He wrote to Joseph Leidy upon the resignation of Hayes Agnew from the position of demonstrator of anatomy at the university in 1870: "I do not conceal my desire to succeed him. You can never know how anxiously I have looked forward to it since 1865 as the means of ending my pecuniary needs, and as a relief from the frets of general practice."[120] Even after he assumed the physiology chair, Allen's scientific work continued to reflect his morphological orientation. Despite a salary of $2,000, with the potential for a salary of $3,500 if there was a surplus from student fees, an income comparable to that of a practitioner, Allen continued to practice medicine. The university did not require him to devote his whole time to physiology.

One writer argued that it was necessary to offer scientists higher salaries to encourage research in America. Contrasting the productivity of German medical scientists with the modest contributions from Americans, he claimed that it was the value placed on scientific research by Germany rather than any intellectual advantage that accounted for the discrepancy between the two nations. The writer proposed that two reforms were necessary if Americans were to make meaningful contributions to medical science: "Professors must be relieved from an excess of labor as teachers, so that they shall have time for research, and must be paid so well that it shall not be necessary for them, as it is now, to eke out a bare living by lecturing, practicing medicine, engineering, etc., etc."[121]

Concerned Americans were increasingly aware of the magnitude of endowment required to sustain a meaningful program of laboratory training and research in the basic medical sciences. In 1882, Mitchell and his fellow reformers initiated a call for contributions to a fund of $100,000 to endow the Joseph Leidy chair of anatomy at the University of Pennsylvania. The fund was to be more than a memorial for one individual: "It is intended to still further enlarge and elevate the [medical] course so that it shall compare favorably with the highest instruction in European schools. Such changes involve increased expenditures, and a temporary reduction in the receipts from tuition fees. Consequently it becomes doubly important to secure endowments for those chairs, which, like that of anatomy, demand the entire time of their occupants."[122] Mitchell was well aware of the difficulties of reconciling a busy practice with a sophisticated and sustained research effort. This dilemma had also frustrated Meigs, Allen, and countless others who were interested in science but, of necessity, made a living as medical practitioners.

Allen had little impact on physiology at the University of Pennsylvania or in Philadelphia. Increasingly interested in the developing clinical field of otolaryngology, he began devoting more time to his medical practice and resigned from the physiology chair in 1885. Although Allen continued to pursue anatomical studies, he lost interest in physiology and did not join the American Physiological Society when it was established two years later. Allen's resignation made it possible for Mitchell and the officers of the university to search for a more appropriate individual to introduce a physiology program that included opportunities for original research. This time there were more candidates, but problems remained. As Agnew had done seven years earlier, now Mitchell expressed bias against foreigners holding faculty positions in the university: "There are possibly men abroad who would credibly fill this chair but to secure them we would need much more money than we can offer and such an equipment of Laboratories as is usually found in connection with great schools abroad. Moreover the success of a foreigner is often doubtful and perhaps it may not be wise to put too many foreigners on our faculty."[123]

The candidates to replace Allen were Edward Reichert and Robert Meade Smith. An 1879 medical graduate of the university, Reichert became interested in pharmacology and physiology as a medical student. The year following his graduation, Reichert edited a new American edition of Michael Foster's physiology text. He also collaborated with Mitchell on a paper on the physiological action of potassium nitrite which was based, in part, on original experiments performed in Horatio Wood's laboratory of experimental therapeutics at the university.[124] In the autumn of 1882, Mitchell invited Reichert, then demonstrator of physiology at the university, to assist him in a new series of experiments on snake venom. The resumption of Mitchell's venom studies in the 1880s was "due chiefly to the fact that I had become sure of the existence in my former papers of many grave errors and defects, due largely to the wants of such means of research as are to be found to-day in every laboratory."[125] Their collaboration resulted in the publication of a highly regarded monograph on venoms in 1886.[126] Reichert also gained sophistication in physiology from study in Europe during an extended period from 1882 to 1885.

Reichert's opponent for the chair was Robert Meade Smith, the son of Francis Gurney Smith, Jr., who had beaten Mitchell for the same chair two decades earlier. Robert Smith had excellent credentials and was qualified to hold the chair. He served as demonstrator in physiology in the university from 1877 to 1884, and during the summers of 1880 and 1883 he studied physiology abroad, spending part of this time with Carl Ludwig. According to Henry Bowditch, Smith was "trained in the best schools of experimental physiology in Europe, [and] has already given proof of his ability to make important contributions to our knowledge of physiological laws."[127] Smith was a formidable candidate. He was trained by several of Europe's most prominent physiologists and was an experienced lecturer, demonstrator, investigator, and author.

Mitchell played a significant role in deciding the contest in favor of Reichert. He complained to his fellow trustees before the election, "The chair of physiology in this school . . . has never been held by a working physiologist."[128] In view of his previous collaboration with Reichert, it is not surprising that Mitchell supported him for the chair. It is tempting to speculate whether Mitchell was unwilling to support the son of the individual to whom he lost the Pennsylvania chair in 1863. Smith became professor of comparative physiology in the new veterinary school at the University of Pennsylvania and published a major monograph on the physiology of domestic animals in 1889. His loss of the physiology chair in the medical school signaled his departure from the mainstream of American physiology, however. Although a founding member of the American Physiological Society, he was never an active participant in its meetings.

Shortly after Reichert's election, Horatio Wood and James Tyson expressed their concerns that the University of Pennsylvania might soon lose its ability to attract and retain high-quality professors because of salary. "The triumphs of the Medical Department of the University have been won chiefly by the sacrifices of its professors," and the higher salaries paid by schools in Baltimore and New York will hamper recruiting and keeping better medical teachers. They wanted "the most brilliant men in the United States," but because salary offers twice that provided by the university were now common, the university would have to be content with "second choice." Wood and Tyson advocated more pay for the assistants as well as for the professors as the solution.[129]

Although the University of Pennsylvania's catalogs described opportunities for laboratory training in the 1880s, the financial outlay for the physiology department beyond the professor's salary was minimal. Despite the acknowledged growing role of the basic sciences in the medical curriculum at Pennsylvania, Wood and Tyson cited in 1886 that the total funds the University expended for the physiology department, exclusive of the professor's salary, were $500. They argued that this was not competitive in an era when other institutions were sharply increasing their support of the basic medical sciences. "It is evident that this state of affairs cannot be permanent. . . . Our supply of scientific apparatus is in many respects pitifully below our needs and the contrast between our laboratories and well-furnished halls of rival institutions is very great—in the opinion of the medical faculty the Medical Department can maintain its prestige only by the further development of its scientific laboratories."[130] They suggested that the income received for medical teaching should be used for faculty salaries and increased support of the laboratories rather than going to the university treasury. Inadequate funding remained a significant problem, however. Reichert complained to Tyson in 1889 that his demonstrator had left and a suitable replacement had not yet been found.

Competition did stimulate a change in the salary system at the University of Pennsylvania. Reichert's salary increased from $3,000 to $6,000 between 1891 and 1896. The perceptions of individuals outside and inside the University of Pennsylvania differed, however, on the commitment of the institution to the research ethic and the advance of medical education reform. In 1895 Henry Bowditch commended William Pepper, who had served as provost of the university from 1880 to 1894, "I have been astonished at the progress in every department of the university that has characterized your administration."[131]

On the other hand, Simon Flexner, professor of pathology at the University of Pennsylvania, held a different view. In 1902 he described the problems and prospects of the school to his former teacher William H. Welch of Johns Hopkins:

> What is, however, important with reference to the future is the position which the medical school is likely to take towards higher medical education and to what extent it will participate in the research movement. With the best of intentions I cannot be enthusiastic or even very hopeful for marked progress in these directions. The medical school is almost without endowment. . . .
> What outlook is there for a group of [research] workers? Chemistry can yield nothing, anatomy is doomed to sterility, and physiology is, I fear, not very promising.[132]

Although he did not win the chair of physiology he so eagerly sought, Weir Mitchell maintained his interest in physiology. William Osler remarked in 1890 that Mitchell's interest in physiology remained strong despite his growing recognition as a leading physician. Comparing Mitchell to William Harvey and John Hunter, Osler claimed that Mitchell "illuminated the dark pathways of practice with the lamp of science." Mentioning Mitchell's "disappointed academic ambitions," Osler suggested they were "now long past, perhaps even forgotten by him."[133]

Mitchell had not forgotten, but he had made the best of the situation. In 1893 he recalled:

> Glancing back over a career which has been, perhaps, one of exceptional success, I see that many things which I began by meaning to be or do I quite utterly failed to be or do. If anyone had told me at the start, or a little later, that I should never reach in all my life the goal I early set before me—a professor's chair—I should have been troubled, perhaps discouraged. That I should secure other prizes as valuable I did not—could not—see. That I should stand here to-day where I once hoped to stand as a professor, and should feel that the fate which deprived me of the chance to teach with the tongue was my best friend—ah, that indeed seems strange to me as I look back and recall the bitterness of defeat.[134]

Mitchell's career was remarkably successful; he became one of the most influential physicians of his generation. His impact on American physiology, though substantial, was blunted by his failure to win one of the Philadelphia chairs in the 1860s. His influence in developing the scientific curriculum at the University of Pennsylvania in the 1870s and 1880s was significant, however. The relative sterility of the Jefferson physiology program in the 1880s and 1890s compared with the University of Pennsylvania program may be explained, at least in part, by Mitchell's influence at the latter institution. Although an amateur physiologist, he played a leading role in the founding, in 1887, of the American Physiological Society, discussed in chapter 5. He was active in the scientific reform movement and lived to see the research ethic adopted by the basic science faculties in America's most prestigious medical schools.

CHAPTER THREE

Henry P. Bowditch

*The Prototypical Full-Time Physiologist
and Educational Reformer*

HENRY PICKERING BOWDITCH (1840–1911) played a critical role in the professionalization of physiology in America. He traveled to Europe for postgraduate training two decades after Dalton and Mitchell had studied under Claude Bernard. Just as they had introduced the French approach to physiology teaching and research into America, Bowditch, a pupil of Carl Ludwig, introduced the German interpretation of this scientific field into the United States. Bowditch's agenda was broader than Dalton's, and his local circumstances were more favorable than Mitchell's. In addition to a personal commitment to writing and research, Bowditch established a laboratory open to medical students as well as advanced workers. According to Weir Mitchell, Bowditch established, in 1871, "the first American physiological laboratory for the use of students, a laboratory which soon proved hospitable to investigators in every phase of experimental medicine."[1] He taught them new techniques of experimental physiology and encouraged them to undertake research. Advanced pupils and physicians with an interest in experimental physiology or the collateral sciences now had a facility in which to pursue their studies under the supervision of a thoroughly trained, full-time physiologist.

Bowditch was born into a prominent, wealthy, and scientifically oriented family. He was the son of Jonathan Ingersoll Bowditch, a successful Boston merchant; the grandson of Nathaniel Bowditch, a world-renowned mathematician and astronomer; and the nephew of Henry Ingersoll Bowditch, an influential Boston physician. On his mother's side, Bowditch was related to Edward and William Pickering, noted astronomers, and Benjamin M. Pierce and his son Charles S. Pierce, mathematicians and scientists. Following graduation from Harvard College in 1861, Bowditch enrolled in the Lawrence Scientific School in Cambridge. There he was exposed to a new departure in American higher education. The Swiss naturalist Louis Agassiz, who had taught at the school since its founding in 1847, encouraged practical laboratory training to supplement traditional didactic lectures. When Bowditch was a pupil there, the Harvard overseers who had responsibility for the school declared, "The course of instruction wisely adopted by Professor Agassiz must in a manner force the students to investigate and observe for themselves, and the result is sure to be the most wholesome and beneficial, both to them and to the cause of science and sound education."[2] While a pupil at the Lawrence School, Bowditch studied chemistry under Charles W. Eliot, whose course included laboratory instruction. Eliot had recently succeeded Ebin Norton Horsford, one of Justus Liebig's earliest American pupils. Although Horsford was responsible for transferring the new German experimental approach to chemistry to America, his efforts at combining a program of teaching with research at the Lawrence Scientific School were unsuccessful.

Bowditch's uncle supported his nephew's plan to devote himself to a scientific career. He had once studied under Horsford, and from that experience concluded American medical students should have laboratory instruction in chemistry. The elder Bowditch found that, although Horsford agreed, he felt the short medical curriculum and the limited funds of most medical students precluded anything more than a cursory chemistry course.[3] The Civil War interrupted young Henry Bowditch's studies at the Lawrence Scientific School. He enlisted in the First Massachusetts Cavalry and, although wounded in 1863, remained in the army until June 1865. He then re-entered the Scientific School and enrolled in courses taught by Jeffries Wyman. In addition to his regular course work, Bowditch collaborated with Wyman on a study of the function of cilia.[4]

In the fall of 1866, Bowditch entered the Harvard Medical School and attended the new course on the physiology and pathology of the nervous system taught by Charles-E. Brown-Séquard, one of the world's leading experimental physiologists. When Brown-Séquard first lectured in Boston fifteen years earlier, Henry's uncle heard and applauded the French physiologist.[5] Brown-Séquard's appointment at Harvard in 1864 acknowledged the growing importance of experimental physiology to medicine. The peripatetic physiologist proposed building at Harvard "a

Physiological and Pathological Institute, combining the most important features of Virchow's, a DuBois-Reymond's and Valentin's Institutes with those of Claude Bernard's laboratory." He vowed to return to America ready to establish such an institute, promising one "on a larger scientific and practical scale than that of any in the Old World." To ensure the fulfillment of his vision he agreed to finance the purchase of the instruments and apparatus.[6] These ambitious plans were not realized due to Brown-Séquard's ill health and the ambivalence of the Harvard faculty regarding the venture. Nevertheless, Brown-Séquard did introduce vivisection in teaching at the Harvard Medical School and stimulated an interest in experimental physiology among several of his pupils.

In his introductory lecture before Bowditch's class, Brown-Séquard argued persuasively for laboratory training and research in physiology. Adequate preliminary scientific training was a critical step in achieving a productive program of research in Brown-Séquard's view. He also told his pupils that the United States needed an "institute" where the philosophy and techniques of scientific research were taught by competent men. Such an institute would do much "to place this country on a level with Europe" in terms of scientific discovery.[7] Brown-Séquard also encouraged his students to devote more time to the basic medical sciences than was customary in American medical schools. Bowditch was inspired by Brown-Séquard's philosophy; forty years later he wrote, "Those who were privileged to listen to him will not readily forget the enthusiasm which he awakened in his listeners for medicine as an experimental science."[8]

Brown-Séquard's presence at Harvard also reflected the consensus that Oliver Wendell Holmes's teaching of physiology in conjunction with anatomy was inadequate.[9] Brown-Séquard's conviction of the utility of physiology was not widely held in the 1860s. Even Holmes warned against undue emphasis on the basic medical sciences, although he did not deny that anatomical and physiological discoveries occasionally resulted in advances in clinical medicine. The poet-anatomist declared in 1867, "I am in little danger of underrating Anatomy or Physiology; but as each of these branches splits up into specialties, any one of which may take up a scientific life-time, I would have them taught with a certain judgment and reserve, so that they shall not crowd the more immediately practical branches."[10] Holmes also argued that the practicing physician should not pursue abstract scientific research. Patients deserved the undivided loyalties of their physicians; there was no place for science in the life of a busy practitioner. Bowditch was familiar with the content of Holmes's lecture and probably was present when it was delivered.[11]

As was the case with Dalton and Mitchell, young Henry Bowditch benefited from the interest leading medical scientists took in him. Although he was a talented and interested pupil, Bowditch was also a member of an influential "Brahmin" Boston family. Holmes's son, Oliver Jr., and Bowditch were classmates at Harvard College, and Holmes was a longtime friend of Henry's uncle with whom he studied in Paris in the 1830s. At that time, Holmes characterized the elder Bowditch as "an excellent fellow, and there are not probably a dozen young men in the country whose name is so powerful an introduction in Europe."[12] Jeffries Wyman and Henry I. Bowditch had also been friends for many years. The elder Bowditch held the naturalist in high regard, and wrote in 1866, "I like him. He is learned, and loves truth. . . . He is such a fund of information."[13]

Bowditch's family had strong ties to Harvard as well. In addition to being a prominent Boston practitioner and pioneer of the public health movement, his uncle was professor of clinical medicine at the Harvard Medical School from 1859 through 1867. Moreover, his father was a member of the Harvard board of overseers. Because his background and contacts placed him in a favorable position Bowditch was not the average American medical student and graduate. As historian William Rothstein has recently emphasized, family background, wealth, social standing, and friendship were of great importance in setting up a successful medical practice, gaining admission to the elite institutions, and attracting a wealthy clientele in nineteenth-century urban America.[14]

In view of the long tradition of postgraduate study in Europe among the Harvard elite, it is not surprising that Bowditch elected to study abroad. His interest in European study was heightened by the enthusiastic appraisal of continental facilities he received from his friend William James. James and Bowditch were fellow students at the Lawrence Scientific School and the Harvard Medical School. Writing to Bowditch from Berlin where he was attending the lectures of Emil Du Bois-Reymond, James exclaimed, "The opportunities for study here are superb, it seems to me. Whatever they may be in Paris, they cannot be better. The physiological laboratory, with its endless array of machinery, frogs, dogs, etc., etc., almost 'bursts my gizzard,' when I go by it, with vexation."[15]

Following his graduation from Harvard Medical School in 1868, Bowditch traveled to Europe hoping to study with Brown-Séquard who had recently returned to Paris. Brown-Séquard was unable to accept any students, however, and he encouraged Bowditch to study with Claude Bernard. In letters to his family and his mentor Jeffries Wyman, Bowditch chronicled the development of his interest in experimental physiology and his decision to forgo medical practice to devote himself to this expanding scientific field. Although he found Bernard a stimulating teacher, he became increasingly frustrated by the inadequacy of the French physiologist's laboratory. He complained to Wyman, "The want of a good laboratory for practical instruction in physiology is seriously felt in Paris. The Frenchmen acknowledge the great advantage the Germans have over them in this respect. Bernard's laboratory, where I work nearly every day, is dark, poorly provided with apparatus, & with no proper arrangements for pupils."[16] Wyman responded, "It has always been my hope that you give your time to the Scientific rather than to the practical side of the profession, & now that you have given a winter to it, I am quite encouraged in the belief that my hope may be realized."[17]

Bowditch informed his father, "I have been devoting myself lately almost entirely to the purely scientific part of my profession which certain has much greater attractions for me than the more practical portion. I wish I could see a real good opening for a purely scientific career . . . & let practice go but pure science in our country is rather hard to live on."[18] Bowditch's concerns were well founded. Speaking of the position of the scientific investigator in this period, the prominent astronomer Benjamin A. Gould complained to members of the American Association for the Advancement of Science, "The scientist is compelled, almost without exception, to earn his bread independently of his vocation, that is to say, by work other than scientific research."[19] Wyman assured Bowditch, however, "Physiology is just beginning to receive the attention that belongs to it, & I am sure there will be openings for places among us, though of course, unless endowed better than they have been heretofore, they will never be very remunerative."[20] As was the case in New York and Philadelphia, some Boston physicians expressed interest in expanding the teaching of physiology in the medical curriculum. One contemporary writer argued that physiology should be studied by vivisection and "should occupy an early and prominent place in our professional studies. By experimental physiology alone, can we learn the laws of functional life, and test the effect of drugs."[21]

Coming from a wealthy family, Bowditch did not have to practice medicine to subsidize his scientific interests as had been the case with Mitchell. In the view of one contemporary writer, physicians with independent means should devote themselves to medical science. This writer argued that the contributions of Americans to technology proved that the nation could produce imaginative and creative individuals. He agreed with others who argued that the pursuit of wealth and "the necessity of a lucrative and rewarding private practice in order to live" discouraged capable individuals from devoting their energy to medical research. He urged wealthy young men who entered medicine "merely for a position" to devote themselves to medical science: "Let those who are wealthy reflect that no happier, and no more useful life can be found than that of a *savant* pursuing the study of medical truth for its own sake, and in the hope of benefitting his fellow men."[22] Henry Bowditch did do just that; he devoted his life to medical science, not medical practice.

Historians of American science have shown the importance of family origins in determining scientific careers. A significant percentage of nineteenth-century American scientists were sons of professional men, often physicians. This group possessed certain economic, social, and educational advantages.[23] Bowditch's father assured him, "I hope you understand . . . that I am in favor of you studying the science of medicine & for taking your chance when you get home—I can help you to keep the 'pot boiling' if it shd be necessary."[24] Writing from Paris, the son revealed, "My only hesitation arose from the feeling that in following pure science I should probably not be able to support myself so soon as in taking a more practical branch. But now, being reassured in this point, I shall push on and aim at getting as thorough a physiological education as possible."[25] Similar practical considerations were of concern to Bowditch's friend William James when he had considered a career in business, science, or medical practice a few years earlier. James informed his mother, "I feel very much the importance of making soon a final choice of my business in life. I stand now at the place where the road forks. . . . I confess I hesitate. . . . I shall confer with Wyman about the prospects of a naturalist and finally decide. I want you to become familiar with the notion that I *may* stick to science, however, and drain away at your property for a few years more."[26] Now, James encouraged Bowditch to persist in his dedication to physiology.

The Harvard Medical School established the position of assistant professor of physiology in 1866. Josiah S. Lombard, an 1864 Harvard medical graduate, was the first to hold this new post. In February 1869 Bowditch learned from his former teacher Wyman that Lombard was not likely to hold the appointment in physiology much longer and, if this was the case, "there will be a good place for somebody." The Harvard naturalist continued, "I have the strong conviction that if you will give yourself to physiology an honourable career is open to you."[27] The following day, Wyman wrote Henry's influential uncle, declaring his conviction that his nephew was "just the person for the professorship in Boston."[28] The letter was passed on to Henry's father who lent strong support to the plan and forwarded the letter to his son in Paris, adding, "I think it very pleasing to have old men take such interest in you & I shall be very glad to have you follow their advice."[29]

Even though medical practice would almost certainly have been a successful venture because of his credentials and family background, his European training reinforced young Henry's belief that it would be possible to specialize in a single medical science. Combined chairs of anatomy and physiology persisted in America, but were now unusual in Europe. Yet the concept of specialization was gaining support in America as well, and Bowditch's father informed him, "A specialty is likely to lead to success in our great & ever increasing country."[30] Even the American Medical Association had recently taken a stand in favor of specialization in medical science.[31]

While Bowditch was in Europe, Harvard was undergoing important developments that would provide the budding scientist with an opportunity to introduce his interpretation of modern experimental physiology upon his return to America. The changes at Harvard related not only to the teaching of physiology, but to the structure and philosophy of all aspects of higher education at the institution. The far-reaching reforms at Harvard were due, in large part, to one man, Charles W. Eliot, who became president of the institution in 1869. Eliot's predecessor, Thomas Hill, a scientifically oriented mathematician and theologian, had served as president of Harvard from 1862 until 1868. While president, Hill encouraged the development of the scientific curriculum at Harvard, among other educational reforms. Compared with the sweeping changes introduced by Eliot, Hill's accomplishments were minor, however.

Charles Eliot was the son of a prominent Harvard graduate who became mayor of Boston in 1837 and was elected to Congress in 1850.[32] As a student at Harvard College, Eliot worked in Josiah Cooke's chemistry laboratory. He gained respect for practical laboratory training and scientific research through this experience and his exposure to other Harvard scientists including Benjamin Pierce, Asa Gray, Louis Agassiz, and Jeffries Wyman. In 1858, five years after his graduation, Eliot was appointed assistant professor in chemistry and mathematics at the Cambridge institution. He hoped to succeed Horsford at the Lawrence Scientific School in 1863, but was not appointed to this position. When his five-year term as assistant professor ended, Eliot did not have a position at Harvard, and he departed for a tour of European institutions. This trip lasted two years and provided him with valuable insight into the newer systems of higher education evolving in France and Germany.

Eliot was invited to return to Boston as a chemistry professor at the new Massachusetts Institute of Technology. William B. Rogers, president of the institute, encouraged Eliot to accept the chair: "I look forward to making these professorships sufficiently remunerative to place the professors at ease in regard to income. But there is much work to be done, and you can greatly aid in doing it. . . . It was with no small satisfaction that I learned a few days since of your determination to hold to your scientific pursuits. I believe you will never regret that decision."[33] Eliot's philosophy of higher education was shaped by his experiences at Harvard, his exposure to numerous European institutions of higher learning, and his participation in the inauguration of instruction at the Massachusetts Institute of Technology.

In 1869, Eliot published his views on higher education in an essay, "The New Education and Its Organization." In this article, he identified several shortcomings of the American system of higher education. He predicted that the emerging American universities would be more than copies of European institutions of higher learning; they would be a "natural outgrowth of American social and political habits, and an expression of the average aims and ambitions of the better educated classes."[34] Eliot realized the European schools of science benefited greatly from government subsidies, but America was different. He explained to William Rogers, "What governments do in Europe individuals must do with us, and ours is infinitely the best way in the long run."[35]

Support for Harvard's president Thomas Hill eroded and concern regarding his administrative abilities grew as his health declined. Many viewed his resignation in 1868 as an opportunity to revitalize Harvard. A writer in the *Nation* saw the appointment of a successor as a matter of national importance: "What we do not want is a mere business man, a fossil man, an ultra-radical man, or a clergyman. What we do want is a man of thorough scholarship . . . and at the same time endowed with sound judgement, shrewd mother-wit, practical good sense."[36] Thirty-five-year-old Charles Eliot was one of the nominees to succeed Hill. Jeffries Wyman explained to his brother Morrill, "Eliot's nomination was somewhat of a surprise, but I feel quite certain the time has come when the burden of the administration of the college must rest on younger shoulders, & I really believe that his are as broad as those of any other candidate—I presume that there will be much opposition, in some quarters, quite bitter. . . . His position will be an arduous one & he must expect many hard rubs from those who do not believe in his educational ideas."[37]

Numerous correspondents kept Henry Bowditch informed of the events at Harvard. He learned the details of Eliot's election from his father, a member of the board of overseers who supported the young chemist. The elder Bowditch informed his son, "I believe Mr. E. will prove to be the right man in the right place."[38] No one expected Eliot to maintain the status quo at Harvard; he was already known as an innovative, energetic, and forceful leader. In his inaugural address, delivered in October 1869, Eliot outlined his agenda for reorganizing Harvard. As a scientist who had recently visited European laboratories, he viewed practical laboratory training as a necessity: "The University recognizes the natural and physical sciences as indispensable branches of education, and has long acted upon this opinion; but it would have science taught in a rational way, objects and instruments in hand—not from books merely, not through the memory chiefly, but by the seeing eye and informing fingers." The Harvard president had broad responsibilities in Eliot's view. He must evaluate and rank requests, seize opportunities to enlarge the institution's endowment, recruit a dedicated and talented faculty, attract qualified scholars, and serve as a spokesman for the cause of higher education. One function of the Harvard president had special relevance for Henry Bowditch. "The most important function of the President," declared Eliot, "is that of advising the Corporation concerning appointments, particularly about appointments of young men who have not had time and opportunity to prove themselves to the public. It is in discharging this duty that the President holds the future of the University in his hands."[39]

More than rhetoric would be necessary, however, if Bowditch was to return to Harvard as a physiologist. Indeed, Eliot cautioned in his introductory address that many demands would be placed upon him as Harvard embarked on a new course; and not all demands could be met. Nevertheless, Eliot's election improved Bowditch's chances for a position at Harvard on the completion of his course of European study. Bowditch decided to devote himself to physiology even before Eliot's election, however. By the spring of 1869, frustrated with the situation in Bernard's laboratory, he planned a course of scientific study in Germany to begin in mid-1869. He had the help of Wilhelm Kühne, a prominent German physiologist who had just assumed the chair of physiology at Amsterdam. Kühne had studied with many of the leading scientists in Germany and was able, therefore, to give Bowditch a firsthand account of the various opportunities then available. He advised the young American to first study physiology for several months with Max Schultze in Bonn. Thereafter, he encouraged Bowditch to spend an entire year with Carl Ludwig at the new Leipzig Physiological Institute and a final year divided between Hermann von Helmholtz and Rudolf Virchow.[40] Bowditch received encouragement for this plan from Wyman and his father. To facilitate his entry into the German laboratories, he obtained letters of introduction from Bernard and Brown-Séquard. By the fall of 1869, when Eliot was inaugurated as Harvard's president, Bowditch had already completed a summer in Bonn studying under Schultze and was working in Ludwig's physiological institute.

The German influence on the development of higher education in America is widely acknowledged. In the early decades of the nineteenth century, *Naturphilosophie* had placed romantic speculation and mysticism before objective analysis and was accompanied by a period of relative stagnation in German science and medicine. Complex social, economic, and political factors during the middle of the nineteenth century, however, shaped higher education in Germany and also led to increased emphasis on science teaching and research. The Revolution of 1848, the culmination of growing instability, affected all aspects of life in the German-speaking lands of Western Europe. The students and faculty of the University of Vienna played a critical role in this revolution, which led to fundamental reforms in the philosophy and structure of higher education in Germany and Austria. As an integral part of German universities, the medical schools were also affected by the reform movement. The university reforms included an increase in state support for salaries, enabling medical professors to devote more time to teaching and research; greater funding for facilities, equipment, and assistants; and a new commitment to academic freedom.

Pioneering scientific laboratories had been established in Germany before the Revolution of 1848. Early laboratories of medical chemistry or physiology founded between 1820 and 1830 included those at the University of Freiburg, directed by Carl Schultze; the University of Breslau, directed by Jan Evangelista Purkinje; and the University of Giessen, directed by Justus von Liebig. The most important figure in the transition from *Naturphilosophie* to the experimental era in German medical science was Johannes Müller who explicitly outlined the application of the methods of chemistry and physics to physiology in the 1830s.[41] Müller's students who placed German biomedical science on a firm footing of experimentation and objective observation included Emil Du Bois-Reymond, Ernst von Brücke, and Hermann von Helmholtz. These three individuals strongly influenced Carl Ludwig, whose laboratory became the training ground for many future leaders of European, British, and American physiology. Carl Ludwig studied medicine at the universities of Erlangen and Marburg and worked in the laboratory of Robert Bunsen, the pioneering chemist. With Du Bois-Reymond, Helmholtz, and Brücke, he skillfully and persuasively articulated the physico-chemical approach to the biomedical sciences. Largely through their efforts, vitalism was overthrown and experimentation replaced speculation in physiology.

Dramatic advances in medical science and medical practice resulted from the intense spirit of inquiry in the German laboratories and clinics during the second half of the nineteenth century. These exciting developments led many American medical graduates to seek additional training in Germany and Austria. Most Americans wanted to develop practical skills that would make them more competitive as medical practitioners upon their return home, but some hoped to study in the German scientific laboratories. Clement Smith, a Harvard College graduate studying in Göttingen, informed his sister in 1866, "I am beginning to think that there are more American students in the German universities studying medicine or chemistry and engineering than any other branch. It is certainly so here. I am the only one studying Philology; there are two theology and one Law student; all the rest work in the dissecting room or in the laboratory."[42]

Ludwig succeeded Ernst Heinrich Weber at the University of Leipzig in 1864 and supervised the construction, equipping, and staffing of a new physiological institute that opened there in 1869. This large and well-equipped facility, built at government expense, was unmatched anywhere in the world for physiological research. Although Ludwig's responsibilities included the instruction of medical students, his major commitment was to training advanced pupils who he hoped would devote themselves to careers in the biomedical sciences. He was aided by several assistants with a sophisticated understanding of the physico-chemical approach to physiology. Advanced workers in Ludwig's laboratory were expected to participate in research under his direction. Ludwig's pupils universally extolled his willingness to advance their careers through consistent encouragement and assistance throughout the entire process of research: from hypothesis, through design and performance of the experiments, to synthesis and interpretation of the data, to publication of the results.

By the time Kühne advised Bowditch to study with Ludwig, he had already heard praise of the great teacher of physiology from his friend

William James. In June 1868, James had informed him, "In Germany the tradition is that Ludwig is 'the best teacher of Physiology'—ask any student and he will tell you so."[43] Bowditch was enthusiastic about his early months at the Leipzig Physiological Institute. In the fall of 1869, he informed Wyman: "I am now fairly started on a course of physiological study under circumstances which leave nothing to be desired. Prof. Ludwig's laboratory is a perfect model for establishments of this sort . . . is furnished with every imaginable sort of apparatus & if any new want arises there seems to be no lack of means to supply it."[44] A month later Bowditch proposed sending a description of Ludwig's institute to the *Boston Medical and Surgical Journal:* "People at home or even in France have very little idea of the way in which physiology is taught and studied in Germany. . . . It seems to me desirable that a description of this model institution should be published in some of our medical journals in order that the medical profession may understand how science is valued here in Europe."[45] His description of the facility, complete with a floor plan, appeared in the Boston journal and was reprinted in the London scientific periodical *Nature.* In this review, Bowditch revealed his enthusiasm for the German approach to research: "The patient, methodical and faithful way in which the phenomena of life are investigated by the German physiologists not only inspires great confidence in their results, but encourages one in the hope that the day is not far distant when physiology will take its proper place as the only true foundation of medical science."[46]

It was in Ludwig's institute that Bowditch's reputation as an experimental physiologist was established. The active participation of advanced students in original research was characteristic of the German institutes and distinguished them from the modestly equipped and poorly endowed French laboratories. Shortly after arriving in Leipzig, Bowditch initiated a study of cardiovascular innervation under Ludwig's direction. Ludwig had a longstanding interest in this subject and, with one of his pupils, Elie de Cyon, had recently described the vasomotor reflexes. Bowditch's research led to the discovery of two fundamental laws of cardiovascular physiology: the all-or-none law of myocardial contraction, which came to be known as "Bowditch's law," and the "treppe" phenomenon of cardiac muscle. These results, derived from experiments performed under Ludwig's guidance, were published in German under Bowditch's name alone, a common practice of Ludwig, designed to facilitate the scientific careers of his pupils.[47]

While Bowditch was in Europe, Charles Eliot was solidifying his position as Harvard's new president. He followed the progress of his former pupil and wanted Bowditch to teach a graduate course at the university in 1870.[48] Eliot began a series of negotiations to lure him away from his proposed long period of European study. Despite Eliot's advice to Bowditch's father that he "had better come home," the young physiologist was determined not to interrupt his Leipzig training. He received further encouragement for continuing his European studies from his former teacher Max Schultze. Calling Eliot's offer "extremely tempting," Bowditch explained to the Harvard president that if he were to return home prematurely he would be "sacrificing a large part of the benefit to be derived from my studies in the German universities."[49]

The significance of Bowditch's decision to decline an offer of a teaching position at his alma mater under the leadership of its new, innovative president is hard to exaggerate. Had he left the Leipzig Institute after his first year, it is likely that the important physiological discoveries he made in conjunction with Ludwig would not have been credited to him. Not only would Bowditch have lost this opportunity to become known in the community of experimental physiologists, his exposure to German physiology and to Ludwig, in particular, also would have been prematurely severed. Moreover, Eliot's offer contained no commitment for research and did not specify any role for Bowditch in the medical school. Bowditch felt confident that a position would be available for him upon his return, even if it was delayed a year. He informed his mother: "I am much obliged to my friends at home who are laying out so much lecture work for me. It seems that I shall not want for employment when I get home. There is a great deal of work to be done in the Boston Medical School before Physiology can be taught as it ought to be."[50]

As did Mitchell and Dalton, Bowditch appreciated the intimate relationship of experimental physiology to the reform of medical education in America. His agenda was too broad for him to be content with a lectureship at Harvard University, however. From Europe, he revealed to his mother: "I have been feeling very happy at the prospect of devoting my whole time to scientific pursuits. I have been building all sorts of laboratories and medical schools in the air. In this labor I have been materially assisted by Coll. Warren, who is quite convinced that something ought to be done to raise the standard of scientific education in our community. I mean, of course, particularly medical science."[51]

Bowditch was not alone in his belief that the curriculum and educational philosophy at the Harvard Medical School required revision. As would be the case at the University of Pennsylvania, the movement to reform the Harvard curriculum was led by the younger, scientifically oriented faculty members. One of the most active participants was James C. White, an 1853 graduate of the medical school. White, as had Eliot, once participated in research and laboratory exercises in Josiah Clarke's chemistry laboratory. White's interest in natural history was inspired by Asa Gray and Jeffries Wyman during his undergraduate years at Harvard. Following postgraduate training in Europe, White returned to Boston and was appointed instructor in chemistry at the Harvard Medical School in 1858. As was the case with most medical school faculty members, White was also in private practice. He had a special interest in young Bowditch's career since he served as an assistant to his uncle, a prominent Boston physician.[52]

White and Eliot, sharing interests in chemistry and medical school reform, developed a special bond. During the 1860s, White contributed a number of editorials to the *Boston Medical and Surgical Journal* on the need for reform in medical education in general, and at Harvard specifically. From White, Eliot learned the inner workings of the Harvard Medical School and the standard excuses offered in response to pleas for reform. White explained that most faculty members believed the brief medical term was necessary and that an extended term would be too costly to prevent the loss of Harvard students to other schools that offered less expensive and shorter courses leading to a medical degree. Nevertheless, White believed that Eliot could play a meaningful role in certain reforms to raise the standard of medical education at Harvard: "Matters are less in the hands of one or two than they have been and with some assistance I hope that these reforms may be accomplished."[53]

White sought Eliot's advice regarding an address he was planning on the status and prospects of American medical education. He proposed including specific suggestions for reform at Harvard and asked Eliot "whether or not it would be well to attempt to answer the tone of Dr. Holmes in his address (three years ago) concerning the folly of pursuing science in the study of medicine?"[54] Eliot apparently supported White's plan since, in November 1870, he delivered the address, including a refutation of Holmes's claim that scientific education should not be expanded in the medical curriculum. White denounced Holmes's emphasis on practical training, and informed the Harvard medical students, "The bedside and the medical lecture-room are no places for you until you have learned all that physiology will teach, and have made yourselves familiar with chemical reagents and their action upon the normal tissues and fluids of the body. . . . These branches are the groundwork of the art of medicine, and it is in these that students generally fail in thoroughness, and therefore as physicians fail to know their art through life." He admonished the students to reject the common claim that "everything can be learned at the bedside."

White concluded his address with a series of prophetic suggestions for improving the quality of medical education at Harvard and in America. He advocated research, noting, "If we cannot with our present means immediately effect so great a change, we can at least and at once take some of the steps above alluded to. . . . We can encourage a love of science and the habit of independent investigation."[55] Although many observers found his comments stimulating, some thought them too revolutionary.

Eliot became the leader in the movement to revise the structure and philosophy of education at the school, but his proposals provoked heated controversy. Philosophical differences regarding the balance between scientific and clinical training, and concern about the financial impact of lengthening the curriculum led several faculty members to resist the proposed changes. The outcome of this dispute had major implications for Henry Bowditch, who was kept informed of developments by his family and friends. In order to introduce successfully the European style of experimental physiology with its emphasis on advanced teaching and research at the Harvard Medical School, several changes were necessary: physiology had to be freed from its traditional sister discipline of anatomy; vivisection had to be tolerated, if not freely encouraged; and research with its implications for space, apparatus, and assistants had to be supported.

Eliot's active involvement in the affairs of the medical school came as little surprise to some of his friends and former colleagues. Announcing Eliot's election, William James informed Bowditch, "His great personal defects, tactlessness, meddlesomeness, and disposition to cherish petty grudges seem pretty universally acknowledged, but his ideas seem good and his economic powers first-rate. So in the absence of any other possible candidate, he went in."[56] Holmes exclaimed to his friend John Motley, "I cannot help being amused at some of the scenes that we have in our Medical Faculty,—this cool, grave young man proposing in the calmest way to turn everything topsy-turvy; taking the reins into his hands and driving as if he were the first man that ever sat on the box."[57]

One of Eliot's concerns was the issue of adequate salaries for the Harvard teaching staff. Eliot's own low salary had once led him to consider giving up his career as a chemistry teacher.[58] Bowditch with his substantial family support would not have to worry about the salary he received from Harvard. Dalton and Mitchell, less fortunate, could not subsidize programs in experimental physiology from family wealth.

Although Eliot expressed concern about the effect repetitive elementary courses had on the morale of the faculty and their opportunities for advanced work, financial considerations led him to favor traditional didactic instruction over the aggressive expansion of research at Harvard in 1869. In his inaugural address, he explained that lack of endowment in America's institutions of higher learning meant that didactic teaching, not research, must be the primary function of the nation's professors. Even well-endowed Harvard had only one fund designated for the support of research—that of the observatory.[59]

During 1870 and 1871, numerous animated meetings and heated debates occurred between Eliot and members of the Harvard medical faculty. The issues included the balance of the scientific versus the clinical branches in the curriculum and the relative value of didactic versus practical teaching. The prominent and powerful surgeon Henry J. Bigelow championed the status quo, with its emphasis on the clinical branches at the expense of the scientific subjects. He was supported by Richard M. Hodges, adjunct professor of surgery, and Oliver Wendell Holmes. Bigelow was not oblivious to medical progress; he witnessed the first operation performed under anesthesia and immediately appreciated the monumental significance of this discovery.[60] Nevertheless, he was a strong proponent of practical training at the expense of the scientific courses.

Eventually, Bigelow reluctantly accepted the reforms proposed by White and Eliot and informed Eliot in April 1871: "Our new move, which has overturned a school eminently successful for this provisional region, was inaugurated from various motives . . . [and] *would have made no headway, except for the earnest support of the president. . . .* If the move proves successful, I for one give you full credit for foresight in the matter."[61]

Bigelow remained skeptical of the reforms, however, and expressed his own philosophy of medical education to members of the Massachusetts Medical Society in June 1871. His comments addressed issues relevant to Henry Bowditch's prospects at the Harvard Medical School. "In an age of science, like the present, there is more danger that the average medical student will be drawn from what is practical, useful, and even essential, by the well-meant enthusiasm of the votaries of less applicable science, than that he will suffer from want of knowledge of these." Although Bigelow acknowledged the value of medical progress, his tone toward physicians who devoted their energies to science rather than to patients was condescending. Bowditch could not expect encouragement from Bigelow for his plan of introducing modern experimental physiology at Harvard. Reflecting his exposure to the French school and study with the British surgeon and pathologist James Paget, Bigelow favored pathological anatomy, "the corner-stone of medicine," over "experimental Physiology, which leads away from broad and safer therapeutic views, and toward a local and exclusive action of chemistry and cells,— uncertain ground for students, for whom the result of large and well-attested medical experience is here the safest teaching, and a habit of mind leading to experiments on patients the most questionable."

One factor that contributed to Bigelow's lack of support for experimental physiology was his abhorrence of vivisection. He repudiated this fundamental component of the new physiology: "How few facts of immediate considerable value to our race have of late years been exhorted from the dreadful sufferings of dumb animals, the cold-blooded cruelties now more and more practised under the authority of Science! The horrors of VIVISECTION . . . are mostly of as little present value to man as the knowledge of a new comet . . . contemptible, compared with the price paid for it in agony and torture." In a statement with direct implications for Bowditch's physiology program at Harvard, he declared, "It is dreadful to think how many poor animals will be submitted to excruciating agony, as one medical college after another becomes penetrated with the idea that vivisection is a part of modern teaching, and that, to hold way with other institutions, they, too, must have their vivisector, their mutilated dogs, their Guinea-pigs, their rabbits, their chamber of torture and of horrors to advertise as a laboratory."

In an obvious reference to Bowditch, Bigelow exclaimed, "He who comes home, fresh from German opportunities, and, impressed with their obvious advantages, attempts to incorporate the German into the accepted American system, will find that this luxuriant growth of another hemisphere is not wholly adapted to our soil or to our requirements." Neither concern for the threat of competition from other medical schools introducing vivisection techniques into teaching nor admiration for the "patient and learned worker in the remote and exact sciences" should alter the balance between the scientific and practical courses in the medical curriculum. The medical student should not "while away his time in the labyrinths of Chemistry and Physiology, when he ought to be learning the difference between hernia and hydrocele."[62]

A large segment of the American medical profession shared Bigelow's belief that the medical curriculum should be brief and clinically oriented in this era. They agreed that students should be exposed to the principles of medical practice, not the vagaries of science. At Harvard, once Eliot and his fellow reformers overcame the conservatives led by Bigelow, the curriculum expanded so that students learned both the science and the practice of medicine. Bigelow was a formidable opponent, however. Once Holmes lent his support to Eliot's plan, he admitted to the Harvard president, "You have undoubtedly seen what is the matter with me. I have been sitting under Dr. Bigelow's thumb so long that I've not been able to get out from under."[63]

The reforms at the Harvard Medical School were substantial and involved more than simple curricular changes. Holmes informed his friend Motley:

> Our new President, Eliot, has turned the whole University over like a flapjack. There never was such a *bouleversement* as that in our Medical Faculty. The Corporation has taken the whole management of it out of our hands and changed everything. We are paid salaries, which I rather like, though I doubt if we gain in pocket by it. We have, partly in consequence of outside pressure, remodeled our whole course of instruction. Consequently we have a smaller class, but better students, each of whom pays more than under the old plan of management.[64]

During the debate over reform at the Harvard Medical School, Henry Bowditch was spending his second year in Carl Ludwig's physiological institute. His decision not to return home prematurely was supported by his father who expressed concern that the young physiologist would not have sufficient independence if he accepted the position of assistant professor while Holmes retained the dual chair of anatomy and physiology traditionally held by the Parkman Professor. His father explained, "I feel satisfied that *at present*, the position you wd occupy would not probably meet yr views—I cannot say more, without mentioning names which I am not at liberty to—All wish for yr services & I wish you to be properly situated when you accept."[65]

Josiah Lombard's resignation, and Bowditch's refusal to return to Harvard, led to the appointment of William T. Lusk as assistant professor of physiology in August 1870. Lusk received medical training at Bellevue Medical College and the Long Island College Hospital where he succeeded his teacher, Austin Flint, Jr., as professor of physiology in 1868. Lusk used vivisections in his course at Harvard and told his students physiology was an independent science based on animal experimentation.[66] Although Lusk's physiology course was a significant advance over Holmes's cursory lectures, Harvard students had no opportunity to participate in laboratory work or undertake research, a possibility only with the construction of a laboratory facility upon Bowditch's return from Europe.

Bowditch's return was eagerly anticipated by several of his friends and other interested observers. James J. Putnam, a former medical student with Bowditch, exclaimed to his father, "How Dr. H[olmes] would open his eyes if he could spend a day or two in Leipzig and see how Physiology is taught there. If they make Henry Professor as soon as he comes home, as they will if they know anything, he will teach the students more than they have been taught for many a year." Putnam was aware of the controversy among the Harvard faculty over vivisection and the balance of scientific and clinical courses: "He expects to meet with a good deal of opposition from the practical men in trying to introduce so much pure science, but I hope that they will soon see that the discovery of as many physiological facts as possible whether apparently important or not, must in the end lead to the discovery of some simple law which put into the hands of practitioners all over the world will benefit two men for every one animal that was slaughtered in the cause."[67]

Among Bowditch's goals in establishing a physiological laboratory at the Harvard Medical School was to provide advanced training for individuals seeking careers in physiology and the related biological sciences. His teacher and mentor Jeffries Wyman appreciated the implications of such a physiology program in Boston. Wyman visited Ludwig's physiological institute in 1870 and explained to his brother, "A physiological laboratory in Boston well fitted out would of course not be self sustaining but would repay the cost by sending out a half dozen well educated physiologists in a year. It will be long I fear before our medical faculty will be willing to supply the means for doing so good a work."[68] A Boston practitioner who had seen Ludwig's institute exclaimed, "Would that Boston had such a physiologic laboratory and such a teacher at its head."[69] Bowditch's physiology program at Harvard, initiated in 1871, was modest compared with that of Ludwig, but represented a major new departure in American physiology. Dalton did not establish a physiological laboratory, and Mitchell was unable to get a medical school position in this science. Bowditch's agenda was broader than Dalton's, and his local circumstances were more favorable than Mitchell's.

Undaunted by his earlier unsuccessful attempts to induce young Bowditch back to Boston, Charles Eliot tried once again in the spring of 1871. This time, Bowditch accepted Eliot's offer. His original plan of comprehensive training in physiology was nearing completion; he was confident of support from several members of the Harvard faculty; and his father was going to provide money for apparatus and supplement his academic salary. In his acceptance, however, Bowditch made it clear that he expected independence and a voice in the affairs of the school. Writing from Leipzig, Bowditch explained to the Harvard president:

> I have for several years past looked forward to studying & teaching physiology as the business of my life and I therefore accept with pleasure the position which you offer me. As you invite me on my return home "to take part in the good work of reforming medical education" in America, you will, I trust, not consider it amiss if I express my opinion, which is also, I think, that of most of the members of the medical faculty, that the professorship of physiology should be an independent chair, as it has long been in nearly all European universities, and that the person who has the responsibility of teaching such an important branch of Medicine should have a voice in the management of the school. This I consider a matter of vital importance for the reputation of the medical school and I trust that among the projected reforms a change of this sort may be included.[70]

Eliot welcomed another scientific faculty member at the Harvard Medical School and viewed the expanded physiology program as a significant component of the larger reforms he was urging at the school. Bowditch shared Eliot's commitment to reforming American medical education. Both believed Harvard should serve as a model for other medical schools. It was not arrogance so much as his dedication to educational reform and his freedom from financial concerns that led Bowditch to inform his father, "If I don't like the way I am treated I can always resign."[71]

Bowditch did not anticipate generous financial support from the Harvard Medical School for his physiological laboratory in Boston, nor did he need it. His father's financial commitment simply shifted from the subsidy of a European education to the equipping of the new Harvard physiological laboratory. The elder Bowditch informed his son, "I wish you to get everything you may need & do not desire you to restrict yourself to the one thousand dollars, but purchase what in your judgement may be necessary."[72] Bowditch responded, "If you see Mr. Eliot you can tell him that I hope he will give me a good laboratory for I am going to bring home quite a quantity of apparatus."[73] Bowditch's father reassured his son that Eliot seemed "well satisfied" with the arrangements, and Calvin Ellis, the dean of the medical faculty, "said you would have all you desired."[74]

Shortly before Bowditch's return to America, Calvin Ellis and James White obtained estimates and plans for the construction of physiological and chemical laboratories in the medical school.[75] A two-room physiological laboratory was built in the attic of the medical school building for $7,000. Half of the money for this construction came from the estate of Bowditch's friend George Swett, who died of diphtheria in 1869 while they were studying abroad.[76] Not only would Bowditch have his laboratory, he would also have an independent department: the Harvard Corporation voted in May 1871 to separate physiology from the Parkman chair. This rearrangement of the professorships at the medical school afforded him control of the physiology program at Harvard.

Bowditch returned from Europe more thoroughly trained in the German approach to physiology than any other American. Although he started his physiology program at the Harvard Medical School without paid assistants, and in a modest two-room laboratory, his career represented a new departure in American medical education. He was a full-time basic medical scientist who believed in the research ethic. Moreover, he sought to train other medical scientists and physicians to undertake research. The combination of personal goals and institutional circumstances distinguished Bowditch from Dalton and Mitchell. Bowditch returned to an institution whose philosophy and structure of medical education were rapidly evolving. The Harvard catalog for 1871–72 proclaimed: "The plan of Study in this School has been radically changed. . . . The course of instruction has been greatly enlarged, to extend over three years. . . . Laboratory work will be substituted for, or added to, the usual didactic lectures, and laboratory work will be as much required of every student as attendance at lectures and recitations."[77]

Just as Dalton and Mitchell had transmitted Claude Bernard's interpretation of experimental physiology to America, Bowditch brought the German laboratory approach to medical science to the United States. He saw the value of teamwork in Ludwig's institute and encouraged qualified individuals to use his Harvard facility. Bowditch also had the institutional base that Mitchell had so earnestly desired only a few years earlier. Having decided not to practice medicine, Bowditch was spared the conflict between medical science and medical practice that plagued virtually every scientifically oriented physician in this era. The opportunity afforded Henry Bowditch at the Harvard Medical School resulted from a unique combination of individual and institutional circumstances. In this context, Bowditch served as a role model for future full-time basic medical scientists whose commitments were to advanced teaching and research and not simply to delivering didactic lectures and writing textbooks.

Bowditch returned to Boston in the summer of 1871 shortly after marrying Selma Knauth, the daughter of a Leipzig banker. He hoped to delay the initiation of his lecture course for two or three months following his return, but a postponement proved impossible. William Lusk had already left Boston to assume the chair of obstetrics at the Bellevue Hospital Medical College in New York; Bowditch had to teach the physiology course. The Harvard physiology department had no paid assistants or mechanics, so Bowditch had to rely on his own resources. In addition to delivering lectures, he arranged, operated, and maintained the apparatus he used in his demonstrations and research.

Soon after his arrival in Boston, Bowditch initiated a series of experiments on the rate of transmission of the nervous impulse and resumed his studies of ciliary motion, a subject he had investigated when he was Wyman's pupil. Bowditch must have felt isolated in his attic laboratory as he recalled the expansive Leipzig institute with its skilled workers and sophisticated apparatus. Nevertheless, he was in a familiar institution and was encouraged by a supportive family and friends who shared his interest in experimental medicine and educational reform. Moreover, he returned to a country in which interest in science was gradually but perceptibly increasing. Surgeon David Cheever announced to Harvard medical students in the fall of 1871, "Physiology, comparatively a modern science, has made great advances of late years, and is still in a transition state. As influencing and correcting the *practice* of medicine it is the most important of either [of] the departments [anatomy and physiology]."[78] Cheever lent his support to the practice of vivisection except when used for simple repetitious experiments.

Bowditch was a full-time physiologist. There was growing awareness that this level of commitment to the rapidly expanding field of physiology was necessary. A contemporary British writer stated it clearly: "No man can become *permanently* attached to any of the great laboratories with the slightest idea of practising medicine and surgery. The teacher of physiology must henceforth be a physiologist and no other thing. His days and nights must be spent in his workshop."[79] Reality was in conflict with this ideal in America, however. "In consequence of deficient endowment, the union of medical practice and medical teaching, even in what are called the non-practical branches, is essential . . . at the present day, and is likely to continue so for some years longer."[80]

These matters did not need to concern Bowditch, however. Financially secure, he was able to devote himself exclusively to an academic career in physiology.

Filled with enthusiasm from his recent European training and committed to encouraging the development of medical science in America, Bowditch embarked on a propaganda campaign in which he reported important discoveries emanating from European research laboratories. Beginning in 1873 and continuing through the decade, he published a periodic "Report in Physiology" and reviews of new publications in physiology in the *Boston Medical and Surgical Journal*. In addition to keeping up with the published European literature on physiology, he received firsthand reports of new developments from colleagues he had met abroad. These friendships formed the basis of an important international network of individuals committed to introducing scientific principles into medicine and encouraging research. For example, E. Ray Lankester, a British scientist who had worked with Bowditch in Ludwig's laboratory, kept him informed of developments in British science and education in the early 1870s. Lankester encouraged Bowditch's dedication to the field of physiology. Reflecting on the growing subdivision of the biological sciences into distinct disciplines, he revealed to his Boston friend, "I am not a pure anything and so I am afraid it will go badly with me in the future."[81] The trend toward division of the basic medical sciences into distinct disciplines was progressing most rapidly in Germany, but it was also occurring in Britain and the United States. No longer would the arrangement of the scientific chairs in American medical schools reflect simply the interests of the individual who held them rather than some intrinsic logic.

Bowditch's first advanced pupils in the Harvard physiological laboratory were not individuals seeking careers in physiology. Most were scientifically oriented recent medical graduates who wanted to use his physiological apparatus and apply new experimental approaches to problems in medicine and the collateral sciences. These individuals paid a fee of $30 a year for the use of the laboratory. Senior medical students were also permitted to pursue research studies in the physiological laboratory. A full year of laboratory training under Bowditch's direction was available to advanced students for a fee of $150.[82]

The reforms at the Harvard Medical School and Bowditch's physiology program attracted widespread attention. A New York writer explained, "In 1871 a physiological laboratory, the need of which had long been felt, was added to the school. . . . Physiology was imperfectly taught before the new system was inaugurated. . . . Dr. Bowditch was appointed Assistant Professor of Physiology under the new system, and, with thorough lectures, recitations, experiments, and a laboratory for students to work in, has done much to develop this previously-neglected branch."[83]

The scope of Bowditch's physiology program necessitated the hiring of an assistant. Bowditch's friend William James, who had also received formal training in physiology in Europe, filled the position. Periodically incapacitated by physical and emotional problems, James had decided not to practice medicine. The appointment reflected their friendship more than James's desire to be a physiologist. He disliked vivisection and five years earlier had informed Bowditch, "I can't be a teacher of physiology . . . for I can't do laboratory work."[84] Bowditch did not suffer the aggressive attacks of the antivivisectionists Dalton confronted in New York. Nevertheless, the Harvard physiologist observed in 1873, "Without entering into a defense of scientific vivisections, which is fortunately quite unnecessary in this community, it may be well to suggest that even the noble desire to prevent cruelty to animals may possibly be pushed to a vicious extreme."[85] James's participation in Bowditch's laboratory came to an end in 1874 when he was appointed head of the Museum of Comparative Anatomy following Jeffries Wyman's death. James did use the physiological principles he learned in Europe and from Bowditch to redirect American psychology and place it on a sounder scientific basis.[86]

Shortly after Bowditch's return from Europe, papers based on research performed in his laboratory began to appear in the medical literature. Bowditch and his colleagues published more than twenty scientific papers between 1873 and 1879. There was no predominant research theme: the publications reported investigations dealing with the physiology of the digestive system, the circulatory system, the lungs, and the nervous system, as well as pharmacological studies. The research in this early period reflected the diverse interests of the workers who used the new Harvard facility.[87] Bacteriology does not appear to have been actively pursued in Bowditch's laboratory in this era. As noted earlier, Dalton became interested in this subject and wrote about it, and H. Newell Martin's laboratory at Johns Hopkins undertook bacteriological studies later in the decade. Although Bowditch viewed the spontaneous generation debate as a subject of great scientific importance, he believed it was "physiological only in the widest sense of the word."[88]

Bowditch's teaching of practical physiology to students and advanced workers in his laboratory was greatly facilitated by the publication of John Burdon-Sanderson's *Handbook for the Physiological Laboratory* in 1873. Bowditch claimed that this well-illustrated manual supplied

> a want which has long been felt by all readers of physiology. Recognizing the fact that physiology is emphatically an experimental science, it furnishes minute instructions for performing a great variety of experiments illustrating all the most improved methods of physiological investigation. . . . The publication of this work may fairly be regarded as marking an important advance in physiological science, for it enables all students and practitioners of medicine to verify for themselves the experimental basis upon which scientific medicine must ultimately be built up.[89]

During the summer of 1875, Bowditch returned to Europe and visited his former teacher Carl Ludwig. At this time he met H. Newell Martin, an Irish pupil of Michael Foster and Thomas H. Huxley, who was studying in Leipzig. He met other British physiologists in Ludwig's laboratory as well; Walter Gaskell and Edward Schäfer were working there at the time.[90] This visit allowed Bowditch to maintain and enlarge his international network of medical scientists. Neither Bowditch nor Martin realized at this time that the young Irishman would soon come to America to inaugurate an experimental physiology program at the Johns Hopkins University. These two professional physiologists would have an enormous impact on the development of their chosen scientific field in the United States. Bowditch's isolation from other sophisticated experimental physiologists was less absolute once Martin came to Johns Hopkins. Shortly after Martin's arrival in Baltimore in 1876, they began corresponding about their mutual interests.

As more workers in the Harvard physiological laboratory completed research projects, Bowditch concluded there was a need for an American journal devoted exclusively to anatomy and physiology. Although Harvard exerted little pressure to encourage Bowditch or his coworkers to publish the results of their investigations, he recognized the importance of disseminating the results from his laboratory to legitimize the physiology program. He had learned this lesson from Ludwig. The German scientific literature was already well developed and served as a model for Bowditch. Martin was initially supportive of Bowditch's plan to establish a scientific journal, but the need was eliminated when Michael Foster founded the *Journal of Physiology* in 1878.[91] Bowditch

and eight of his co-workers in the Harvard physiological laboratory contributed several papers to Foster's journal during its first decade. The
regular appearance of publications from Bowditch's laboratory in this
prestigious scientific periodical assured international recognition of his
Harvard program.

Bowditch's department also gained in stature as his scientific pupils
matured and visited or worked in other institutions. He encouraged several of his students to study abroad, particularly with Carl Ludwig.
Charles S. Minot, following a year as Bowditch's assistant, went to Europe for additional postgraduate scientific training. He informed Bowditch, "Your introduction secured for me a most kindly welcome. . . .
Everyone is ready with your praises, Zühlsdorf . . . tells me of your industry, Kronecker of your ingenuity (which has given him a high opinion of Yankees), Ludwig of your abilities."[92]

The Harvard reforms and Bowditch's physiology program attracted attention in North America as well. William Osler, following
visits to the Harvard Medical School in 1876 and 1877, published an account of the institution in which he characterized it as the most progressive medical school on the continent. At the time of his visit to Boston,
Osler was professor of the institutes of medicine at McGill University
and pathologist to the Montreal General Hospital. Osler had first met
Henry Bowditch in 1875, and the two became close friends. When a new
physiological laboratory was constructed at McGill five years later, it
was partially patterned after Bowditch's Harvard facility. In his description of the Harvard Medical School, Osler applauded Bowditch's
physiology program and noted that the professor devoted his whole time
to the subject. He also reported that he had observed a class of medical
students performing experiments on frogs in order to elucidate the physiology of reflex action.[93]

Beginning with the 1876–77 term, junior students as well as seniors
at the Harvard Medical School were admitted to Bowditch's laboratory
and, if they desired, could participate in research projects.[94] The success
of the laboratory resulted in the need for additional space within three
years of Bowditch's return from Leipzig. At a meeting to promote the
erection of a new building for the medical school in 1874, Eliot explained, "Five years ago there was no physiological laboratory in the
school, none whatever, and no microscopical room except one fifteen
feet square, with very little daylight in it. Now we have laboratories of
physiology and microscopy, which are resorted to by the students with
great assiduity. But the changes in the system of instruction have ren-

dered these rooms inadequate to the daily wants of the school." The
Harvard president asked for financial support from the community:

> The medical faculty of the university is leading in a reform in
> medical education which is of the utmost consequence, not only to
> this community, but to the country. . . . The community, as a
> whole, has a great stake in the advancement of medical education.
> The public health is a matter of the utmost concern, even to our
> new communities. . . . In order to enlarge the range of medical
> knowledge it is absolutely essential that there should be investiga-
> tors in medical science—men who have received the best training
> that the world can give; who are gifted by nature with the quali-
> ties which investigation demands, and who are enabled to live in
> the prosecution of investigation. For this purpose we need salaries,
> laboratories, working places, museums, for such men.[95]

Such a commitment required a substantial endowment, however.
A fundamental change in the salary structure and philosophy for the
professors of the basic medical sciences was necessary as well. Oliver
Wendell Holmes pointed out the problems inherent in a system in which
the professors' salaries were dependent on students' fees: "We must hope
that in due time the more important professorships, if not all of them,
will be endowed, so that the existence of the school will not under any
circumstances depend on its being able to attract large classes by accom-
modating its standard of teaching to a popular average, and making its
degree too easy of attainment."[96]

In this era of the nation's Centennial, writers expressed a growing
concern about the lack of support for scientific research and for individuals interested in devoting themselves to careers in science. They attributed the gap between expectation and reality in American scientific education to the lack of funds for this purpose. One writer explained,
"Experimental facilities are expensive. . . . This is a potent reason why
there is so much sham in so-called scientific education."[97] Medical science was particularly important. Eliot's former chemistry teacher,
Josiah P. Cooke, informed his Harvard students in 1875, "No educated
man can expect to realize his best possibilities of usefulness without a
practical knowledge of the methods of experimental science. If he is to
be a physician, his whole success will depend on the skill with which he
can use these great tools of modern civilization." Cooke, a strong advocate of the research ethic in higher education, declared:

> The time has passed when we can afford to limit the work of our
> higher institutions of learning to teaching knowledge already ac-

quired. Henceforth the investigation of unsolved problems, and
the discovery of new truth, should be one of the main objects at
our American universities, and no cost grudged, which is required
to maintain at them the most active minds, in every branch of
knowledge which the country can be stimulated to produce. I
could urge this on the self-interest of the nation as an obvious
dictate of political economy.[98]

During the 1874 meeting to explore the options for the construction
of a new laboratory at the Harvard Medical School, a building committee was selected that included Henry Bowditch and James White. They
agreed that the new curriculum at the Harvard Medical School with its
emphasis on laboratory training necessitated a new facility; the dilemma was how to pay for it. Bowditch, White, and Eliot did not want
to make the same mistake that the officials at the University of Pennsylvania had made. They sought to erect a building that would be suitable
for several decades, not obsolete in a few short years. Their elaborate
plans were expensive, however, and construction did not begin until the
summer of 1881.

Space limitations affected the scope of Bowditch's physiology program during its first decade. Practical laboratory instruction, although
advertised in the Harvard catalogs, was actually quite modest. When
Bowditch's laboratory consisted of two attic rooms, instruction in physiology was limited mainly to lectures and demonstrations. Although opportunities for advanced work were available, relatively few students
took advantage of them. Frederick W. Ellis, a member of the medical
school class of 1881, later recalled that Bowditch taught primarily by
lectures illustrated with demonstrations and by conferences. Ellis's class
did receive a small amount of practical laboratory training in Bowditch's attic laboratory, but it was not a prominent part of the Harvard
physiology course.[99]

Although the Harvard physiology program was more sophisticated
than that offered by any other American medical school in this era, some
observers thought that more could, and should, be done. A harsh assessment of physiology teaching at Harvard came from Alonzo B. Palmer,
professor of medicine at the University of Michigan. After visiting Harvard in 1877 and seeing Bowditch's attic laboratory, he informed James
B. Angell, present of the University of Michigan, that he was disappointed at the number of Harvard students at work in the physiological
laboratory and the condition of the apparatus. Palmer believed that
Michigan could (and must) do better, but he cautioned that students
were less interested in experimental physiology and medical research

than they were in microscopy.[100] He was right. The immediate practical
value of a knowledge of microscopy to a medical practitioner was
greater than familarity with the techniques of experimental physiology;
even Bowditch would not dispute that. But, with limited space and fi-
nite resources, Bowditch devoted his attention to advanced workers and
to research, much as his teacher Ludwig had done in Leipzig. Another
Michigan faculty member, Henry S. Cheever, who taught physiology
among his other responsibilities, was more optimistic about the interest
students had in physiology. Cheever had previously taught physiology at
Long Island College Hospital where he used vivisections as well as lectures in his course. In a comprehensive analysis of the status and prospects of physiology at the University of Michigan written in 1876,
Cheever informed Angell this approach was warmly received at Long
Island. Practical laboratory training and research in physiology depended on the interest and availability of the professor in Cheever's
opinion. "For a long time there had been a gradually increasing demand
for the same kind of experimentation in connection with the course of
physiological instruction here [at Michigan] though the want of it was
less felt owing to the most admirable teaching qualities of Prof. Ford to
whose chair physiology was many years since attached. This demand it
was impossible for Prof. Ford to meet owing to the superior claims of
anatomy to his attention."

Cheever revealed that the Michigan dean and members of the medical faculty had asked him to deliver an illustrated course of lectures similar to the one he had recently completed in Brooklyn and establish a
physiological laboratory for practical exercises and research. This broad
agenda was impossible, however, because of a "want of means and
time." Not only did Cheever teach several different courses, he also
practiced medicine. Things had to change if the University of Michigan
was to maintain its image as a progressive school. Cheever declared, "In
the first place the demand for illustrated instruction in physiology and
the establishment of a physiological laboratory in an institution like this
is so great that in our present circumstance we cannot well ignore it. In
the second place it requires for a proper presentation of this subject the
time of a full chair and hence no one chair can give it requisite time in
connection with any other topic." Cheever advocated a separate chair of
physiology to be filled by an individual capable of performing research,
directing others in this undertaking, and lecturing using vivisections and
other demonstrations. Anticipating the shortcomings Palmer would describe in Bowditch's department the following year, Cheever asserted,
"In truth the laboratory cannot be expected to spring up mushroomlike

into full growth at once but must gradually and steadily develop into being with a rapidity proportioned to the energy of the man in charge and the liberality of the Board of Regents."[101]

Physiological laboratories did not become common in America's medical schools for more than a decade. The opening of a physiological laboratory required a dedicated professor trained in the techniques of modern experimental physiology, the financial support of his institution, and a sustained demand by students or advanced workers for such a facility. In most instances it was a physiologist who urged his institution to establish a physiological laboratory. America's medical students, still poorly prepared for a scientific education, were not in a position to demand practical training in physiology or request opportunities to perform research. Nevertheless, advocates of experimental physiology sensed a trend that reflected society's growing interest in the scientific side of medicine. In 1874, members of the American Medical Association heard Elias Gray of Bloomington, Illinois, recount the practical advances in man's understanding of the pathophysiology of many diseases because of experimentation. A pioneer of public health, Gray declared, "The practice of medicine, resting as it does, and as it must to be completely successful, upon physiology, is making progress, *pari passu*, with the advance of physiological science, becoming more and more rational and scientific."[102]

Although the importance of the scientific branches of medicine was becoming more widely acknowledged, and the need to teach them by practical methods in the laboratory was gaining support, economics dictated the pace with which reforms could be introduced into the curricula of America's medical schools. Until adequate endowments or other means of financial support replaced students' fees as the main source of income, there was little opportunity for rapid expansion of the full-time system or the research ethic, personified in Henry Bowditch. Potential Harvard students were concerned about the increased cost of a medical education the expanded curriculum required. Letters to the dean of the Harvard Medical School in the mid-1870s reflected this concern. Prospective students complained that they had little money and needed scholarships or would have to work during their medical training. Several candidates expressed the hope that the required courses could be completed in as short a time as possible. Nevertheless, they were eager to get the Harvard degree, which they viewed as having great prestige. One potential student asked, "Having studied medicine during three years under the direction of a Doctor and taken advantage of every opportunity which his practice afforded—after that—will, a term of nine

months at Harvard having passed the required examination, entitle me
to a diploma? If not, how long is the shortest time? Should it take three
years, in Boston, as I have heard, I propose going to New York."[103]

Although Bowditch's laboratory was successful by American standards of the 1870s, its initial impact was modest. His efforts would not
have their full effect for a generation. Of the thousands of young physicians who annually graduated from the numerous American medical
schools, only a handful had personal experience in physiological laboratories in the 1870s. One medical editor from Philadelphia, complained
in 1877, "There is not to-day and there never has been on this continent
a well-organized physiological or pathological laboratory steadily fruit-
ful in good work." He attributed this lack "to our system of medical education, which does not require the professor of a scientific medical
branch to be anything more than a popular orator, or to have any other
than a book-knowledge of the branch he teaches." Other factors responsible in his view included the utilitarian outlook of Americans and the
lack of opportunities for individuals who wanted to pursue scientific careers:

> There have been men who at thirty have accomplished as much of
> original work in the medical sciences as have at the same age the
> most illustrious of our European *confrères*. The promise of the
> morning, however, is not fulfilled by the noon of life. The reasons
> of this are not so much intrinsic to the individual as extrinsic.
> There are no facilities for work provided; there is no active *esprit
> de corps* to stimulate to sustained effort; there is no career offered
> which, whilst affording a modicum of substantial reward, shall
> give the reputation and influence which atone with many for a
> pecuniary compensation less than that afforded by the more lucra-
> tive professions.

The writer made an important distinction between teachers of the
natural or physical sciences and the medical sciences. He explained that
the naturalist or astronomer did not have a lucrative alternative for the
application of his talents, whereas "the physiologist, who has probably
always retained some hold on practical medicine, finds it very easy to
slide into a life whose rewards are so immediate, and for whose success
the previously-earned reputation makes a most excellent foundation."
The solution, he asserted, was to establish endowed chairs, fellowships,
and well-furnished laboratories. Suggesting a salary of five thousand
dollars as a minimum (which was greater than the average physician's
income in this era), he argued that the professor should be required to

refrain from medical practice and only individuals who had demonstrated commitment to and productivity in research should be hired.[104]

This Philadelphia writer was apparently unfamiliar with the activities in Bowditch's department, formed only six years earlier. Another contemporary writer J.R.W. Hitchcock, who was knowledgable about the situation at Harvard, held similar views about the emphasis on teaching, however. After listing the research work that had been published from Bowditch's department, he decried the disproportionate emphasis on teaching at most American institutions of higher learning. He attributed this imbalance to the targeting of most endowments for the support of teaching rather than research. Even at Harvard, "no research fund exists, and aside from the stated work of the university, many of the instructors devote a portion of their time to private instruction, which . . . drains upon the time and energy of the professors [and] render the more surprising and creditable that so much original research is being constantly carried on in the different departments of the university."[105] In this writer's opinion, individuals might wish to pursue research, but institutional and local circumstances often made it difficult or impossible to do so.

The officials at the Harvard Medical School, like their counterparts at the College of Physicians and Surgeons of New York and the University of Pennsylvania, understood the problem. They also believed they knew the solution: endowment. The reorganization of the Harvard Medical School placed it in an unusual position; the professors no longer profited from it directly. Harvard's president Charles Eliot argued that as long as medical schools were proprietary and run solely to benefit their physician-owners there was no justification for their requesting financial support from the community. In 1871, however, after the Harvard Medical School became an integral part of the university, it was no longer set up simply to bring profits to the professors. For this reason, Eliot believed the institution could request support from the community. Like Eliot, others argued that mankind would benefit from the endowment of medical education. "Whatever motives induce benevolent persons to endow institutions which teach the humanities or theology should also avail for the endowment of medical education" was the claim of one Boston writer in 1882. "The seed and the fruit, the planting and the harvesting, may be different in kind; but these various cultures all have in view a common end, namely, the improvement of man's estate."[106]

The opportunities for laboratory teaching and research in physiology at Harvard did increase as a result of bequests and gifts for the completion of the new medical school building in 1883. Extensive laboratory facilities in this building bore witness to the palpable shift in the philosophy of medical education that had occurred at Harvard in the brief span of fifteen years since the election of Charles Eliot as president of the university. The research ethic was now acknowledged at the Harvard Medical School. Joseph W. Warren, who became Bowditch's assistant in 1881, described the purpose of the new physiological laboratory: "It is intended to serve primarily as a laboratory of research, and secondarily as an adjunct to the lectures on physiology in the preparation of suitable apparatus and experiments. Courses in 'practical physiology' are also given in the laboratory to the class in sections of a convenient size."[107] Warren's comments, the configuration of the medical school laboratories, and the curriculum at Harvard reflected the emphasis Bowditch placed on lectures including demonstrations and original research. Bowditch's agenda did not include extensive student participation in laboratory exercises. This approach would not become part of the Harvard physiology curriculum for another decade.

Bowditch was anxious to have the Harvard physiological laboratory compare favorably with the new facilities at Johns Hopkins that opened in 1884. Warren's detailed description of Bowditch's laboratory appeared in *Science* just five months after the publication of a similar review proclaiming the merits of Martin's biological laboratory at Johns Hopkins in the same journal.[108] William Osler wrote to Edward Schäfer late in 1883, on the eve of the British physiologist's visit to America: "You will be interested in Bowditch's & Martin's Laboratories, the only good ones on the continent."[109] G. Stanley Hall, who worked with both Bowditch and Martin, exclaimed after touring the new Hopkins facility, "Why! I had no idea of this—why! it is ever so much better than Bowditch's new laboratory!"[110] Bowditch toured Martin's laboratory in 1884 and declared to his wife, "He has very fine new quarters & beautiful apparatus, everything in fact, to make glad the heart of a physiologist."[111] Other physiologists and scientifically oriented physicians also visited Bowditch's new laboratory, including John C. Dalton. John Shaw Billings and Weir Mitchell were frequent visitors to the new Harvard laboratory and followed the activities in it and the Harvard reform movement with great interest.[112]

On the occasion of the one hundredth anniversary of the Harvard Medical School and the opening of its new building, Oliver Wendell Holmes explained:

> You will see extensive apartments destined for the practical study
> of chemistry and of physiology. But these branches are no longer

studied as of old by merely listening to lectures. . . . Physiology, as now studied, involves the use of much delicate and complex machinery. . . . Never was the human body as a machine so well understood; never did it give such an account of itself as it now does in the legible handwriting of the cardiograph, the sphygmograph, the myograph, and other self-registering contrivances, with all of which the student of to-day is expected to be practically familiar.[113]

In another address on the same occasion, Holmes appealed for financial support from the community for the new Harvard curriculum and the ambitious program of research. Holmes's comments reveal that he now accepted the philosophy of medical education espoused by Eliot, White, and Bowditch. He was no longer persuaded by Bigelow's argument for practical medical education. The poet-anatomist claimed, "A medical school has to teach much that seems incidental to medical practice, but only in this way can it send forth fully equipped practitioners. It begins with chemistry, anatomy, physiology, and thus prepares its students for study at the bedside and in the operating-room."[114]

Bowditch was interested in the reform of American medical education before he was a Harvard faculty member. His opportunity to influence this movement both at Harvard and nationally increased in 1883 when he was selected to succeed Calvin Ellis as dean of the medical faculty. Bowditch was not Eliot's first choice for dean, however. The Harvard president favored Francis Minot, the Hersey Professor of Medicine. Minot raised an issue of growing importance in his letter to Eliot in which he declined to accept the position: the role of the full-time faculty member as administrator.

I think Dr. Bowditch would make an admirable Dean. He is well versed in the affairs of the School, is methodical and industrious, and will be at the College a large part of the day and accessible to the students and others. Moreover he teaches the First Class, and has thereby a better acquaintance with the whole body of students than one who merely lectures to the third year men. I am much gratified by your expressed preference for me to fill such an important office, but I am very unwilling to take it unless it is absolutely necessary for the welfare of the School. I am sure Dr. Bowditch is much better qualified for it than I am. While the incessant interruptions incident to my practice would seriously interfere with the punctual discharge of the duties of a Dean.[115]

Thus, the demands of practice could now be viewed as an obstacle to serving as an administrator in a medical school in addition to being an impediment to teaching the basic medical sciences.

Bowditch's appointment resulted from a consensus of the medical faculty. They may have recognized more than Eliot the difficulty of combining practice with the increasingly important administrative tasks of a medical school dean. This situation was especially true with the lengthening of the curriculum, the enlargement of the faculty and facilities, and the growing importance of endowment to sustain the reform movement. Other leading medical schools also placed full-time basic scientists in charge of their faculties in this era: John Dalton was selected as president of the College of Physicians and Surgeons of New York in 1883; Victor Vaughan, a physiological chemist, was elected dean at the University of Michigan Medical School in 1891; and William Welch, a pathologist, became dean of the Johns Hopkins School of Medicine upon its opening in 1893. Eliot's biographer, Henry James, commented on the significance of Bowditch's appointment as dean, "Nothing could have proved more pointedly that the School had become an institution for the teaching of medical science instead of one which an association of practitioners conducted for the purpose of licensing men cheaply to go out and learn the art of healing at the bedsides of their patients."[116]

Bowditch devoted his later years to the larger concerns of reform in medical education. One of those with whom he shared this interest was John Shaw Billings who invited the Harvard physiologist to chair the section on medical education at the ninth International Medical Congress planned for Washington in 1887.[117] Billings, secretary-general of the congress, explained:

> You are selected to be Chairman of this section for the reason that you are the Dean of the Harvard Medical School; that you have been interested in the subject of buildings for Medical Schools, are well acquainted abroad with those who have been foremost with making improvements in the methods of teaching, and your school is taken at present as the Representative of advanced medical education in this country. . . . I think you are eminently fitted to preside over this section and in fact I do not know of anyone else in this country who can do it.[118]

A major political struggle for control of the congress led to mass resignations and Bowditch did not participate, however.

As Billings claimed, Bowditch was a nationally and internationally recognized authority on medical education as well as a leader of American physiology. Bowditch retired from the position of dean in 1894, "having by his clear judicial mind and impartial spirit contributed more than any other to guide the School safely through the experimental stages of the new system of education."[119] While Bowditch's contributions to the advancement of medical education were receiving increasing attention, his department of physiology remained productive as well. In 1888, two of his former teachers expressed their admiration for what he had accomplished. Brown-Séquard declared he was proud of Bowditch, and Carl Ludwig exclaimed, "You have founded a physiological institute."[120]

Bowditch was spared the intense and unrelenting attack of the antivivisectionists Dalton had to endure throughout his career, but he was occasionally threatened by members of the humane movement. Like Dalton and Mitchell, he believed that animal experimentation was crucial for the advance of medicine. As a leading spokesman for scientific medicine and the reform of medical teaching in America, Bowditch chose the subject of vivisection for his address to the Massachusetts Medical Society in 1896. His conclusions reflected the philosophy of his European teachers Bernard and Ludwig: "Enough has been said, I trust, to demonstrate the expediency of permitting physiological research to go on unchecked, and even of encouraging it, in every possible way, as the only legitimate basis of scientific medicine."[121]

Bowditch continued to refine his vision of the ideal American medical school. By the turn of the century, he was still addressing the critical questions of preliminary education, the balance between didactic and laboratory training, and the proper preparation of medical school teachers.[122] As had Dalton, Bowditch dedicated his final years to the financial concerns of medical education and science. In 1901, he helped secure a gift in excess of one million dollars from J. Pierpont Morgan for new facilities at the Harvard Medical School.[123] A revolution in the teaching of the scientific branches of medicine in American medical schools occurred during Bowditch's thirty-year career as a professional physiologist. He served as a role model for future full-time basic medical scientists who accepted the research ethic and sought to make medicine more scientific by encouraging an appreciation of science among medical students and physicians.

Bowditch's contributions to physiology and medical education were summarized in his obituaries. In the *Lancet* he was characterized as "the *doyen*, and in reality the founder, of the American School of Physiologists."[124] William Osler told Bowditch's widow:

Think of what the Harvard Medical School was when he joined and what it was when he resigned, and his energy and the confidence he inspired were the motive powers in the great transformation. In those early days he brought the knowledge of how things should be, and fortunately he had the organizing capacity necessary to mold the old school in new lines. Then as the father of the American School of Physiology he brought a new spirit into the science of medicine. It was always delightful to recognize the affection which the younger men had for him, and he did much to set the standard high in scientific work."[125]

CHAPTER FOUR

H. Newell Martin

*Johns Hopkins
and the Research Ethic*

ARLIER CHAPTERS HAVE demonstrated the importance of institutional factors in the careers of three pioneers of American physiology. Bowditch was the most successful of the three because of the
special personal and institutional factors that made it possible for him to
devote his career to teaching, research, and the training of other
full-time medical scientists. H. Newell Martin (1848–1896), the fourth
major contributor to the maturation of American physiology, did not
have the strong family and institutional ties that made it relatively easy
for Bowditch to become Harvard's first full-time physiologist. Martin
was a foreigner, was not independently wealthy, and was virtually unknown to American physicians and scientists when he was hired in 1876
to inaugurate the biology program at the new Johns Hopkins University
in Baltimore. Mitchell's career demonstrated how an individual could
make major contributions to the development of physiology without an
institution. At Johns Hopkins, the institutional context was more important than the individual. Martin's broad agenda for research and teaching with emphasis on graduate training was facilitated by the unique
philosophy and financial strength of the new Baltimore university.

In order to appreciate H. Newell Martin's role in the development
of American physiology, it is necessary to demonstrate how the Johns
Hopkins University came to place such emphasis on research and on
physiology. It is important to consider briefly the origins of the university, the attitudes of its first president, Daniel Coit Gilman, and those of
John Shaw Billings, Gilman's main adviser for the medical aspects of

Johns Hopkins. The contributions of this university to the development of graduate and medical education in America are widely acknowledged.[1] Factors that led to the early success of the Johns Hopkins University included an unprecedented endowment; the freedom from tradition of a new institution; a group of dedicated and open-minded trustees; a young and energetic faculty who shared a commitment to the research ethic; the vision of John Shaw Billings; and a president who was committed to elevating the standard of higher education in America.

Endowment, a theme that has arisen repeatedly in earlier chapters, was not a problem for the new university in Baltimore. When it opened in 1876, Johns Hopkins had an unprecedented endowment. The university's founder and namesake, Johns Hopkins, was a Quaker merchant whose adult life was spent in Baltimore. When he died in 1873, he left a bequest of nearly seven million dollars to found a university and a hospital. Johns Hopkins's decision to endow higher education was inspired, in part, by George Peabody, a merchant and financier, who established the Peabody Institute in Baltimore in 1857. There was growing recognition of the need for private support of higher education in America; significant government funding seemed unlikely and, in the minds of some observers, undesirable.[2]

There was precedent in America for the endowment of institutions of higher learning that emphasized science in their curriculum: the Lawrence Scientific School, the Sheffield Scientific School, and Cornell University owed their existence to the generosity of wealthy citizens. Although he personally selected the boards of trustees for his university and hospital, Johns Hopkins did not explicitly define the character of his proposed institutions. Half of the trustees were, like the founder, Quakers, but the university's first president, Daniel Coit Gilman, claimed, "I never knew ecclesiastical preferences to govern the action of a single member of the board."[3]

The makeup of the university board of trustees was typical of other institutional boards of the period; it included seven businessmen, four lawyers, and one physician. Three board members were especially influential in defining the scientific emphasis of the new university. George Dobbin, a lawyer and dean of the law faculty at the University of Maryland, was, of all the original trustees, perhaps the most interested in science. He had an avocational interest in photography and astronomy but, according to Gilman, he watched "the progress of chemistry, physics, astronomy and biology . . . with an intelligent and comprehensive interest."[4] Reverdy Johnson, Jr., a lawyer who had studied in Heidelberg, was also interested in science and was one of the most influential

trustees. The third trustee who was, with Gilman, responsible for outlining the plan of instruction and developing the philosophy of education at the university was James Carey Thomas, a prominent Baltimore
physician and the sole medical representative on the board. The Johns
Hopkins trustees took their responsibility seriously. In addition to reviewing nearly two dozen recent publications relating to educational
philosophy, they elicited the opinions of several American leaders of
higher education.

Among the most important events in the formation of the university
were the interviews of the trustees with three young university presidents: Andrew D. White, Charles W. Eliot, and James B. Angell.
White, the president of Cornell University, first met Gilman when they
were students at Yale College in the early 1850s.[5] White accompanied
Gilman on an extended trip to Europe in 1853. Although they were as-
signed to the American Embassy in Russia, the recent Yale graduates
had an opportunity to visit many institutions of higher learning in Great
Britain and Western Europe. White, a historian, credited Gilman with
stimulating his interest in science and scientific education. Three years
before he was invited to advise the Johns Hopkins trustees, White had
revealed his dedication to the research ethic in higher education and his
interest in science. At the farewell celebration for British scientist John
Tyndall, whose American lecture tour had come to an end, White declared, "I maintain that the true spirit of scientific research . . . is, at
this moment, one of the most needed elements in the political progress of
our country."[6] As president of Cornell University, White established
laboratories for practical training in the natural and physical sciences.
He informed the Hopkins trustees of the advantages of this form of practical education and encouraged them to build laboratories as soon as
possible.[7]

The recent reforms of Charles Eliot at Harvard stimulated great
interest among all observers of American higher education. During his
meeting with the trustees, Eliot emphasized the need for an institution
in America that would provide high-quality graduate training. His
background as a chemist made him especially sensitive to the need for
more opportunities for adequate scientific training in America. Anticipating a problem the Hopkins officials would confront in recruiting
their first faculty, Eliot declared, "There is in this country, already, a
very considerable body of teachers who know how to teach Latin and
Greek, and the elements of language; but if you are in search of teachers
to teach botany, chemistry, physics and so on, you cannot find them.
They do not exist . . . and this difficulty is a very serious one. A body of

teachers not existing for the scientific method, you are apt to get poor teachers, or teachers trained in another system."[8] Indeed, the University of Pennsylvania appointed anatomist Harrison Allen to the physiology chair in the absence of a more suitable American candidate.

James B. Angell, president of the University of Michigan, identified Baltimore as a great industrial city and encouraged the trustees to emphasize the practical applications of science in their university.[9] As White had urged, Angell advised the trustees to construct laboratories as soon as possible. Although the three university presidents addressed many aspects of higher education, each emphasized the opportunities for advancing scientific education possessed by the new, well-endowed Baltimore institution. White, Eliot, and Angell had each visited Europe where they witnessed dramatic advances in higher education. The three university presidents were active reformers and sought to encourage research and better scientific teaching. They were anxious to have an ally in their struggle to reform American higher education appointed to the Hopkins presidency. All three encouraged the trustees to select Daniel Coit Gilman as the university's first president.

Gilman's role in shaping Johns Hopkins is difficult to overemphasize.[10] His interest in science was stimulated while he was a student at Yale College beginning in 1848. There, he came under the influence of the prominent scientists Benjamin Silliman, his son Benjamin Silliman, Jr., and James Dwight Dana. Following graduation from Yale, he made a survey of the scientific schools of Europe at the request of Henry Barnard, the pioneering American educator, and found that many Europeans believed scientific and technical education had benefits for their society. Gilman agreed: "The material prosperity of many European countries is manifestly dependent upon the extent and character of their systems of scientific education." He argued that the demand for scientific training in the United States was demonstrated by the number of American students who were beginning to go to Europe for advanced training in science, the success of the Lawrence Scientific School of Harvard, and the popular new courses in engineering and applied chemistry at Yale. Economics played a role in this trend toward education in the sciences: "The young men of this country, as the professions of law, medicine, and theology become crowded, are eager for the proper training to excel in other sciences, and also because the producers of every kind, are rapidly learning that for a long and successful competition with the manufacturers of Europe, the same union must be established in this country which exists abroad, between Applied and Theoretical Science." Gilman incorporated the themes of competition, overcrowded professions leading to shifts in careers, and growing nationalism into his essay.[11]

Gilman's review revealed his sophisticated understanding of the means of scientific training and his philosophy of the role of education in the advance of American society. Elementary science was already taught in institutions throughout the United States and some opportunities for experimental work existed, "but, more than this is needed. We need higher courses of instruction, which, alone, will secure our continued advancement, or even our permanent prosperity. . . . A school which, rising above those common places which are universally known, should supply an education of the most elevated order, and should stimulate original inquiries and investigations."[12] Gilman would contribute to the creation of such a school in Baltimore two decades later.

Following his return from Europe, Gilman was responsible for raising funds for the development of the new scientific school at Yale. His views of scientific education were reflected in the appeals of Yale president Theodore Woolsey and Yale scientist James Dana for economic support for the school.[13] Gilman was elected professor of physical geography at the Yale Scientific School in 1863. He maintained his interest in educational issues and published a review of six recent pamphlets on higher education and the Morrill land grant act four years later. In this review, he emphasized the strong sense of nationalism that resulted from the Civil War. In his opinion, the Rebellion resulted in the withdrawal of "extreme sectional men" from Congress, and their withdrawal facilitated the passage of legislation to benefit "the national welfare." In this context, Gilman proposed the development of "National Schools of Science," which would encourage research and advanced courses in the physical and natural sciences.

Gilman was an early and zealous advocate of the research ethic and specialization. At Johns Hopkins, he would implement the philosophy articulated in his 1867 review: "Where there is a university organization, the constant effort should be made to educate men of science, able to investigate, competent to teach, proficient in specialties." Nearly a decade before Gilman hired H. Newell Martin, he argued, "It is the men who make the college. . . . A corps of instructors, young, manly, thorough, truth-loving, able to teach, speak, and economize, will do more to give character and success to a foundation which is still dependent upon the favor of the people, than a corps of older men, who may have been titular professors for a quarter of a century, but who are not possessed with the spirit of modern inquiry."[14]

Although he had turned down the same position two years earlier,

Gilman accepted the presidency of the University of California in 1870. He left New Haven hoping a milder climate would benefit one of his frail children, and because he was concerned that Yale's new president, Noah Porter, a conservative theologian, would not encourage the further development of science at Yale.[15] In his California inaugural address, Gilman again emphasized the critical role of the faculty in building a university. Arguing for specialization in view of the "vast expansion of science," Gilman told his California audience, "The versatile and facile American must learn to admit that there is a difference between ability to do anything and ability to do everything." The goals Gilman set for the new University of California were clear: "The question is, how to secure the best sort of instruction, the fittest sequence and relation of studies, the most eminent teachers, the most complete laboratories, and the best apparatus; and likewise how to encourage that special proficiency which is indispensable to success in modern scientific professions."[16]

Political controversies regarding the organization and operation of the University of California intensified during Gilman's presidency. An astute observer of American higher education, he was aware of the plans to found the Johns Hopkins University. Writing to his friend Andrew White in April 1874, he revealed his impatience with the California situation: "I should be strongly tempted to accept a good call to go hence. . . . I confess that the *Baltimore* scheme has ofttimes suggested itself to me."[17] Thus, even before he was interviewed by the Hopkins trustees, White was aware of his friend's desire to relocate and his interest in the new university. After Gilman's trip to New York in the summer of 1874, the two university presidents further discussed the Baltimore opportunity.[18] Gilman also received encouragement from Eliot who wrote in July 1874, "Don't you want to go to Baltimore and start the Johns Hopkins University there? . . . They wanted some advice from me last month and I went there to look into their affairs a little bit. I should say that the chance of doing a useful work was a good one."[19]

In November 1874, the Johns Hopkins trustees invited Daniel Gilman to become the first president of the new Baltimore university. Enthusiastic, but cautious, Gilman informed White that he wanted a personal interview before accepting the position.[20] Reflecting his frustration with the circumstances he confronted in his final months at Yale and during his brief tenure in California, he expressed pleasure that the Hopkins trustees "are responsible neither to ecclesiastical nor legislative supervision; but simply to their own convictions of duty and the enlightened judgement of their fellow men. . . . Their means are ample; their authority complete; their purposes enlightened. Is not this opportunity without parallel in the history of our country?"[21]

Gilman met the Hopkins trustees in December 1874. The summary of this interview, published in the *Nation*, outlined his agenda for Johns Hopkins: seeking leading professors, emphasizing research, and requiring regular publication to demonstrate productivity in research. Gilman was aware of the conflict between routine teaching and research and recognized that increased scientific productivity could only be gained by minimizing the teaching responsibilities of the professors. He decried the current state of American higher education: men were generally "employed at small salaries in existing colleges, whose work in certain fields of research would be of inestimable value to the science and literature of the world, but who are compelled, in order to earn their livelihood, to pass most of their time teaching the rudiments to boys, or preparing school-books."[22] In fact, this predicament describes the circumstances John Call Dalton faced at the College of Physicians and Surgeons of New York, as noted earlier. Gilman emphasized a philosophy of education at Johns Hopkins that would facilitate the development of a program of research and advanced training in physiology, rather than elementary instruction.

Gilman arrived in Baltimore in the spring of 1875, more than a year before the anticipated inauguration of instruction. He soon made several visits to discuss the organization of the new university with American leaders of science and higher education. Among others, Gilman met with Joseph Henry and Spencer Baird of the Smithsonian Institution, Ferdinand Hayden of the Geological Survey, and John Shaw Billings of the Surgeon General's Office. Henry was enthusiastic about the promise of the Johns Hopkins University which, with its ample endowment, could encourage scientific research to an unprecedented degree among American institutions. At the farewell banquet for John Tyndall in 1873, Henry outlined the factors that retarded the growth of science in America. In Henry's opinion, the need to "subdue" the continent and the utilitarian nature of the American people were largely responsible for the lack of interest in scientific research in the United States. He was cautiously optimistic, however, and believed the growing wealth and educational attainments of Americans would soon lead to increased interest in science and research. Henry shared Gilman's views on the needs of higher education and advocated the endowment of universities to permit liberal support for faculty and equipment, the hiring of a learned faculty with a deep commitment to research, and the acquisition of the necessary apparatus to undertake this research.[23]

Henry wrote to Gilman in August 1875:

> I take a deep interest in the University over which you have been
> appointed to preside and I think it offers the best opportunity ever
> presented for elevating the character of the literature and the
> science of our country. It has ample means and can afford to em-
> ploy the best men that can be found and establish chairs which
> shall be looked up to as the most desirable positions to be filled
> only by those who have achieved a high reputation: it is not de-
> pendent upon public favor and may be the means of forming and
> directing instead of following popular opinions. I take the liberty
> of expressing these sentiments to you since I have been informed
> that they coincide with your own, and to assure you that it will
> give me pleasure at all times to enforce and defend them.[24]

He expressed his "confident hope" to the Hopkins trustees that their
well-endowed university "will be so managed as to advance the best interests of sound learning and promote original science in this country."[25]

Gilman elicited advice from old friends and new acquaintances; he
wanted to take full advantage of his opportunity to organize a major
American university. Charles Eliot continued to be a valuable consultant. Shortly after arriving in Baltimore, Gilman informed the Harvard
president, "The Trustees are in excellent spirits, full of devotion & cooperation, somewhat conservative but not *set* for or against any particular
scheme. . . . Before we go very far in plans, I shall want very much to
have a good talk with you."[26] Although Gilman had some knowledge of
medical education from his role in the development of the innovative
premedical course at the Sheffield Scientific School and his involvement
in the merger of the Toland Medical College with the University of California, he was anxious to have help in developing plans for medical
teaching at Johns Hopkins. His most influential adviser on medical matters was John Shaw Billings.[27]

Although Billings's activities on behalf of Johns Hopkins related primarily to the hospital and medical education, they are relevant to the
development of the scientific curriculum at the university. Billings
entered the Medical College of Ohio after graduating from Miami University of Ohio in 1857. Although this medical school was founded by
Daniel Drake, a champion of medical education reform, its curriculum
was no different from other contemporary medical institutions: the requirements for graduation consisted of two five-month terms of didactic
lectures with minimal exposure to patients.[28] As was the case with Weir
Mitchell, Billings's career took an important turn when he enlisted as a
medical officer in the Union Army in 1861. While stationed at the Army

General Hospital in West Philadelphia, Billings came under the influence of Joseph Leidy from whom he received training in microscopy.
Billings's interest in microscopy matured with the assistance of his
colleagues Edward Curtis and Joseph J. Woodward, and he used the
microscope in research that led to several publications. These experiences signaled the beginning of Billings's lifelong devotion to scientific
medicine.

It was not Billings's microscopical work, but his extensive monograph on the construction and operation of barracks and hospitals, published in 1870, that brought him to the attention of the Johns Hopkins
trustees. On the basis of this highly regarded study, Billings's friend
Alfred Woodhull suggested to the Hopkins trustees that they enlist the
young army surgeon as their consultant for the planning and construction of the Johns Hopkins Hospital.[29] In March 1875, the trustees invited
five men with experience in hospital design to submit plans for the proposed hospital.

Billings's proposal included his views on the current status and
needs of American medical education. In addition to suggesting a higher
standard of admission and a more rigorous curriculum, Billings asserted:
"An important feature of the school should be a first-class Physiological Laboratory, with ample facilities for chemical and microscopical
work. . . . If we are ever to advance in accurate knowledge of the laws
of health and disease, it will be by the application of instruments of precision and of graphic measurement to the secretions and motions of the
body." Billings declared it was the responsibility of the Johns Hopkins
Hospital and Medical School "to promote discoveries in the science and
art in medicine. . . . In this country it is too much the case that scientific
and medical men who are qualified and have the desire to make original
investigations, and thus increase our stock of knowledge, want either the
means or the time to do so."[30] Billings and Gilman shared the conviction
that the new university and its medical department must have a major
commitment to research. The trustees were responsive to these suggestions, and with the opening of the Johns Hopkins University an American institution offered an unprecedented degree of support for advanced
teaching and research with emphasis on the scientific curriculum.

Billings was formally selected as adviser to the trustees for the construction of the Johns Hopkins Hospital in July 1876. His first printed
report to the trustees included themes relevant to the university as a
whole, however. Reminiscent of Gilman, Billings declared that the faculty would be more important than buildings and that, although adequate salaries were necessary to attract them, "we can much more cer-

tainly secure men who will minutely and patiently investigate . . . by showing them that they shall have space and apparatus to work with, that the resources of modern science and mechanical skill shall be at their command, and that any discoveries which they may make shall be properly published, than by simply offering double pay."[31]

Although financial considerations delayed the opening of the Johns Hopkins Hospital and Medical School for several years, it was necessary to select the original faculty for the university scheduled to open in the fall of 1876. The commitment of Gilman, Billings, and the Hopkins trustees to research, specialization, and adequate salaries that made it unnecessary for teachers to supplement their university income set the new university apart from other institutions of higher learning in the United States. Because the medical school was considered a critical component of the Johns Hopkins institutions, and because of Gilman's deep interest in science, one of the most important appointments in the new university was the chair of biology. Initially, physiology at Johns Hopkins would be taught in the "biology" department. The choice of the name biology rather than physiology reflected the scope of subjects taught and studied in this department and Thomas H. Huxley's input into its structure and philosophy.

As news of the philosophy of the Baltimore institution spread, Gilman and the trustees received encouragement. A writer in the *Boston Medical and Surgical Journal* exclaimed in 1875:

> If accounts be true our countrymen have every reason to be grateful to the late Johns Hopkins, whose munificent bequest has put it in the power of Baltimore to found a university on a scale such as has not hitherto been attempted in this country. . . . A seat of learning which will not only undertake to give a good medical education, but will also make it possible for our best men to devote their lives to teaching and scientific work will be surely a novelty with us, and will, we doubt not, be highly appreciated by the American medical profession.[32]

Thus, the significance of the opening of the Johns Hopkins University was appreciated even in Boston, where Charles Eliot had recently reformed teaching at Harvard, and Henry Bowditch had established a physiological laboratory in which interested individuals could do research.

Gilman sailed abroad in 1875 to observe recent developments in universities in England and on the continent and to solicit suggestions for faculty members. The trustees encouraged Gilman's trip; he would also serve as an ambassador for the new Baltimore institution. When he arrived, Gilman found scientists and educators anxious to hear about the plans for the new university. In England, Gilman met with several members of the "X-club," a group of leading British advocates of scientific education and research who met socially, including Thomas H. Huxley, Herbert Spencer, and John Tyndall. One of the most important individuals Gilman met during his visit to England was Huxley, a leading British scientist and vocal spokesman for the advancement of scientific education.[33] He valued Huxley's opinions and incorporated the British scientist's ideas into his own conceptualization of how science should be taught at Hopkins. Recounting his experience in Germany, Gilman informed the trustees that he found several leaders of German science "already aware of the Johns Hopkins foundation and very eager to know how its plans are to be developed."[34]

When Weir Mitchell tried to win an academic chair in Philadelphia in the 1860s, he was thwarted, in part, by the failure of influential individuals in that city to recognize the growing differentiation of the natural sciences. There was more recognition of the value of specialization in science a decade later. A leading proponent of specialization in science, Huxley declared in 1874, "There is a scientific superstition that Physiology is largely aided by Comparative Anatomy—a superstition which, like most superstitions, once had a grain of truth at bottom; but the grain has become homoeopathic, since Physiology took its modern experimental development, and became what it is now, the application of the principles of Physics and Chemistry to the elucidation of the phænomena of life."[35] Huxley believed practical laboratory work was indispensable for science teaching; and an adequate staff was necessary for it to be successful. He had formulated his views of scientific education over more than two decades. As early as 1854, his opinions reflected those of the continental experimental physiologists. In that year Huxley claimed, "Physiology is *the* experimental science *par excellence* of all the sciences" and its methods and results were as exact as those of mathematics or physics.[36]

By December 1875, with the opening of the university less than a year away, Gilman's search for professors intensified. In an essay on the selection of professors prepared for the Hopkins trustees, he contrasted the peripatetic students and teachers of the German universities with their American counterparts who were often bound to a single institution by ecclesiastical, geographical, or personal ties. In his opinion, the regionalism of Americans would interfere with his attempts to attract a distinguished faculty to Baltimore. He told the trustees, "I cannot imagine any circumstances as likely to arise which would bring here some of those persons whose names are foremost on our lips when we speak of the leading teachers in this country." He was emphatic that adequate salaries were necessary so professors would not be forced to "eke out their support by extra-professional work which takes away a part of the energy which they ought to expend in the appropriate duties of the professorship." He informed the Hopkins trustees that the most promising teachers would be found among recent graduates and young instructors "who have twenty years before them rather than twenty years behind them." He was aware of the benefits of having a prominent scientist and teacher such as Louis Agassiz on the faculty whose mere presence would attract talented students to the university. Nevertheless, reality dictated that the first faculty would be comprised of younger men, free to relocate to Baltimore.[37]

Gilman initially sought qualified Americans for faculty positions at Johns Hopkins. It is likely that he tried to recruit Henry Bowditch for the Hopkins chair of biology. William Welch wrote to his friend New York surgeon Frederic Dennis in 1875, "It must be he [Bowditch] whom Gilman told you they thought of selecting for professor of physiology in Baltimore."[38] But Bowditch, a Boston native, was well established at the Harvard Medical School by 1875. Charles Eliot, impressed by high salaries offered by Johns Hopkins, informed his friend Gilman, "Please don't think that I feel in the least annoyed at proposals made by you to Harvard men. On the contrary, I should have thought it very odd if there had been no men here whom you cared to try for."[39]

Initially, the Johns Hopkins Medical School was to open shortly after the university. Because the scientific faculty of the university was expected to play an important role in the planning and operation of the medical school, Gilman took the responsibility of selecting the professor of biology especially seriously. This individual would be responsible for teaching physiology to the medical students as well as directing the biology program at the university. The successful candidate for this chair was H. Newell Martin whose appointment was strongly encouraged by Huxley. Martin was born in Newry, County Down, Ireland, in 1848, the eldest of twelve children of a Congregational minister and schoolmaster.[40] Following preliminary education from tutors, Martin entered University College, London, at the age of fifteen. At this time, he was also apprenticed to James A. McDonough, a Dublin native who lectured on anatomy in that city before his removal to London where he established a general practice. Although McDonough may have encouraged Martin's interest in the basic medical sciences, a more important stimulus was his exposure to the faculty of University College who placed greater emphasis on science than the faculty of any other British medical school.

At University College, Martin was a pupil of William Sharpey who revitalized the teaching of physiology in England. With his lifelong friend Edward Schäfer, Martin was among the earliest pupils of Michael Foster, who began teaching practical physiology and histology at the institution in 1867. It was from Foster that Martin learned the techniques of modern experimental physiology.[41] Foster was a medical graduate of University College who entered practice with his father, a prominent surgeon, after two years of postgraduate study in Paris. A decade later, Foster was selected to succeed George Harley as teacher of the practical physiology and histology course at his alma mater. Foster's subsequent appointment at Trinity College, Cambridge, was made possible, to a significant degree, by the influence of Huxley who developed a friendship with Foster in the mid-1850s. Before accepting the Cambridge position in 1870, Foster toured German laboratories of experimental science with William Sharpey. Foster's physiology department at Cambridge was modeled, in many respects, after Carl Ludwig's program at the Leipzig Physiological Institute.

Foster immediately recognized Martin's abilities and invited him to serve as his demonstrator—first at University College and subsequently at Cambridge University. Martin also served as Huxley's assistant in his course on elementary biology at the Royal College of Science in London and helped Huxley prepare his popular textbook of elementary biology that first appeared in 1875.[42] Foster and Huxley were grateful to Martin for his contributions to the organization and operation of their laboratory courses. These responsibilities, and Martin's need to supplement his income by teaching, limited his time for research. When Huxley proposed Martin to Gilman as a candidate for the Hopkins chair, the young Irishman's sole publication was a brief paper on the olfactory membrane.

Huxley gave Martin an enthusiastic endorsement. He pointed out to Gilman that Martin was well trained in physiology and general biology, was energetic, and was highly regarded by Michael Foster as well as himself. Huxley concluded, "I am very glad to find that my plan of teaching finds favour on your side of the water—and it would be very gratifying to me to know that its development was in such hands as Martin's."[43] In contrast to the University of Pennsylvania's reluctance about hiring foreigners to fill vacant chairs, Gilman was quite willing to recruit faculty members from abroad. The Hopkins president promptly responded to Huxley's suggestion, and forwarded a letter through him to

Martin opening negotiations for the biology chair. He also took this opportunity to invite Huxley to participate in the ceremony marking the inauguration of instruction at Hopkins scheduled for the fall of 1876.[44]

Just as Henry Bowditch had received coaching from his family and scientific friends in Boston when he negotiated his return to Harvard with Charles Eliot, Martin benefited from Huxley's counsel as he discussed various aspects of the Hopkins position with Gilman. In response to Gilman's first offer, Martin explained:

> I must decline your offer; chiefly for the reason that, others being at present partly dependent upon me, I cannot afford the pecuniary loss which acceptance of your offer would entail. Another point which has influenced me is that you mention one room as being set apart for a biological laboratory. . . . I could not undertake to direct the whole biological teaching of the university, as well as the encouragement and assistance of the more promising students in original research, with such scanty accomodation [sic].

Martin then proceeded to outline the terms that would lead to his acceptance, explaining that these were developed in collaboration with his "scientific friends" in England. In addition to an annual salary of 800 pounds, the promise of the construction of a biological laboratory, and the title of professor, Martin demanded (reminiscent of Bowditch), "with the rest of the teaching staff, a direct voice in the arrangement of the curriculum and studies of the university."[45]

Martin got sufficient concessions from Gilman and the Hopkins trustees that he accepted the Baltimore position. Huxley reassured Gilman, "I am sure that Martin will . . . be a very valuable colleague. . . . I have a great regard and esteem for him and it is a great pleasure for me to know that he has secured so excellent a position."[46] The hiring of foreigners to fill some chairs at Johns Hopkins heightened the interest in the university among British and European observers of higher education and science. A writer in *Nature* declared, "Some compensation for Dr. Martin's loss at Cambridge may be found in the thought that biology in the United States will gain by the presence of a man so well versed in European methods, and especially in the systems of instruction worked out by Prof. Huxley, Dr. Foster, and others in England."[47]

Gilman delivered his inaugural address in February 1876, declaring:

> In our scheme of the university, great prominence should be given to the studies which bear upon life—the group now called biologi-

cal sciences. Such facilities as are now afforded under Huxley in London, and Rolleston at Oxford, and Foster at Cambridge, and in the best German universities, should here be introduced. They would serve us in the training of naturalists, but they would serve us still more in the training of physicians. By the time we are ready to open a school of medicine, we might hope to have a superior, if not a numerous, body of aspirants for one of the noblest callings to which the heart and head can be devoted.

Martin read Gilman's inaugural address before accepting the Baltimore position and was concerned about an apparent contradiction between Gilman's stated philosophy of laboratory accommodations and the actual facilities planned for the university during its early years. In his address Gilman declared, "At present laboratories are demanded on a scale and in a variety hitherto unknown," but instruction would begin in two converted houses and one small building, Hopkins Hall, erected for the university.[48] Gilman learned of Martin's concerns through Huxley and reassured the young Irish physiologist that the biology program at Johns Hopkins would receive adequate support.[49] Modern experimental physiology required more than space, however. Martin informed Gilman of the need of importing sophisticated physiological instruments from Europe. The apparatus Martin listed was similar to that in Foster's Cambridge laboratory, and the Hopkins trustees approved the purchases. Thus, Martin came to an American institution that provided him with a salary to be a full-time physiologist and with apparatus and advanced students to inaugurate a sophisticated program of research and advanced training in physiology.

The circumstances at Johns Hopkins were ideal for the introduction of a physiology program that emphasized graduate training and research. Martin's agenda reflected the broad commitment of Gilman and the Hopkins trustees to these activities and to the sciences. Martin was to teach in a university where physiology was a subject worthy of special study, not simply a course preliminary to more practical clinical subjects. The name of the department at Johns Hopkins—the biology department—reflected the broader agenda necessitated by the recent spectacular growth of the life sciences in the European and British universities. A well-endowed university could support such a program; a proprietary medical school could not.

Philosophical as well as economic factors distinguished the circumstances of Johns Hopkins from those at Harvard and less progressive American institutions of higher learning. Although Bowditch had the support of Eliot, several faculty members, and his family, dissenters such as Bigelow discouraged the expansion of physiology teaching at Harvard. Martin joined a new institution that defined its mission at a time when science was gaining in prestige, and the experimental method was growing in importance and acceptance. Perhaps most important, the institution had the resources to implement the ideals that he and Gilman shared. It was Bowditch's independent wealth that made it possible for him to establish the Harvard physiological laboratory. The endowment at Johns Hopkins enabled Gilman to select a capable and motivated individual without concern for his financial status.

Although Martin had served as an apprentice to a physician and obtained a medical degree in London, he expressed no interest in practicing medicine. By 1876, the concept of the full-time basic medical scientist was well established in Germany and was gaining proponents in England. That year, Scottish physiologist John G. McKendrick informed members of the British Association for the Advancement of Science that research into the pathophysiology of disease

> cannot, in the present condition of society, be thoroughly investigated by a practitioner, who is often too busy a man to engage in this kind of work. Such labour must be handed over, to a large extent, to a special class of men. They must investigate, experiment, and work up the subject in the laboratory—either the physiological laboratory of the university or school of medicine, or of the hospital or infirmary—as the business of their lives. . . . Many of the best contributions to physiological and pathological science, during the past twenty years, have been from men busy in practice . . . but in the future, much scientific work, as a basis of the practical treatment of disease, must be done by men specially devoted to the laboratory, the pathological theatre, and the clinical ward. . . . Such stupendous work can scarcely be left to individual effort. To carry it on requires men, time, and money; and these can only be supplied by the aid of governments, or municipalities, or by private munificence.[50]

Martin departed for America on 27 July 1876, accompanied by Huxley who, during a lecture tour of America, would deliver the opening address at Johns Hopkins. Before Martin's arrival, a university announcement described the courses and opportunities for research in the biology department. Reflecting the views of Huxley, Foster, and Martin, it asserted an emphasis on practical laboratory training. Even the elementary course in biology would include extensive practical instruction "so that the students, besides acquiring a knowledge of the leading ideas of modern biology, will gain an acquaintance with the methods and instruments employed in biological research." This exposure of undergraduates to the philosophy and techniques of modern biological research was unique among American institutions of higher learning in this period.

It was not the elementary laboratory courses that represented the most significant contribution of Johns Hopkins to the advance of physiology and the related life sciences during the final decades of the nineteenth century, however. The opportunities for postgraduate training and research in biology were unparalleled in North America. A preliminary Hopkins circular proclaimed that the laboratory "will be very completely fitted up, and so far at least as regards physiology will present facilities for work unequalled, it is believed, in this country, and excelled by but few laboratories abroad. . . . The collection of instruments for experimental physiology will be very complete, including the best used in every department of physiological work."[51]

Huxley delivered his inaugural address in September 1876 to an audience of more than two thousand people. It reveals his influence on the educational philosophy and plan of instruction at Johns Hopkins. He repeated several themes he had presented in earlier lectures and papers: physiology was based on physics and chemistry; specialization within the sciences was necessary for their full development; teaching and research were mutually beneficial for professors; and adequate endowment was imperative to sustain a program of advanced scientific training and research. Huxley also publicly congratulated Gilman and the Hopkins officials for the emphasis they placed on research in organizing the university.[52]

Martin was a sincere advocate of Huxley's views on science and education. In his introductory lecture, delivered the day before the inauguration of formal instruction at Johns Hopkins, Martin emphasized his dedication to pure science and revealed his enthusiasm about his new program and the future of biology in America. He declared, "To those who are in any degree acquainted with the state of the scientific world, the present must seem a specially opportune time for founding a biological school. At no previous period has such an interest been taken in biological problems, or have so many earnest workers been in the field— never before has so rich a harvest been in view." Martin encouraged his pupils and informed them: "The only absolutely necessary faculties for the scientific investigator are love of his work, perseverance, and truthfulness. . . . What we want here, then, is men with the requisite zeal and training for investigation—we care not whether classification, or morphology, or physiology, or any other branch of biology is their specialty; all we claim is that they shall be able to work, shall mean to work, and shall work—we shall give no quarter to the indolent or ignorant." If this plan were to be followed, Martin predicted, "we [might] look forward with confidence to the time when we [should] find ourselves in the condition of such laboratories as those of some of the German universities, where, on account of the high class of work done in them, the ablest young men from all over the world beg for admission."[53] Martin's address received favorable reviews. A writer in the *Popular Science Monthly* applauded his ideas, commenting that the combination of practical training and original work was "full of promise." He urged other scientific teachers to attempt to incorporate Martin's methods into their own courses.[54]

The research program at Johns Hopkins received much publicity, and by the inauguration of formal instruction on 24 October 1876 local physicians and advanced students were already working on projects in the biological laboratory. Martin's program was successful; Gilman informed him early in 1877, "There is throughout the University a hearty appreciation of what you are doing."[55] Martin soon came to realize, however, that the local practitioners who first used his laboratory were inadequately prepared for sophisticated physiological research. Fifteen years later, he expressed remorse to Henry Bowditch about the quality of the first publication from his laboratory. Martin had rewritten a paper based on research performed by a Baltimore physician, but ultimately came to believe the paper unworthy of publication.[56]

Martin assessed his first few months in America in a letter to his friend Edward Schäfer:

> I am now getting settled down here very well and like my quarters. The University authorities are very liberal in providing all I ask for and so in that direction I have nothing to complain of; and now that I am beginning to know the people here I like many of them extremely. . . . My present laboratory accommodation consists of one large room which I use for general classwork: and six smaller ones: one of which is my private room: another fitted up as a chemical laboratory and the rest for special work on research: or rather will be when there is anyone fit to put into them.[57]

He also informed his former British colleague that he feared an attack by the antivivisectionists.

Martin intended to use vivisection in teaching, although he emphasized that anesthetics would always be employed in demonstrations. He was fully cognizant of the potential threat of the antivivisectionists to his program in experimental physiology. Shortly before his departure from England, Martin had attended the inaugural meeting of the Physiological Society which was founded, in large part, in response to the growing antivivisection sentiment in that country.[58] The antivivisection movement in America was a decade old, and Martin realized he might face legal curtailment of experimentation. Such was the effect in England of the passage of the Cruelty to Animals Act in 1876.

Martin's methods contrasted with the teaching of physiology at the College of Physicians and Surgeons of New York, the Philadelphia schools, and even Bowditch's program at Harvard. He encouraged the routine participation of students in original and repetitive experiments in the laboratory in preference to demonstrations. Billings believed the opportunities for students to participate in laboratory exercises in Baltimore exceeded those of students in Ludwig's institute in Leipzig. In November 1876, Billings informed Gilman that after touring the laboratories and other facilities of the medical department of the University of Leipzig he was impressed, but also somewhat disappointed. He concluded that the physiological laboratory was designed primarily for research rather than for the instruction of students, and it was not easy for pupils to take advantage of the apparatus and facilities.[59]

An unusual feature, designed to insure a corps of qualified advanced students at Johns Hopkins, was the establishment of a program of fellowships. One of the ten fellowships with an annual stipend of $500 was available to support a graduate student in the biology department. Billings conferred with Gilman regarding the proposal for fellowships and scholarships at the university and declared, "How I should have jumped at such an opportunity 15 years ago.[60] In response to the receipt of ten applications for every available fellowship, the trustees doubled the number of awards.

Inspired by his mentor Huxley's commitment to widespread teaching of science in the British schools, Martin introduced a biology class for schoolteachers in the fall of 1877. This class, patterned after one he had taught with Huxley in London in 1871, would have the direct benefit of familiarizing the schoolteachers of Baltimore and other eastern cities with advanced methods of teaching biology. Huxley and his fellow reformers believed that a fundamental requirement for the ultimate advance of science through research was to increase the number of young individuals exposed to the philosophy and techniques of modern science during their elementary education. An indirect, but undoubtedly anticipated benefit was to enlarge the base of support for the scientific activities of the new university. Martin believed that the teachers would provide him with allies if the antivivisection movement gathered momentum in Baltimore. He was pleased with the teachers' response to his course, and they appreciated his efforts on their behalf.[61]

Research was a major component of Martin's biology program. Shortly after his arrival in Baltimore, the young scientist began to investigate the physiology of respiration. He soon published two papers on this subject in the new *Journal of Physiology* edited by his teacher Michael Foster. With Henry Bowditch and Horatio C. Wood, Jr., Martin served as an American editor of the journal which Foster sought to make "a common medium for English speaking physiologists."[62] Martin and several of his fellows and graduate students made contributions to Foster's journal over the next two decades. Their publications enhanced the image of Martin's department as a productive research unit.

As Martin's program took shape and a new premedical curriculum was planned for the fall of 1878, he became impatient for better facilities. He informed Gilman that the premedical course would necessitate additional staff and space. Returning to a concern he had expressed before his departure from England, Martin urged Gilman and the trustees to provide a new, more suitable building for his biological laboratory or "institute" as soon as possible. In Martin's opinion, the present building had several shortcomings including the lack of a private entrance and ground floor rooms for sensitive instruments.[63] Martin's concern regarding the entrance to the laboratory was related to the antivivisection threat; anyone could see the delivery and disposal of animals used in vivisection. He explained to Gilman that his department should include, in addition to the professor of biology, an associate in each of the subdivisions of comparative anatomy and zoology, physiology, human anatomy, botany, as well as a curator of a natural history museum.

Despite the unprecedented endowment of Johns Hopkins, Gilman had to determine priorities among his faculty's requests. The scope of instruction at the university was broad, and Martin was not alone in desiring to reap benefits from the liberality of Gilman and the trustees. Ira Remsen, professor of chemistry, shared Martin's frustration at the delay in construction of a suitable laboratory facility.[64] Although Martin and Remsen received consistent support from the university for the development of their research-oriented programs in biology and chemistry, it would be more than five years before a new laboratory building was constructed.

The medical school and hospital were to open shortly after the university, and John Shaw Billings remained active as a consultant to Gilman and the trustees. The army surgeon delivered a series of twenty lectures on medical education in Baltimore in 1878. He emphasized the need to improve clinical instruction in American medical schools, but argued:

> The second existing demand is for the promotion of original research and discovery in Medicine, including the making known of these discoveries. In this field, we do not find any organized effort being made in this Country. In no University or College, Hospital or Asylum, do we find going on systematic and scientific investigations in Physiology, Pathology or Therapeutics, such as are being made in Germany—and, less generally and systematically, yet still to a great extent and with good results, in France and Great Britain.[65]

Billings ignored the activities of Henry Bowditch and his colleagues at the Harvard Medical School and its physiological laboratory established seven years earlier. He urged a more extensive program of advanced training and research in the basic medical sciences.

Billings's comments on American medical education were based, in part, on his recent exposure to hospitals, medical schools, and institutions of higher learning in continental Europe and England. During his travels abroad in the fall of 1876, he interviewed several leaders of science including Martin's teachers Huxley and Foster, as well as John Burdon-Sanderson, T. Lauder Brunton, and Norman Lockyer.[66] Moreover, he received news of the developments in medical education at several leading American medical schools from his friends in the medical reform movement, and learned the details of reform attempts at the University of Pennsylvania in the mid-1870s from Horatio Wood, Jr. and Weir Mitchell. James Chadwick and Edward Cowles kept Billings posted on developments at the Harvard Medical School. Edward Curtis, John G. Curtis's older brother, and Abraham Jacobi reported events in New York.[67]

In the course of Billings's twenty lectures on medical education, which were delivered to an average audience of fifty students and physicians, he emphasized and reemphasized the important role research should play in medicine.

> When I reflect upon how much in Medicine is as yet only conjecture and theory, with no firm basis of observation and experiment, and when in examining the medical literature of the day, I see how few thoroughly skilled Chemists and Physicists are really at work upon the problems presented by the living body in health and in disease, and how slight are the probabilities that for many

years to come any Institution in this country will systematically
undertake work of this character,—I find it difficult to reason
coolly and dispassionately as to what is best to be done.[68]

He believed the medical department at Johns Hopkins, when inaugurated, should encourage research and, moreover, must train individuals
who would continue to perform research once they left Baltimore. He
acknowledged that practical results would ultimately result from sustained medical research, but believed investigation should be undertaken for its own sake. Billings was a persuasive advocate for the research ethic in higher education, and in medical education in particular.

He hoped that the published version of his lectures on medical education could be distributed among scientifically oriented physicians and
basic medical scientists for their comments. The list of individuals prepared by Billings sheds light on his network of medical reformers in the
late 1870s. In addition to Martin and Remsen from Hopkins, Billings
wanted his comments circulated to John C. Dalton, Austin Flint [Sr.],
Weir Mitchell, Reginald Fitz, William Pepper, [Edward] Curtis, Christopher Johnston, and Henry [P.] Bowditch. Billings encouraged Gilman
to publish the responses of these individuals along with his paper. "It is
by what your university does for the natural (and social) sciences and for
medicine that you must stand or fall."[69]

Billings reviewed American medical education in 1878 in the
widely circulated *American Journal of the Medical Sciences* at the request of its editor, Minis Hays. An 1868 medical graduate of the University of Pennsylvania, Hays watched the reform movement at his alma
mater with interest. In the context of the recent reforms in medical education at Pennsylvania led by Mitchell, Tyson, Pepper, and Wood, Hays
informed Billings, "The times seem right for a review on the subject of
medical education. . . . As you have paid a good deal of attention to the
subject I have thought it might be agreeable to you to prepare such a
review."[70] Billings's review included an indictment of the state of American medical education. He urged reform and closed his essay on the
hopeful note that the Johns Hopkins University would succeed in the
"production of men qualified to teach medicine and the cognate sciences, and to carry on original research."[71] Until the opening of the
medical school, Martin's department would be the site of research relevant to medicine at Johns Hopkins.

Following the publication of Billings's review of medical education, the new university in Baltimore attracted increased attention from
the medical community. The circulation of a brochure describing the

university's proposed preliminary medical course heightened this interest. A Philadelphia writer exclaimed, "There is no institution in the United States which is watched, by those who are interested in the advancement of medical science among us, with as much of mingled hope and fear as is Johns Hopkins University."[72]

Some observers misunderstood the relationship between the proposed university premedical course and the medical curriculum, to begin when the medical school opened. In a letter to a Philadelphia medical journal, Martin explained the need for, and purpose of, the Johns Hopkins premedical course:

> Ever since our University has been opened we have received applications for admission—to its scientific departments especially— from students from all parts of the country, who either intend to take up the medical profession or who have already studied one or two sessions in a medical school; in many cases from men also who have just taken the M.D. degree. These candidates have imagined, rightly or wrongly, that the instruction which a university with endowed laboratories can give on such subjects, so essential as a foundation of scientific medicine, is likely to be more complete than that which can be obtained at most medical schools, where the professors are often men whose time is largely otherwise occupied, and in which practical instruction is, with few exceptions . . . very deficient.

Although Martin was unable to describe the medical course envisioned at the university fully since it had not been implemented, he did explain that "laboratories and endowed chairs will be founded . . . so that the professors may be relieved from the cares of practice, and be able to devote their whole time and energies to the subjects they teach."[73]

In this brief statement Martin outlined the agenda of the scientific reformers. Laboratory instruction in the basic medical sciences—physiology, in particular—was an "essential foundation of scientific medicine." Moreover, full-time scientists should supervise the instruction in endowed laboratories. He characterized the typical contemporary American medical school course in physiology as "emasculated." His letter reflected the convictions he shared with Gilman and Billings: the adoption of the full-time system and the research ethic by the nation's elite medical schools was necessary if American medicine was to become scientific. Few medical schools in American could implement this plan, however. Events at the College of Physicians and Surgeons of New York, the University of Pennsylvania, and the Harvard Medical School demonstrated that a special combination of individual and institutional cir-

cumstances was necessary for the hiring of a full-time physiologist imbued with the research ethic. The professor must be willing to give up
medical practice to devote himself to physiology, and the institution
must be able and willing to support a program of research and advanced
training as well as elementary teaching. Moreover, the research ethic
and vivisection had to be accepted by the institutional authorities and
the community. Only one American institution met all these criteria in
the 1870s—the Johns Hopkins University.

In 1878, New York medical editor George Shrady published a perceptive review of the goals of the Johns Hopkins preliminary medical
course and its relationship to the traditional medical curriculum at
America's medical schools.

> If the above-mentioned seat of learning at Baltimore has gained a
> reputation for any one thing in particular at this early stage of its
> growth, it is for doing thoroughly whatever it undertakes. The
> excellence and completeness of its academical and scientific
> courses are already matters of history. . . . We hope that the wise
> example afforded by the trustees of the Johns Hopkins Medical
> College will be speedily followed by other great medical schools—
> Bellevue, Harvard and the University of Pennsylvania. Let them
> establish preliminary courses of medical education, and require of
> their matriculates the knowledge which Johns Hopkins school will
> strive to inculcate.[74]

The concept of a formalized premedical curriculum was unknown
to most American physicians, although Gilman and his colleagues had
established such a course at the Sheffield Scientific School several years
earlier. Most Americans entered medical school directly from high
school; there were essentially no educational requirements for admission
to the majority of the nation's medical schools. One American editor,
commenting on Rudolf Virchow's 1879 address on medical education,
explained that the German pathologist "discussed especially the kind of
preliminary training which the medical student should have had. He
sketched out a preliminary course in the classics and the physical and
natural sciences, which would be likely to quite paralyze the average
American plow-boy ambitious to deal in pills."[75] Gilman informed the
Hopkins trustees in 1878 that American medical schools were "receiving
young men who could not enter the lowest class of a respectable college,
and young men who have had no preliminary training in scientific principles and who have done no work in scientific laboratories." Gilman,
Billings, and Martin sought to improve this situation.

Gilman was pleased with what had been accomplished at Johns Hopkins in such a short time. He told the trustees:

> The student has great advantages who pursues his scientific work in this University. There is here an atmosphere of study, exhilarating and strengthening. It is a place where many men of diverse pursuits, coming from every part of the country and from many different colleges, are engaged in advanced intellectual work. The best of books and journals and instruments are procured as required, and are freely accessible. Diligence, perseverance and earnestness are expected from all. . . . There is an abundance of encouragement for laboratory research.[76]

By 1879, Martin was teaching courses in general biology and animal physiology, was providing occasional demonstrations to Baltimore medical students, was performing research, was giving a Saturday course for biology teachers, was supervising several graduate students, and was delivering a public lecture series in general biology.[77] In addition to these activities, he made a concerted effort to meet the medical practitioners of Baltimore and of Maryland. An opportunity arose for Martin to address the members of the Medical and Chirurgical Faculty of Maryland in the spring of 1879 when the scheduled lecturer, John Woodworth, died unexpectedly. Martin's invitation was encouraged by Christopher Johnston, a member of the executive committee of the Medical and Chirurgical Faculty, who had previously held the chair of anatomy and physiology at the University of Maryland. Johnston, a strong advocate of Martin and Johns Hopkins, had with S. Weir Mitchell, studied under Claude Bernard, and "early manifested a strong taste for scientific studies and research, and this continued up to the last days of his life."[78]

Martin urged his audience of physicians to consider the value of physiological research and enlisted their aid in what he considered an inevitable challenge from the antivivisectionists. Alluding to the British experience, he exclaimed, "Should similar circumstances arise here, it rests with you, exerting that vast influence upon public opinion and enlightenment which the medical man possesses, to secure the freedom and advance of physiology, the triumph of reason over prejudice—of knowledge over ignorance."[79] He realized the vulnerability of his program to the antivivisectionists and the importance of gaining the backing of the medical community. Because Johns Hopkins had as yet no medical faculty Martin did not have any physicians with direct ties to his program or his institution who might help him combat the antivivisectionists should they become active. John Dalton recognized the importance of gaining a broad base of support among the medical profession for vivisection. Carl Ludwig also appreciated the need to win medical support for the practice. The German physiologist, in the opinion of one of his American pupils, G. Stanley Hall, had come to believe that it was "very fortunate . . . that physiology did not go into the *philosophical* faculty as he was at one time inclined to wish. For if it had, the medical men would not have stood by him so effectively in this vivisection war as they had done."[80] Vivisection played a central role in the expanding research program in physiology at Johns Hopkins. Martin would not risk an attack by the antivivisectionists without forming a coalition to respond to their charges.

The Hopkins biology department included a remarkable group of advanced workers by the early 1880s. Martin's department awarded the first doctorate to Henry Sewall in 1879. As an undergraduate at Wesleyan College, Sewall had read Huxley's *Physiology* and had come under the influence of William North Rice who had known Gilman in New Haven. Sewall had originally hoped to enter Harvard Medical School, but financial circumstances precluded his doing so. James Carey Thomas, a member of the Hopkins board of trustees, introduced Sewall, who grew up in Baltimore, to Martin. Martin appointed Sewall associate in biology to help with the teaching of the nearly two dozen students who were participating in laboratory exercises in microscopy and practical physiology. Writing to Edward Schäfer more than half a century later, Sewall recalled, "You will not be surprised to know that the bent of my whole life has been determined by the inspiration of those 5 or 6 years of teaching and research in Physiology with dear Martin."[81] In addition to Sewall and William K. Brooks, a pupil of Louis Agassiz who was hired to take charge of the morphological work, the department included William T. Sedgwick, who began a fellowship in Martin's department in 1878 following his graduation from Yale, and William H. Howell, who entered Hopkins in 1879. These individuals had access to the most comprehensive collection of physiological apparatus in North America and were successful in their early efforts at research.[82]

By 1880, Johns Hopkins provided the most satisfactory opportunity for advanced instruction and research in the biological sciences in the United States. Morale among the young faculty and advanced students in Martin's department was high. William Sedgwick conveyed his appreciation to Gilman, "I am glad of an opportunity to express my gratitude to the faculty as a whole, and to yourself and Prof. Martin in particular, for the freedom and opportunities for work which I have never, before, so fully enjoyed; and, also, for the general guidance and advice which has been so freely sought and yet more freely given."[83] Gilman and his young faculty sought to redirect scientific teaching in America in an atmosphere charged with excitement for research. Publications from Martin's department began appearing regularly in the *Journal of Physiology* and *Studies from the Biological Laboratory of the Johns Hopkins University*, first issued in 1879.

A writer in *Scribner's Monthly* identified the circumstances at Johns Hopkins that contributed to its success:

> A student, working for several hours each day, in the physical, physiological, or chemical laboratory, working with and without his professors, surrounded by other young men interested in special lines of inquiry, has an exceptional opportunity for individual growth. . . . A great incentive to original research on the part of the associates is offered by the publications of the university. All original work of value finds its way to the public, without having to conquer the difficulties and struggle above the obscurity which so often discourage young and unknown men. This work, under the fostering care and censorship of the university, reaches the outside world indorsed, and at that same time serves to add dignity to the institution itself.[84]

A vital component of the research ethic is the desire of investigators and their sponsoring institutions to publish the results of their research. Bowditch and Martin understood the importance of publishing papers from their laboratories to show the scientific world they had established departments in which sophisticated research was taking place.

The Johns Hopkins University, with its unusual emphasis on science, was gaining increasing recognition from the medical profession. It was "favorably received by the medical profession of Baltimore, many of whom countenance the lectures and patronize the scientific courses. Almost any day practitioners may be seen in the laboratories."[85] In 1881, George Shrady enthusiastically proclaimed the virtues of the university: "The opportunities for physiological and morphological study and research at the university in question are probably the best to be found in this country. And it is a centre which has already shown evidences of good scientific work. The medical profession should feel gratified that opportunities for such original work now exist in this country."[86]

Reviewing the activities of his department during its first five years, Martin declared that one of his aims was "to train men as specialists in Physiology, so that they might not only be qualified to teach it, but to add to our knowledge of the working of the living body. . . . Physiology has only recently begun to advance into that fortunate position . . . to be pursued for its own sake."[87] He was proud of what had been accomplished, but he was impatient and sought more support for his program. In a report to the Hopkins trustees, Martin explained that he wanted "a Physiological Institute not surpassed by any in the world," and requested additional funding for the construction of a special building for the biology department. He argued that the emphasis in the department should remain upon animal physiology: "It would be a pity to devote funds which may be approved for the biological department of the University to the further development of the Marine Laboratory until the physiological work in Baltimore has been placed on the best possible footing: it is best to first do one thing thoroughly well; and then take up the next."[88]

Martin emphasized animal physiology in his department. Five years earlier, when he was negotiating with Gilman about taking the Hopkins chair, he had recommended the hiring of an assistant with special interest and training in morphology. This advice led to the appointment of William K. Brooks as a fellow in 1876.[89] Brooks was responsible for most of the teaching and laboratory work in morphology in Martin's department. Martin cited two factors that led to the decision to stress physiology at Johns Hopkins. The founder wanted his university and hospital to cooperate in advancing medical education and medical science. Moreover, he hoped that his institutions would place emphasis on subjects for which advanced programs in teaching and research were not yet well established in the United States.[90]

The proponents of the basic medical sciences continued to gain momentum in the 1880s. A coalition of pure scientists, educators, medical editors, and scientifically oriented medical teachers and practitioners was forming. It represented an extension of the network Mitchell had called upon twenty years earlier to help him try to achieve his goal of obtaining an academic chair of physiology. The medical and academic communities, and society at large were gradually accepting the ideals of the reformers. Americans were beginning to acknowledge the importance of research, the benefits of specialization in science, and the critical role of endowments in elevating the standards of higher education—including the training of physicians. Only by pursuing these goals could the United States hope to compete with the increasingly productive and sophisticated scientific institutions in Europe.

The reformers who sought to make medicine scientific extended the argument Dalton had used to justify vivisection, and it became a crucial part of their platform. Advocates of the full-time system and the research ethic asserted that the health of the population was directly dependent on advances in medical knowledge that could be achieved only through experimentation. The early success of the Johns Hopkins University lent credibility to the claims of the reformers who advocated several changes in American medical education. Among these were the improvement and standardization of preliminary training of medical students so they entered the professional school literate and with a background in chemistry and physics; the expansion of the medical curriculum to include extensive practical experience in the laboratory and at the bedside; the hiring of full-time biomedical scientists who could teach using new methods and perform research; and the support of laboratory facilities, apparatus, and personnel required for original investigation.

In 1881, thousands of physicians, including many of the leaders of American scientific medicine, attended the International Medical Congress in London where several speakers expressed their views on the value of research. Thomas Huxley recited his now familiar theme of the importance of scientific training for medical practitioners. At the same meeting, James Paget emphasized the need for specialization in science, and Rudolf Virchow outlined the critical role played by vivisection in the advance of medical science.[91] Their rhetoric was persuasive, but unless there were jobs for full-time basic medical scientists and financial support for their research, Americans would contribute little to the development of the new scientific medicine. Martin, like Bowditch, was eager to find jobs for his scientific pupils. The University of Michigan provided one opportunity in the early 1880s. Science courses had been encouraged at the University of Michigan since its establishment more than a quarter of a century earlier.

Alonzo Palmer, dean of the Michigan medical faculty, was enthusiastic about laboratory training and had tried to obtain funding for a physiological laboratory from the Michigan legislature in 1877. He argued that physiology teaching at the University of Michigan had to be reorganized to reflect the growing trend toward practical laboratory training. One writer claimed in 1880 that the physiological laboratory at Michigan was "positively overrun with students from the beginning to the end of the year."[92] This same year, James B. Angell, president of the university, the board of regents, and the medical faculty, decided that a full-time physiologist should be hired. The university sought an individual trained in the techniques of modern experimental physiology who wanted to devote himself exclusively to this science.

The two departments in North America training advanced workers in experimental physiology were Henry Bowditch's in physiology at the Harvard Medical School and Newell Martin's in biology at the Johns Hopkins University. In view of the scarcity—indeed, the virtual nonexistence—of full-time physiology positions in America in this era, it is not surprising that both Bowditch and Martin proposed candidates for the Michigan chair. A writer in the *American* commented: "There is at present no encouragement to the medical scientist in this country; indeed, because a medical scientific career is practically impossible to any one who is not willing to exist as a pauper or has not been born to wealth."[93]

Henry Sewall, Martin's first doctorate recipient, applied for the chair of physiology at the University of Michigan in 1881. Angell had watched the development of Johns Hopkins with interest. Moreover, Sewall, through Martin, represented a direct link with British physiology. The British interpretation of physiology was familiar to students in Ann Arbor where an estimated 450 copies of Michael Foster's textbook of physiology were sold in 1880.[94]

As noted earlier, the University of Michigan officials were aware of Bowditch's physiology program at the Harvard Medical School. Charles Sedgwick Minot, the candidate from Harvard, became Bowditch's first graduate student following his graduation from the Massachusetts Institute of Technology in 1872. With Bowditch's encouragement, Minot studied with Carl Ludwig in Leipzig during 1873 and 1874. Following additional postgraduate training abroad·that emphasized embryology, histology, and anatomy, Minot returned to Bowditch's laboratory and received a doctorate of science from Harvard in 1878.[95] Minot was unsuccessful in his attempts to find an academic position on at least two earlier occasions. When he failed to win a chair at Vassar, the prominent naturalist Alpheus Packard, Jr., reassured him: "If you don't get this place don't be discouraged—you will be provided for somehow."[96] With the encouragement of Weir Mitchell, Minot applied for the chair of comparative anatomy and zoology in the auxiliary faculty of medicine at the University of Pennsylvania in 1879, but did not win the post.[97] Minot also failed to win the Michigan chair and remained at Harvard where he became head of the new histology department in the medical school in 1883.

Henry Sewall, highly recommended to the faculty by Martin, was the successful candidate for the Michigan chair. Victor Vaughan later recalled:

> Professor Martin took a deep personal interest in the matter. He
> was intent not only on building up his own department in Balti-

more, but in seeing the seeds of the new school of physiology then just coming into bloom in England . . . planted and nourished in the universities of America. I may add parenthetically that I then regarded that movement as the first real awakening of scientific medicine, and I have since had no occasion to reverse my opinion on this matter.[98]

The university delayed Sewall's appointment for a year because of an unexpected deficiency in its finances, which demonstrates the financial instability of institutions of higher learning and the vulnerability of programs in the biomedical sciences in this era. Although generally supported quite liberally by the legislature, the University of Michigan did not have the financial strength of the Johns Hopkins University with its enormous endowment. Nor did Henry Sewall have a patron as did Henry Bowditch, whose wealthy family subsidized his department and his academic career at Harvard. After Sewall's arrival in Ann Arbor, he wrote Gilman, "I am making it my business at present to try & show Faculty, Regents & Legislature that the physiological department is a worthy beggar."[99] Sewall informed the Michigan faculty of the need for an expanded and better equipped physiological laboratory: "I submit to you that the necessities of science, and the great opportunities afforded here, urge the establishment of a Physiological Laboratory, a place where practical Physiology may be taught and original investigation prosecuted. No scientific man will deny that such places are the very fountainheads of scientific knowledge."[100]

Angell, who had encouraged the Hopkins trustees to build laboratories when they had interviewed him nearly a decade earlier, supported Sewall's request and urged the Michigan regents to provide additional funds for the physiology program.[101] Sewall's career at Michigan was brief, however. He contracted tuberculosis and resigned in 1889 to move to the supposedly healthier climate of Colorado.[102]

Although careers were only gradually opening up for individuals who wished to devote themselves exclusively to physiology or one of the other basic medical sciences, a trend in this direction was emerging. John Shaw Billings claimed at the International Medical Congress held in London in 1881:

Seven years ago, Professor Huxley declared that, if a student in his own branch showed power and originality, he dared not advise him to adopt a scientific career, for he could not give him the assurance that any amount of proficiency in the biological sciences would be convertible into the most modest bread and cheese. To-day I think he might be bolder, for such a fear would hardly be

>justifiable—at all events, in America—where such a man as is
>referred to could almost certainly find a place, bearing in mind
>the professor's remark that it is no impediment to an original in-
>vestigator to have to devote a moderate portion of his time to
>giving instruction either in the laboratory or in the lecture-
>room.[103]

Perhaps patriotism stimulated Billings to portray the situation in America in a more favorable light than was really the case. Although a trend
toward full-time scientific careers was slowly developing in the United
States, few institutions could provide facilities for research or salaries for
full-time biomedical scientists in 1881. Billings's assessment of the
chances of a scientific graduate finding a position reflected the small
number of individuals seeking full-time careers in the basic medical sciences rather than the number of opportunities.

By 1882, Martin's research program was well established and was
focused on circulatory physiology. Together with his pupils William
Howell and Frank Donaldson, Jr., he developed a unique isolated mammalian heart preparation that greatly facilitated their experiments in
cardiac physiology and pharmacology. Many workers have used modi-
fied versions of Martin's isolated heart preparation over the past century
to study the physiology and pharmacology of the heart. The development of this technique was an important stimulus for research in his department, which by July 1882 included six faculty members, three fellows, and twenty-six graduate students.[104] In assessing the significance
of Martin's isolated heart preparation, Gilman asserted that its use "in
the thorough study of cardiac physiology will supply abundant work for
many hands for several years, numerous problems which have hitherto
been unattacked being now rendered available for investigation."[105]

In an address to Baltimore physicians on the influence of variations
of arterial and venous pressure and temperature on the heart rate,
Martin cleverly linked his scientific observations to medical practice in
an effort to demonstrate the clinical relevance of his research: "A practitioner may, nowadays, when making a professional visit, omit to say
'Put out your tongue' without being thought to have neglected his duty,
but the family doctor who fails to feel his patient's pulse seriously risks
losing the confidence of mater-familias. . . . I therefore venture to hope
that what little I may be able to add to your knowledge of the causes
which influence the rate of beat of the heart may not be unwelcome."[106]

In addition to publishing numerous papers reporting the results of
his research, Martin wrote several textbooks on elementary biology,

anatomy, and physiology that received favorable reviews.[107] Scientific
publications and presentations by Hopkins faculty members and advanced workers resulted in increased interest in the university at the local, national, and international levels. One writer in the *Boston Medical
and Surgical Journal* declared in 1883: "The influence of the Johns
Hopkins University is beginning to be felt, and the spirit of original research and true scientific investigation have been fully aroused in the
medical profession."[108]

Martin grew impatient as his requests failed to result in the laboratory building he desired. He argued that if the momentum of his program was to be maintained, more adequate facilities were mandatory.
In anticipation of a new building program at the university and the construction of the Johns Hopkins Hospital, Gilman and Billings visited European laboratories and hospitals in 1881. Gilman's early commitment
to attracting a first-rate faculty was now matched by his concern for
more adequate laboratory accommodations. The Hopkins president
noted the competition that his university had inspired among other
American institutions of higher learning and asserted, "It is all important in the race before us that we do not underestimate the building side
of the question. . . . We can well afford to erect . . . buildings for study
& work, as we need them, upon a liberal & wise scale, in keeping with &
as a part of the great future which is before us."[109]

The science professors at Johns Hopkins forwarded their suggestions for new laboratories to the board of trustees in January 1882, and
construction began in the spring of that year.[110] Upon completion of the
new laboratory building in 1883, Gilman proudly announced:

> The size of the rooms, their light, ventilation, apparatus, and
> furniture, give ample facilities for the study of physiology and
> comparative anatomy, in accordance with the best known meth-
> ods, and the scientific power of the university is much increased
> by this addition to its material resources. The significance of this
> laboratory in relation to medical education is obvious. Students
> expecting at a later day to take up the courses in medicine, may
> here acquaint themselves, not only with the use of the microscope
> and the modern instruments of physiological research, but may
> also have ample opportunities to study the normal and healthy
> forms and functions of living beings, before proceeding to the
> study of disease and its treatment.[111]

In his address at the dedication of the laboratory, Martin proudly
proclaimed: "For its purpose [it is] unrivaled in the United States and
not surpassed in the world." He reasserted the dominance of physiology

in the biology program at Hopkins: "It is a biological laboratory deliber-
ately planned that physiology in it shall be queen, and the rest her hand-
maids." In an assessment reminiscent of Mitchell's evaluation of American contributions to physiology published more than a quarter of a
century earlier, Martin decried the paucity of physiological research
that had been undertaken in the United States. "Considering the accumulated wealth of this country, the energy which throbs through it, and
the number of its medical schools," Martin asserted, "it has not done its
fair share in advancing physiological knowledge." He sought to explain
what physiology had done to benefit mankind during the preceding half
century to justify the money and time spent on this science. His argument incorporated several themes put forth by Dalton in his essays on
behalf of vivisection.

As examples of the benefits of physiology to mankind, Martin listed
the overthrow of the vitalistic philosophy, the establishment of the cell
doctrine, and the development of the germ theory of disease. He emphasized that these three advances in medical thought developed from basic
research without any initial concern for practical applications of the discoveries. A strong supporter of basic research, Martin asserted: "Even
the special practical art of medicine itself is to-day far more indebted to
the purely scientific researches of the German students than those of the
French, undertaken with a specific practical end in view." Concluding
his address, he claimed that the objects of the new laboratory were "to
advance our knowledge of the laws of life and health; to inquire into the
phenomena and causes of diseases; to train investigators in pathology,
therapeutics, and sanitary science; to fit men to undertake the study of
the art of medicine."[112]

The opening of the new biological laboratory at Johns Hopkins trig-
gered two attacks on Martin and his program. The emphasis on physiology that he outlined in his 1881 report to the trustees and reaffirmed in
this 1884 address elicited a harsh response from the prominent naturalists Alpheus S. Packard, Jr., and Edward D. Cope. They protested his
emphasis on physiology, which they believed was to the detriment of
morphology.[113] The opening of the laboratory also precipitated a hostile
attack on Martin by the antivivisectionists. Martin was deeply disturbed
by this assault and expended a great deal of energy attempting to blunt
the effect the antivivisectionists might have on his physiology program.

The new laboratory was praised by scientifically oriented physicians as well as by physiologists. The American medical community was
gradually accepting the assertion that laboratory training was an important part of medical education. Announcing the opening of the new bio-

logical laboratory at Johns Hopkins, a Boston writer emphasized the importance of a sound medical education. It should include practical training in the laboratory and at the bedside: "The student must be brought face to face with the phenomena he is to study, he must have a personal acquaintance with the means by which a scientific law is demonstrated, and accordingly laboratories have been established for the instruction of students." The writer continued:

> The modern laboratory is a new thing, the invaluable culmination of that immense intellectual revolution which has nearly freed us from the thraldom of dead authority. Indeed, the progress of scientific education may be approximately measured by the number and character of the laboratories at its disposal. There is no more hopeful indication of the gradual elevation of our medical schools than is given by the improvement and multiplication of their laboratories.[114]

Although interest in laboratory facilities and practical instruction was growing in the medical, scientific, and lay communities, appreciation of the significance of this movement for the reform of medical education was not universal. In a comprehensive survey of medical schools and their curricula published by the Illinois State Board of Health in 1884, laboratory facilities received scant attention.[115] The fundamental impediment to the more widespread introduction of laboratory training in medical schools remained the lack of endowment to cover the cost of building, equipping, and staffing such facilities.

During the 1880s, opportunities gradually arose for American physiologists to assume full-time positions in medical schools and other institutions of higher learning. The year after Henry Sewall left Martin's department to become head of physiology at the University of Michigan, William Sedgwick left Hopkins to introduce a biology course at the Massachusetts Institute of Technology modeled after the one developed by Martin in Baltimore. These departures had significant implications for the continuity of the research and advanced teaching in Martin's department, however. In a letter to Gilman, Martin revealed his ambivalence about Sedgwick's departure; to have a pupil assume a position of importance in a major Boston institution was gratifying, but it meant that Martin had to assume the elementary teaching duties until a suitable replacement for Sedgwick could be trained.[116] In his letter, Martin also pointed out that the paucity of opportunities for teachers of general biology discouraged many potential scientists from entering into or completing training that would prepare them for careers in biology or physiology.

Martin was not opposed to delivering lectures as part of his duties at Johns Hopkins. He was disturbed, however, by the amount of elementary teaching he would be forced to do upon Sedgwick's departure. His colleague Henry Rowland, professor of physics, acknowledged the value and necessity of a university professor combining teaching with research. Nevertheless, he recognized, as did Martin, that the critical balance between these two activities could be upset by an inadequate support staff. Rowland declared, "I know of no institution in this country where assistants are supplied to aid directly in research. Yet why should it not be so? And even the absence of assistant professors and assistants of all kinds to aid in teaching is very noticeable, and must be remedied before we can expect much."[117] As Martin did, Rowland believed that adequate laboratory facilities were crucial for a successful program of advanced teaching and research. Although laboratories of chemistry and biology were built at Johns Hopkins, the construction of Rowland's physics laboratory was delayed. Asking Gilman where this matter stood with the trustees, Rowland testily remarked, "Should no plans have been arrived at—I would suggest that notice of the inadequate accommodations be published in a suitable place so that students may know what to expect before coming here. In a short time when the new laboratories at Harvard, Yale & Cornell are completed we shall probably not be troubled with them."[118] Thus, even at the well-endowed Johns Hopkins University, the professors confronted at least temporary obstacles to the full realization of their plans for training advanced workers in science and maintaining a sophisticated research program.

Although Martin had his new laboratory, he was frustrated that the university was reluctant to pay his staff salaries sufficient to keep them at Johns Hopkins. The integrity and productivity of Martin's department were again threatened in 1886 by the possible departure of William Howell because of a salary dispute. Revealing his anger and dismay, Martin complained to Gilman that Howell would probably leave if his salary was not increased. Since Martin had to assume additional elementary teaching responsibilities with Sedgwick's departure, he was dismayed to consider the impact of the loss of yet another skilled assistant. These departures left him with "little time or energy for research or post graduate instruction—and none for the preparation of advanced courses." Moreover, Martin protested that he was being pressured by James Carey Thomas, an influential trustee, to develop the research program further "so as to keep up with the new laboratories now going up all over the country." His letter was written in a plaintive, almost desperate tone. He concluded that the rapid turnover among junior faculty members in his department and the implications of these departures were "unjust to me and harmful to the University."[119]

Martin did not attempt to disguise his anger; he believed that the agenda he and Gilman had established for physiology at the university was threatened. He realized that his research program, however productive it had been in the early 1880s, was a fragile enterprise. A spacious laboratory and state-of-the-art equipment were not the most critical component of a successful research program: well-trained, innovative, and dedicated associates were the essential factor. They, however, required an ongoing investment on the part of the university which had just expended a large sum of money on laboratory buildings. Moreover, the financial situation of the university had recently deteriorated. Most of the university's endowment was invested in Baltimore and Ohio Railroad stock which did not pay any dividends for several years beginning in 1886.[120]

Despite these internal problems at Johns Hopkins, the prestige of the university and the image of its scientific programs continued to grow. Carl Ludwig, writing to his former pupil Franklin P. Mall, now a fellow in pathology at Johns Hopkins, remarked in 1886, "What you write me of Baltimore was in part new, in part well-known. The effectiveness and ability of Newell Martin have long won my admiration; his example and that of his pupils will not be lost in America."[121] Writing to Gilman the following year, Charles Eliot remarked, "I read carefully your report on the first ten years of the University . . . and was much impressed by the amount of work accomplished and by its original quality. You have every reason to be highly content with the achievement."[122]

Although the Hopkins trustees approved a salary increase for Howell which kept the young physiologist at Hopkins for two more years, it was only a temporary solution. By 1889, Howell was thirty-nine years old and, as one of the best trained and most productive experimental physiologists in America, he was a logical target for the recruiting efforts of other institutions seeking to enlarge the scope and enhance the image of their physiology programs. In rhetoric reminiscent of Martin's complaints to Gilman, Howell voiced his frustration that excessive teaching responsibilities at Johns Hopkins left him with little time for research. For this reason, Howell accepted the chair of physiology at the University of Michigan left vacant by the departure of Henry Sewall in 1889.[123] The departure of fellows and junior faculty members from Martin's program took their toll on both the man and his department. Experimental work employing his isolated heart preparation declined in the closing years of the decade, and fewer individuals who had, or would seek, medical degrees entered Martin's laboratory once they had the option of studying pathology or bacteriology with William Welch.

Martin's health deteriorated as a result of alcoholism and neurasthenia, and his resignation was requested in 1893 on the eve of the long-delayed opening of the Johns Hopkins Medical School. Acknowledging the decline in the Hopkins physiology program, William Howell, who was now at Harvard with Bowditch, informed Gilman, "I was sorely disappointed to learn that no fellow was appointed in physiology. I feel it to be a real disaster to the graduate study of physiology at the Johns Hopkins and more to be regretted because heretofore the Hopkins has been recognized as the one place in the country where graduate work in animal physiology was encouraged. I should be sorry to see it lose this prestige."[124]

The success of Martin's department was due to a combination of his special training and abilities, the encouragement of Gilman, the relatively generous support of the trustees, and the outstanding pupils who were attracted to the biology program at Johns Hopkins. Martin's role was important, but after more than fifteen years his department could go on without him, or so the Hopkins officials believed. The impending opening of the Johns Hopkins Medical School forced the issue of Martin's alcoholism and its consequences. Gilman informed Martin, "We have all great sympathy for you in your affliction. We grieve over what has followed in its train. But you must allow me both to personally & officially to appeal to all that is manliest in your nature—to persevere and recover your usefulness, for you know as well as I that the work of a great university engaged in the instruction of youth must not be allowed to suffer by the failure of any individual if one can possibly prevent it."[125]

It became apparent that Martin could not be counted on to remain sober or regain his health, and he was encouraged to resign by William Osler, who, with Weir Mitchell, cared for him. William Welch informed Franklin Mall of Martin's resignation, noting, "Martin in his day did a great work for this University and for physiology in this country and his case now is one of the saddest, I think the saddest, I ever knew. He has completely succumbed to alcohol and is no longer capable of making the slightest effort to resist it. . . . Fortunately there was no public scandal and the newspapers all gave excellent reviews of his work."[126]

William Howell was recruited to succeed his teacher Martin but the momentum in the biology department at the university had shifted toward morphology.[127] When the Johns Hopkins Medical School opened in 1893, a new department of physiology was established in connection with that branch of the university, and William Brooks became head of the original biology department whose focus was now on morphology and embryology.

Martin was only forty-five at the time of his retirement from Johns Hopkins, and in his late thirties when his pupils Howell and Sewall detected a distinct decline in his enthusiasm and energy. Nevertheless, he had played a critical role in the establishment of physiology as a discipline in America. Gilman recalled:

[Martin] established the first American biological laboratory. A score of successors followed. . . . Martin gave a noteworthy impulse [to the study of biology], and the methods which he introduced were soon followed in other parts of the country. In the Johns Hopkins University it was soon determined that no one should be encouraged to enter upon the study of medicine without a careful previous training in a physiological laboratory. The improvements now common in medical schools are largely based upon the recognition of the principle that living creatures, in their normal and healthy aspects, should be studied before the phenomena and treatment of disease, and credit should always be given to Dr. Martin for the skill with which he introduced among Americans the best methods of study.[128]

CHAPTER FIVE

The American
Physiological Society

A Profession Defines Itself

T HE CONTRIBUTIONS OF Dalton, Mitchell, Bowditch, and Martin to American physiology were substantial. Their accomplishments drew widespread acclaim from scientists and reform-minded physicians in America and abroad. Nevertheless, the isolated efforts of these four pioneers did not prove to the world that American physiology was a distinct discipline. Their mutual efforts in organizing a society devoted to their science did, however.

The American Physiological Society was established through the efforts of Weir Mitchell, Henry Bowditch, and Newell Martin. These individuals called an organizational meeting in the new physiological laboratory at the College of Physicians and Surgeons of New York in 1887. It is not surprising that Bowditch and Martin played an active role in forming the American Physiological Society. Productive programs in experimental physiology were well established at the Harvard Medical School and the Johns Hopkins University by the mid-1880s. More than a score of advanced workers had published papers based on research undertaken in the physiological laboratories of these two institutions since their inception a decade earlier. Pupils of Bowditch and Martin held full-time positions in physiology, biology, and related scientific fields, and some of their current pupils also hoped to enter full-time scientific careers.

Potential physiologists of a century ago could not assume they would find favorable institutional circumstances like those that facilitated the careers of Bowditch and Martin, however. The founders of the

American Physiological Society realized the future of their science could not be left to the whims of individual institutional officers, or to the promise of independent wealth. If the field of physiology was to grow, a stable job market had to exist. There were three main ways that occupational opportunities for experimental physiologists could be expanded: new institutions or departments could be created; additional positions could be established within existing departments; and the qualifications for those who sought to fill the existing (or new) positions could be redefined. The most realistic short-term solution was to convince medical school officials to revise the requirements for physiology teachers.

The American Physiological Society could establish the credentials required for an individual to become a member. By so doing, the society implicitly defined the criteria one had to meet to call oneself a physiologist, although it could not enforce adherence to this definition, or demand that medical schools accept it. Nevertheless, as was the case with other contemporary professional societies, membership in the organization representing physiologists lent stature to those individuals who belonged. The fundamental requirement for election to membership was the candidate's experience in, and commitment to, physiological research using the new instruments and approaches developed in the leading European laboratories of experimental medicine.

The founding of the American Physiological Society led to a greater distinction between amateur and professional physiologists in this country. Virtually all traditional physician-physiologists were excluded from membership in the society. No longer could practicing physicians lay claim to the nation's chairs of physiology. The formation of the society both acknowledged and encouraged the demise of the part-time physiologist-practitioner. If such individuals were no longer suitable candidates for the chairs of physiology in America's medical schools, the younger members of the American Physiological Society, who were full-time scientists imbued with the research ethic, stood a better chance of finding employment. Although these two features of German medical education had been introduced in a few American institutions before 1887, the physiologists hoped they could achieve the widespread adoption of these reforms more rapidly by uniting.

Individual efforts to articulate these principles had accomplished relatively little, whereas a national organization lent authority to the opinions and demands of the physiologists. First, they had to formalize the loose network of medical scientists so there was a recognizable profession of physiology in the United States. Then, they could crystallize their goals and concerns into an agenda for America's basic medical scientists. The physiologists' reasons for forming a society were similar to those of other individuals in many fields who sought to define themselves as specialists in the final decades of the nineteenth century. In addition, however, issues of special relevance for the physiologists encouraged the formation of the American Physiological Society. One of these related to the fundamental technique of experimental physiology—vivisection. Individuals who hoped to become professional physiologists could anticipate attacks by the antivivisectionists when they introduced this technique into their teaching and research. A society could coordinate the response of the scientific and medical communities to the claims of the antivivisectionists.

Americans had formed societies and institutions designed to promote social and intellectual intercourse among individuals interested in science since colonial times. Often, the American societies were patterned after European models, but they also reflected the cultural and scientific circumstances of the United States when they were founded. During the middle third of the nineteenth century, some Americans tried to establish national societies with broad agendas that included the popularization of science in the United States, the promotion of scientific research, and the encouragement of changes in American institutions of higher learning that would lead to the creation of full-time scientific careers. Two early attempts failed: the American Institute for the Cultivation of Science founded in 1838 and the National Institute for the Promotion of Science established two years later. Speaking at the 1844 meeting of the National Institute, scientist Alexander Bache declared, "There is no cause half so depressing to American science as the want of an American feeling in regard to it."[1]

Although those organizations were short-lived, one society formed to encourage science in the United States was more successful. The Association of American Geologists and Naturalists, founded in 1840, within a decade, evolved into the American Association for the Advancement of Science. The first formal meeting of this organization was held in Philadelphia in 1848, and Weir Mitchell's father, John K. Mitchell, was on the local arrangements committee. Building on the membership of the Association of American Geologists and Naturalists, the new association boasted more than 450 members in its first year.[2]

In the 1850s, a small group of influential scientists sought to achieve more than an appreciation of science in America: they wanted financial support for scientific careers and research. The "scientific Lazzaroni," as they came to be called, included fewer than a dozen men, but their impact was substantial. They came from varied institutional backgrounds, different scientific disciplines, and held diverse philosophical positions regarding the needs of American science and higher education. Through their efforts, the National Academy of Sciences was established in 1863. The stated mission of the academy was to identify a body of experts who, on the basis of personal knowledge, experimentation, or investigation could provide insight into any aspect of science that might be of interest to the government.

Although individuals interested in the physical sciences outnumbered naturalists by nearly two to one, the fifty original members of the academy included influential representatives of the life sciences. Jeffries Wyman, Asa Gray, Joseph Leidy, and Louis Agassiz were among the original members. In acknowledgment of their contributions to physiology, John Call Dalton, Jr., and S. Weir Mitchell were invited to join in 1865. Membership in, and support by other members of, the National Academy of Sciences did not help Mitchell win the physiology chair at Jefferson Medical College three years later, however. It would be more than two decades before a society was established in America that addressed the issue of what criteria determined a candidate's claim to a physiology chair in an American medical school.

The Physiological Society formed in England in 1876 served as a model for the establishment of the American Physiological Society eleven years later. The [British] Physiological Society was proposed by John Burdon-Sanderson to coordinate the medical and scientific response to the aggressive British antivivisection movement.[3] Although he was not present at the organizational meeting, Newell Martin was a founding member of the Physiological Society and attended the first regular meeting. He maintained his membership in the British society following his move to the United States and returned to England to participate in the 1882 meeting to present a paper on his isolated heart preparation. Although the Physiological Society meetings included scientific presentations, members paid much attention to political issues such as the role the society should play in thwarting the attempts of the antivivisectionists to suppress animal experimentation.

Several Americans interested in physiology and experimental medicine were familiar with the goals and activities of the Physiological Society. The society extended an invitation to continental and American physiologists to meet with their British counterparts on the occasion of the International Medical Congress to be held in London in 1881. Henry Bowditch and Horatio Wood, Jr., accepted the invitation and heard members of the society encourage publications elaborating the value of vivisection, the aims of physiological research, and the benefits of these activities to mankind.[4] These themes were familiar to the Americans who were well aware of the harsh attacks of Bergh and the eloquent rebuttals of Dalton.

Several speakers emphasized the value of vivisection at the 1881 International Medical Congress. Mitchell's friend Wood was quoted in the British press as claiming: "Without vivisection, there could be no physiology; and the value of the method was scarcely less to the clinician. Even in America it was fully recognised that, except in certain surgical directions, no further progress was to be made in scientific medicine except by the aid of experiments upon the lower animals." Wood's comments provide insight into the methods used by physiologists in the United States to combat the antivivisectionists. He explained that the Americans worked through the "family physicians of the various members of the legislative bodies, and . . . [used] them in obtaining a private hearing from those individuals composing the Legislature. The same measures were taken with regard to the editors of the daily papers and popular magazines."[5]

The articulate and persuasive arguments advanced by Dalton during the 1860s and 1870s, and his willingness to participate in the political arena, limited the impact of Henry Bergh and the antivivisectionists in America. During the 1880s, as vivisection became more widespread in teaching and research, the American antivivisection campaign intensified, however. The *Vivisectors' Directory*, an alphabetized listing of experimenters who used this technique, was published in 1884.[6] It included the address, institutional background, and professional affiliations of each vivisector as well as references to, and extracts from, their publications. Americans listed in this comprehensive directory included Roberts Bartholow, Henry Bowditch, Austin Flint, Jr., H. Newell Martin, S. Weir Mitchell, Isaac Ott, T. Mitchell Prudden, James J. Putnam, William T. Sedgwick, Henry Sewall, Christian Sihler, and George Sternberg. This directory was just one of a growing number of publications of the antivivisectionists designed to enrage the public and encourage legislators to abolish, or at least restrict, animal experimentation.

The smoldering American antivivisection movement burst forth once again in the 1880s and threatened the few programs that encouraged experimental physiology. John Curtis had joined Dalton's fight against the antivivisectionists in the 1870s and became progressively involved in this debate over the next quarter century. Representing the committee on experimental medicine of the Medical Society of the State of New York, Curtis submitted a resolution in 1883 declaring "the supreme importance, to the art of medicine, of scientific experiments upon living animals."[7]

As I have shown, the Jefferson Medical College had no significant program in experimental physiology and the University of Pennsylvania conducted only a small amount of research using vivisection in the early 1880s. Nevertheless, this modest level of activity attracted the attention of the antivivisectionists. Supporters of vivisection and the experimental method found it necessary to argue that these techniques were little used rather than appeal for their widespread adoption. One Philadelphia writer claimed in 1884:

> In the University of Pennsylvania the laboratories for physiology are used by four persons, or at most five, at somewhat long intervals. Students are never alone in the laboratory. Third course students are not permitted to conduct researches and employ animals in aid of these, without the most careful supervision. If they wish to engage in such pursuits, they must apply to the Professor or his Demonstrator, and show that the object in view is desirable, and that they are competent. . . . In fact the University discourages physiological work by students, and it is therefore uncommon.[8]

This writer concluded that vivisection was not abused in America, and, citing the British experience, asserted that legal restraint of the practice would be devastating to the cause of scientific medicine.

Mitchell served as chairman of a committee of the Medical Society of the State of Pennsylvania that addressed the antivivisection agitation in the mid-1880s. His approach was similar to that of Dalton and Curtis in New York. Mitchell's committee reaffirmed the central role of animal experimentation in the advance of practical and scientific medicine, and the society forwarded a strong statement to the Pennsylvania legislature defending the value of this experimental approach.[9] Mitchell called on his fellow practitioners in Pennsylvania to urge the legislature to vote down the restrictive legislation proposed by the antivivisectionists: "To make sure that it does not pass becomes your duty, and we ask you to make it your business on your return from this meeting to urge on your Senators and Representatives the need to vote against all such legislation as the Antivivisection Society contemplates. With your help we can always defeat any such measures; without it, you might find your great schools crippled as they have been in England."[10] Mitchell was also responsible for outlining rules governing vivisection adopted by the University of Pennsylvania trustees in 1885.[11] This same year, Martin prepared guidelines for animal experimentation in his laboratory that were adopted by the Johns Hopkins trustees.[12]

The medical community was not united in supporting vivisection. In America, as in England, a few physicians spoke out in opposition to the practice. Henry Bigelow had done so in Boston fifteen years earlier, and now, in Philadelphia, Thomas Morton and Frank Woodbury attempted to undermine the unanimity among the medical profession that Mitchell felt was critical if the antivivisectionists were to be defeated. Woodbury, as editor of the *Philadelphia Medical Times*, had a vehicle through which to publish his views. Responding to this breach, and the threat it represented, Mitchell and several of his reform-minded Philadelphia colleagues circulated a "Dear Doctor" letter on the University of Pennsylvania letterhead in January 1885. They characterized the antivivisection bill before the legislature as "a monstrous instrument" and declared: "If, therefore, you have any desire that the science of medicine should continue on its path to perfection, that the University of Pennsylvania and other medical institutions in your State should not be crippled and their students driven to other places, we appeal to you to help to smother the present bill in committee. . . . Immediate action is necessary to prevent the strangling of physiology in Pennsylvania."[13] Responding to the events in Philadelphia, George Shrady of New York decried the participation of physicians in the antivivisection cause: "Original work in experimental science is just beginning in America; and it is very unfortunate that any medical men should assist in a movement designed to impede its progress."[14]

Martin vividly described his vivisection techniques in a paper on the effect of temperature variations on the heart rate which Michael Foster presented before the Royal Society of London in 1883. The paper was subsequently published in the *Philosophical Transactions* and provoked an angry response from the *Zoophilist*, a recently founded British antivivisection periodical.[15] In a printed rebuttal to this article Martin strenuously defended his work and made an impassioned plea for experimental science. He denigrated the motives of the antivivisectionists and implored his readers to ignore their rhetoric and "vindicate my University from the charge of having placed one of its most important departments under the direction of a callous brute." Martin sought exoneration by his lay readers and support from his scientific colleagues:

> Friends and fellow-townsmen, I have placed before you a statement of facts which makes it clear that any assertion proceeding

from those persons who desire to prohibit experiments on animals is open to suspicion as regards its truthfulness. I have lived and worked among you for nearly nine years in good repute, and now that a foreign journal is circulated through this community, describing me as a monster glorying in the useless torment of helpless victims, you may deem it needless for me to notice the charge. But, in view of the nature of this attack, the source whence it proceeds, and the movement it is designed to initiate, I have felt it my duty to lay the matter before you. Hereafter, when you may be assailed by charges of inhumanity brought against me and those who work with me, if you feel the least doubt as to the falsity of such accusations, I beg you to visit my laboratory and judge for yourselves of what goes on within its walls.[16]

Few Americans who performed animal experimentation were spared the attacks of the antivivisectionists. The movement was not confined to the eastern cities; it arose wherever vivisection was employed in teaching or research. James B. Herrick, a Chicago practitioner and teacher at Rush Medical College, used vivisection in a classroom demonstration in 1886 and was promptly threatened with legal action.[17]

Philadelphia became a center for antivivisection activity during the 1880s. The American Society for the Restriction of Vivisection, based there, circulated graphically illustrated publications depicting animals being subjected to experiments. Accompanying the illustrations, reproduced from the texts of European physiologists, were quotations from physicians, scientists, and laymen decrying the "horrors" of vivisection.[18] The arguments against vivisection expanded as the issue of cruelty to animals was insufficient to cause legislators to outlaw the practice. Cannon Wilberforce, a visiting British antivivisectionist, assailed the character of individuals practicing vivisection in 1887. He urged a Philadelphia audience to rise up against vivisection: "Those persons who begin by ill treating or being unkind to animals, and neglect their duties toward animals, invariably learn to neglect their duties to their fellow men, and become bad citizens and worthless people."[19]

Although neither the constitution of the [British] Physiological Society nor the charter of the American Physiological Society has an explicit statement regarding the antivivisectionists, the conclusion is inescapable that among the factors that led Mitchell, Bowditch, and Martin to propose the formation of the society in 1887 was their belief that a unified organization representing the interests of experimental physiology could blunt the attacks of the antivivisectionists by coordinating the medical response to their propaganda. Although an occasional physician leant support to the antivivisection campaign, the growing consensus among doctors was that animal experimentation was vitally important for the advance of medicine. Antivivisectionists had threatened Dalton, Curtis, Martin, Mitchell, and Bowditch. An organization representing all medical scientists who used this technique would serve to shift the focus of the antivivisectionists' attacks away from these prominent physiologists to a larger body of experimentalists.

Other factors contributed to the founding of the American Physiological Society. Following the Civil War, a mania for organizing special societies swept America. In medicine and science, Europeans had already established organizations reflecting the progressive subdivision of large fields into smaller disciplines. John Billings claimed in 1886, "A marked feature of the present day, in medicine as in other things, is the tendency to specialisation in study and practice."[20] Americans followed the European example and established a number of medical societies based on specific organs or new diagnostic instruments. Clinical specialties acknowledged as distinct fields by the formation of societies in America during the second half of the nineteenth century included ophthalmology, otology, neurology, dermatology, gynecology, and orthopedics, among others.

Others zealously founded scientific societies. In his presidential address before the inaugural meeting of the American Chemical Society in 1876, John W. Draper explained that the present age was favorable for the advance of science and scientific societies. He remarked that the horizons of science were steadily expanding, the number of investigators increasing, and the productivity of these workers improving each year. Draper was optimistic about the future of science in America and emphasized the important role educational institutions and scientific societies would play in the advance of this area of knowledge and endeavor.[21]

The establishment of specialty societies created some problems for contemporary scientists and practitioners. William Osler discussed the dilemma posed by unrelenting specialization among the relatively small number of scientific workers in America in 1878. That year, at the meeting of the American Association for the Advancement of Science, a subsection devoted to physiology and anatomy was proposed. Osler, then professor of the institutes of medicine at McGill, explained that there were too few individuals interested in these subjects to justify the formation of a special section, however. The current system mixed papers on anatomy and physiology with those on geology, biology, anthropology, and other subjects. In Osler's opinion, this arrangement discouraged individuals from presenting papers on physiology at the meeting.[22] He noted that very few of the 125 papers presented were of medical interest; the majority related to chemical or geological subjects. Circumstances for the creation of a biological section in the association were more favorable two years later, when one was established at the Boston meeting. Others agreed with Osler that this section would lead to an increase in the number of medical science papers presented at the association's meetings.[23]

Several leading American physiologists met in 1884 at the Montreal meeting of the British Association for the Advancement of Science. This meeting was well attended, and the British and American scientists formed a subsection of physiology. The physiological section met in two sessions in the new physiological laboratory at the McGill Medical School. Osler published a summary of the meeting which included presentations by Newell Martin, William Howell, Henry Bowditch, and Charles Minot.[24]

Scientists, as did physicians, formed new societies that acknowledged the narrower focus of their interests. In 1883, the Society of Naturalists of the Eastern United States was founded to facilitate communication and cooperation among "working naturalists." The officers of the new society included Alpheus Hyatt, curator of the Boston Society of Natural History as president; Newell Martin as one of the vice-presidents; and Martin's former pupil Samuel Clarke as secretary. Clarke was the individual most responsible for founding the society. He was one of Martin's first fellows and remained at Johns Hopkins for five years until he was appointed professor of natural history at Williams College. Clarke's sense of isolation from scientific colleagues kindled his interest in establishing a society of naturalists.[25] Martin and Bowditch were active in this society and both served as its president in the 1890s, even after they founded the American Physiological Society.

The agenda of the Society of Naturalists was broader than the simple presentation of scientific papers. Social, political, and economic concerns animated the naturalists who wanted to see their field grow in numbers and influence. The prominent naturalists Alpheus Packard, Jr., and Edward Cope described the organization's first meeting:

The papers read related to the means rather than the ends of the scientific career, no discussion of subjects of pure science being in order. The questions discussed may be classified as follows: (1) The method of original research. (2) The methods of teaching. (3) The constitution of societies and academies of science. (4) The

employment of competent specialists by the educational institutions of the country. . . . The relations of the original investigator
to the public, and the necessity of maintaining academies and
institutions for original research.[26]

The society, which had just over one hundred original members, sought
to expand its geographical scope by changing its name to the American
Society of Naturalists in 1886.

"Working" American scientists had their professional status acknowledged by election as fellows of the American Association for the
Advancement of Science. Although membership in the association did
not require any scientific credentials, fellowship could be attained only
by individuals who were "professionally engaged in science, or have by
their labors aided in advancing science."[27] Nearly a quarter of the original members of the American Physiological Society were fellows of the
association and attended the 1884 meeting held in Philadelphia. (A list
of the original members of the American Physiological Society is in appendix 1. The original members who attended the 1884 meeting of the
American Association for the Advancement of Science were Henry
Beyer, Henry Bowditch, Russell Chittenden, Newell Martin, Charles
Minot, and William Osler.) More than fifty papers were read at the biology section of the Philadelphia meeting. Reminiscent of Osler's complaints about the 1878 Montreal meeting of the association, the scope of
topics presented at the 1884 meeting was broad, however, and included
botany, comparative anatomy, and morphology as well as physiology.
Moreover, most of the papers were based on descriptive rather than experimental techniques. The need for a society that addressed the special
needs of the physiologists was becoming more apparent.

Although several factors set the stage for the formation of the American Physiological Society in the mid-1880s, the catalyst was a political
fight within the American Medical Association. In 1884, the AMA selected eight members including Austin Flint, Sr., and John S. Billings to
discuss with officials of the International Medical Congress in Copenhagen the possibility of holding the 1887 International Congress in the
United States. This proposal was accepted, and, upon their return to
America, thirty-four additional physicians were invited to join in the
planning of the congress. Resentment over the composition of the larger
committee led the AMA to appoint a new committee of thirty-eight physicians to replace the original group. Not surprisingly, substantial ani-
mosity resulted between members of the original committee, comprised
of many of the leaders of scientific medicine, and the new committee,
made up primarily of practitioners.[28]

The original officers of the International Medical Congress of 1887 included Austin Flint, Sr., Henry I. Bowditch, John S. Billings, John C. Dalton, Jr., Francis Delafield, Christopher Johnston, Joseph Leidy, S. Weir Mitchell, and Horatio C. Wood, Jr. They hoped the congress would provide an opportunity for American physiologists and other basic scientists to present their work before an international audience. The original section on physiology included Dalton as president, Martin as one of three vice-presidents, and John G. Curtis as secretary. As noted earlier, Billings invited Bowditch to serve as president of the section on medical education, legislation, and registration. After the original planning committee was replaced, most of the men who would soon become founding members of the American Physiological Society declined any office in connection with the congress. All three founders of the American Physiological Society (Mitchell, Bowditch, and Martin), along with Dalton and Curtis, withdrew their support from the congress and refused to participate in any capacity. The withdrawal of America's most productive physiologists from the congress eliminated an opportunity for these individuals to meet to discuss their mutual interests in scientific medicine, and to demonstrate to the world that American medical science was coming of age.

The actions of the AMA in reconstituting the leadership of the 1887 congress and the resultant resignation of many of the leaders of American medical science precipitated harsh criticism. Among the complaints was that "the changes made by the Committee in the appointees of the Congress are not of a character to inspire the very highest order of scientific work. . . . This action will have but one result, that of lowering the standard of scientific work in this country and of introducing into the ranks of the profession an element of discord and disturbance which cannot be effaced during the next generation."[29] The international congress was held, and the chairman of the physiology section was John H. Callender, an alienist who held the chair of physiology and psychology at the University of Nashville.[30]

Several American physiologists participated in the newly formed scientific and medical societies. Some scientifically oriented physicians who had resigned from the international congress collaborated to organize the Congress of American Physicians and Surgeons.[31] Billings was elected president of the congress at the organizational meeting held in November 1887, and the participants decided that the congress would be held in Washington in September 1888.

Claudius Mastin, an Alabama surgeon with a "keen interest in the advance of medical science," had proposed the formation of the Congress of American Physicians and Surgeons at the 1886 meeting of the American Surgical Association. Practical as well as intellectual concerns stimulated Mastin. He was impressed by the recent growth of special medical societies, and recognized that many leaders of American medicine and medical science held memberships in several of these societies. Unless the meetings of the organizations were coordinated, many interested members would be unable to attend some of the gatherings because of the distance, time, and expense involved in participating in several meetings. The solution, Mastin argued, was to establish a congress comprised of the members of the leading specialty societies. This congress, which would meet triennially in Washington, was to be an elite gathering with membership limited to individuals who were fellows of one of the recognized specialty societies.[32]

The congress was to focus on medical science, not medical politics. The AMA was viewed as a political organization, and, even before the revolt of the mid-1880s, some individuals questioned whether its meetings were a good forum for the promotion of scientific medicine. One such person was Bowditch's uncle, Henry I. Bowditch, who was president of the AMA in 1877. Although he believed the AMA a useful organization, the elder Bowditch told its members in his presidential address:

> How, I would ask, is it possible for an association which meets
> only once a year, which migrates from Maine to San Francisco,
> which annually changes its officers, which allows every one to be
> a contributor to its transactions, instead of seeking the noblest
> minds of the profession and winning them to labor for it,—how is
> it possible for such a society to have any real scientific work done
> at its meetings? It seems to me vain to hope that any such society
> can, of itself, carry on, to any great extent, fine scientific work.[33]

Victor Vaughan, a founding member of the American Physiological Society, remarked on an effect of the shortcomings of the association: "In the eighties the sections of the American Medical Association were so barren in scientific interests that many special societies came into existence. In some of these I found most nourishing intellectual food."[34]

In order for the physiologists to be represented at the 1888 Congress of American Physicians and Surgeons, they had to form a society. Participation in the congress was limited to "members of the nine Societies . . . and of such other societies as may be elected by a unanimous vote of the Executive Committee."[35] Although he could participate as a member of either the Association of American Physicians or the American Neurological Association (he was a founding member of both), Weir Mitchell suggested the formation of a national organization of physiologists. It is likely that Mitchell learned of the plans for the congress from his close friend William Pepper, who was chairman of its executive committee. Mitchell probably viewed the proposed congress as an opportunity for America's experimental physiologists to join together as they had hoped to do at the International Congress which they would now boycott. Mitchell proposed the organization of a society for physiologists to Henry Bowditch, and Mitchell's name appeared first on a mimeographed circular sent out from Bowditch's laboratory on 10 November 1887 inviting interested individuals to participate in the formation of a "National Physiological Society."[36]

In the summer of 1887, Bowditch and Mitchell had discussed the timing of the organizational meeting of the new physiological society. The Harvard physiologist informed the Philadelphia neurologist, "There seems to be a good deal of difference of opinion about the best time for a preliminary meeting. It has been suggested that we postpone the meeting until the Christmas recess & then have it either in New Haven or New York just before or just after the meeting of the Soc. of Naturalists. How does this strike you? I think it is very important to have the meeting when both you & Martin can be present."[37] Several original members of the American Physiological Society were already members of the Society of Naturalists, such as Bowditch and Martin, and Bowditch's suggestion reflects this fact. Bowditch, Martin, and Mitchell decided to hold their organizational meeting in New York during the Christmas break to coincide with the naturalists' meeting. Although their backgrounds, institutional circumstances, and daily activities differed, these three individuals shared an interest in the promotion of scientific medicine and the encouragement and protection of research. They now had an opportunity to formalize the network of experimentalists that had gradually developed in American medical science in part because of their efforts.

Membership in the American Physiological Society would be restricted to individuals trained in modern experimental physiology. Contemporary scientists were becoming aware of the distinction between amateurs and professionals. Charles S. Minot, a founding member of both the Society of Naturalists and the American Physiological Society, claimed the former society was the first national scientific organization in America whose membership was restricted to "professional scientific investigators." It set an example, Minot argued, for several other scientific societies formed during the next quarter century.[38] A reviewer of the 1886 meeting of the Society of Naturalists pointed out the significance of the criteria for membership: "The strict enforcement of the rule limiting membership to persons 'who regularly devote a considerable portion of their time to the advancement of natural history' allows only a slow growth to the society, but it insures the illumination of the association by its members, rather than the reverse."[39]

The American Physiological Society was formed in the context of several identifiable trends, and in response to certain specific events in the United States. Specialization was increasingly common in postbellum America, and its advocates were winning converts in the closing years of the nineteenth century. Not only were disciplines developing within medicine and the broad areas of physical and natural science; there was progressive specialization in business, manufacturing, agriculture, and virtually every segment of American society. Scientists and physicians witnessed these trends at home and abroad.

Although it was a highly regarded organization, the Society of Naturalists did not address the specific needs of the physiologists. In 1884, when he reaffirmed the dominant position of physiology in his biology program at Johns Hopkins, Martin was confronted by a hostile response from leading naturalists who were reluctant to see physiology developed at the expense of morphology and related descriptive sciences. The techniques, apparatus, and approaches used by the naturalists were becoming increasingly irrelevant to the experimental physiologists. Moreover, the naturalists did not share the physiologists' commitment to medical reform; naturalists did not seek employment in medical schools; physiologists did. A new organization that addressed the specific needs of experimental physiologists seemed both appropriate and necessary.

By 1887, the research ethic that characterized the Johns Hopkins University from its inception was being adopted by many leading American institutions of higher learning, but few medical schools. Things were changing, however. As a result of the persistent efforts of reformers such as Mitchell and Bowditch, who sought more emphasis on science in the medical curriculum, career opportunities in the basic medical sciences were gradually appearing. Medical scientists such as Henry Bowditch and Newell Martin, scientifically oriented practitioners such as Weir Mitchell and William Osler, editors such as George Shrady and Minis Hays, and educators such as Daniel Gilman, Charles Eliot, and James Angell had formed a coalition for the encouragement of medical science whose impact was beginning to be felt in the leading medical schools of the United States.

By organizing the American Physiological Society, the three founders—Mitchell, Bowditch, and Martin—had an opportunity to establish the society's agenda, set the standards of admission, and solidify their informal network of scientists into the first national organization for experimental physiologists.[40] The formation of such an organization would also yield practical benefits. Members could look to the society to aid them in fending off the repeated attacks of the antivivisectionists. Equally important, the society could serve to promote the professional interests of its members.

As was true of many scientific organizations formed in this era, amateurs were not encouraged to join the American Physiological Society. The increasing sophistication of experimental techniques and apparatus now made it difficult for amateur physiologists to compete in the field of experimental physiology. Membership in the American Physiological Society served to distinguish the new professional physiologists from the practitioner-teachers who usually had little commitment to (or at least little opportunity to perform) research. Although there were still very few professional physiologists, there were indications that career opportunities would increase. Bowditch and Martin had been training advanced workers in science for more than a decade and helped some of their pupils find full-time positions in physiology or related scientific fields. More jobs were needed, however. Medical schools had to be convinced that their chairs of physiology should be held by experimentalists who were willing to devote their whole time to teaching and research in this scientific discipline.

The American Physiological Society provided its members with an opportunity to meet with other basic medical scientists with mutual intellectual interests and political concerns. Members received a list of fellow scientists who shared their ambitions, fears, and frustrations. The society's scientific program made it possible for participants to present results based on their research, claim priority for discovery, and elicit comments from knowledgeable peers before publication. As was true with the naturalists, the physiologists believed their society should provide a forum for discussing technical problems related to the methods they used in their research. Because the annual meetings were to be held in different cities, it would be possible for the physiologists to see their colleagues' facilities and apparatus and meet their pupils. Demonstrations of equipment and techniques became a standard part of the meetings. Moreover, local physicians and medical school faculty members and officers could see that American physiology was now represented by a group of sophisticated and productive scientists, most of whom devoted their whole time to this endeavor.

The meetings also served an important social function. In 1887, there were few experimental physiologists in America, and, as Samuel Clarke had found when he went to Williams College, intellectual isolation was a problem. A decade earlier, Newell Martin had written to Henry Bowditch acknowledging William James's visit to Baltimore: "It is a great pleasure to me here to meet anyone with whom I can talk a little physiological 'shop.' "[41] The job market for full-time experimental physiologists was gradually expanding as more institutions included practical laboratory exercises in physiology in their curricula or built physiological laboratories for demonstrations and research. The meetings of the American Physiological Society provided an opportunity for recent graduates of scientific training programs to meet seasoned researchers and individuals with institutional contacts who might facilitate their goal of finding employment.

Regular meetings also provided an opportunity for the physiologists to plan an agenda. The issues might include stimulating the development of a job market for newly trained physiologists, encouraging officials of medical schools and institutions of higher learning to adopt the research ethic and the full-time concept for teachers of the basic medical sciences, encouraging philanthropists to support research, organizing against the antivivisectionists, developing an American-based specialty publication in physiology, and finally, demonstrating to European scientists that a profession of physiology was now established in the United States. Although the original members of the American Physiological Society had done many of these things individually for several years, they would now have the encouragement and support of a group who shared their goals.

The three founders were well established in their careers by the time they organized the American Physiological Society in 1887. Mitchell, although largely occupied in the practice of neurology, continued to publish occasional papers based upon research in toxicology, the lifelong focus of his interest in physiology. Martin's program in Baltimore had produced several biomedical scientists. The publications that came from his department were highly regarded in the international scientific community. Like Martin's, Bowditch's physiology department at Harvard, established more than fifteen years earlier, was held in high regard by American and foreign scientists. All three were active in several societies. Bowditch was a founding member of the Boston Society of Medical Sciences organized in December 1887. The object of that society was "the promotion of the sciences connected with medicine."[42]

The organizational meeting of the American Physiological Society was held in December 1887 in the new physiological laboratory of the

College of Physicians and Surgeons of New York. Although he was invited to be a founding member of the society, John Dalton did not participate in this meeting. Weir Mitchell noted that before Dalton's death in February 1889 he had suffered "a long and painful illness . . . and one by one he fell out of the public and social relations which made life valuable to others and pleasant to both them and himself."[43] By the time the American Physiological Society was formed, John Curtis had held the physiology chair at the College of Physicians and Surgeons for four years and Dalton's professional activities were confined largely to his duties as president of the institution. Curtis had recently acquired an extensive collection of modern physiological apparatus that would have been of interest to individuals attending the first meeting of the new society. Although Curtis did not share the deep personal commitment to research of Mitchell, Bowditch, Martin, or his teacher and predecessor Dalton, he acknowledged the importance of this activity and encouraged it.

The constitution of the American Physiological Society drew heavily on that of the Physiological Society in England.[44] The stated goal in organizing the American Physiological Society was "to promote the advance of Physiology and to facilitate personal intercourse between American Physiologists." Eligibility for election as an ordinary member of the society was restricted to residents of North America who had "conducted and published an original research in Physiology or Histology (including Pathology and experimental Therapeutics and experimental research and Hygiene), or who has promoted and encouraged Physiological research." This rule, although it does not sound particularly restrictive, was used to exclude from membership individuals who did not have a sincere commitment to research.

Upon Martin's premature death in 1896, Bowditch declared:

> Probably few of the younger members of the Society are aware of the great debt which we owe to Doctor Martin for establishing the high standard which the Society has always maintained with regard to the qualifications of the members. It was always Doctor Martin's contention that a candidate for admission to our ranks should be required to demonstrate his power to enlarge the bounds of our chosen science, and not merely to display an interest in the subject and an ability to teach text-book physiology to medical students. To his wise counsel in this matter the present prosperity of the Society is, I think, largely to be attributed.[45]

Although most individuals nominated for membership in the American Physiological Society during its early years were elected, some were not. Weir Mitchell and Horatio Wood proposed their fellow Philadel-phian Frances Emily White for membership in 1895. The council of the (all male) society, consisting of Henry Bowditch, Russell Chittenden, William Howell, and Frederic Lee, rejected the candidate "on the grounds that the publications submitted by the candidate did not fulfill, from the standpoint of original research, the qualifications of member-ship demanded by the society."[46]

As was true of the American Society of Naturalists, the restrictions placed on membership in the American Physiological Society had im-plications for the size and rate of growth of this specialty organization. Although the society was founded to acknowledge the existence of a discipline whose fundamental method was experimentation on living animals, the original members had a wide range of scientific interests. William Howell, who was present at the organizational meeting of the society, later recalled, "It was only possible to get together about two dozen who could qualify, even counting the embryo-physiologists of the new laboratories and the near physiologists of the medical profession."[47] Another founder, Frederick Ellis, recalled at the society's semicenten-nial, "In those days almost all the real physiologists in the country could be counted on the fingers and toes, and a number of the gentlemen present at the first meeting did not claim to be physiologists, but were interested in closely related subjects."[48]

The influence of Martin and Bowditch, and to a lesser degree Mitchell, on the original membership of the American Physiological Society is dramatic.[49] Of the twenty-eight founding members, two-thirds were affiliated, at the time the society was organized, with Johns Hopkins, Harvard, the University of Pennsylvania, or the College of Physicians and Surgeons of New York. (See appendix 2.) The largest number, 21 percent, were affiliated with Johns Hopkins. Of those indi-viduals elected to membership between 1888 and 1899, Johns Hopkins and Harvard affiliates were most numerous. Among the individuals who were not at Johns Hopkins or Harvard when they were elected to mem-bership, many had previously received scientific training at those insti-tutions. The prominence of Johns Hopkins and Harvard affiliates in the membership roll of the society during its first decade is not surprising. At this time, these two institutions afforded the greatest opportunities for graduate work in experimental physiology in the United States.

Other characteristics of the original members of the society are of interest. The members were young: the average age of the twenty-eight founders was thirty-seven years. The geographic origins of the founders reflected the continued dominance of the Northeast in the "production" of scientists.[50] With the exception of those associated with Johns Hopkins, the institutional affiliations in 1887 of the founders reflected their state of birth: all of the original members associated with the University of Pennsylvania or Jefferson Medical College were born in Pennsylvania; and all of those affiliated with Harvard were born in Massachusetts. The three foreign-born founders (Henry Beyer, Joseph Jastrow, and Newell Martin) were affiliated with Johns Hopkins, as were individuals born in Massachusetts, Connecticut, and New York. The geographic heterogeneity of the Hopkins affiliates reflected the philosophy of Gilman and the Hopkins trustees. Unlike traditional American institutions of higher learning that drew their faculty and pupils from the local geographic area, Johns Hopkins attracted qualified faculty members and advanced workers from the entire continent and abroad.

It is interesting to compare the Association of American Anatomists, organized in 1888, with the American Physiological Society. Although formed at the same time, and devoted to the two traditional medical sciences, these organizations had different goals. The founders of the Association of American Anatomists claimed their object was "the advancement of anatomical sciences," but they did not restrict their membership to individuals committed to research. Charles Bardeen described the association as it existed in 1891: "There were 84 members. Of these 44 were professors and instructors in various medical schools, scarcely half a dozen of whom could properly be called scientific investigators."[51] Philadelphia had long been a stronghold for anatomy and morphology. It is not surprising, therefore, that the Association of American Anatomists included a disproportionate number of individuals from Pennsylvania, especially Philadelphia. Only one member came from Maryland compared with nineteen from Pennsylvania.

The diversity of scientific interests among the founders of the American Physiological Society has been mentioned. Publications that appeared from the physiological laboratories at Harvard, Johns Hopkins, the College of Physicians and Surgeons of New York, and the University of Pennsylvania in this era reflected the broad range of subjects studied in these facilities. Sophisticated physiological apparatus available in these laboratories could be used to investigate a wide range of problems. Moreover, these early laboratories often served as the institutional focal point for individuals interested in biomedical research, whether their area was experimental physiology, pharmacology, or bacteriology.

Although the scope of investigations undertaken in these pioneering experimental physiological laboratories was broad, each facility had one or two dominant themes. These usually reflected the interest of the professor. At Harvard, cardiovascular physiology and neurophysiology predominated, interests Bowditch had developed while he was Carl Ludwig's pupil. At Johns Hopkins, cardiovascular physiology was the main research theme after Martin had developed the isolated mammalian heart preparation. Moreover, cardiovascular physiology was the major focus of research in Foster's laboratory, where Martin became a physiologist. Mitchell's interest in toxicology influenced the orientation of the University of Pennsylvania group. Hobart Hare, Edward Reichert, and Horatio Wood pursued studies that would now be considered pharmacology.[52] This group's interest in drugs can also be traced to the influence of George B. Wood, an American pioneer of materia medica and therapeutics.

In 1887, physiology was *the* experimental medical science in the United States. Consequently, individuals who eventually came to be identified with other basic medical sciences became members of the American Physiological Society. It gave them an opportunity to join with other Americans who were imbued with the research ethic and who sought to encourage the adoption of the full-time system in the basic medical sciences. The original members acknowledged the importance of the approach that was embodied in experimental physiology. Founders Victor Vaughan and Russell Chittenden shared an interest in physiological chemistry, a field with origins in medical chemistry that had been transformed by experimental approaches adapted from modern physiology. Chittenden, who served as the society's president from 1896 to 1904, explained that physiological chemistry was considered part of physiology in this era: "It was not to be set apart as a thing by itself, neither was it to be looked on as distinctly chemical. The main purpose of physiological chemistry is to study and explain, so far as possible, the chemical functions of the living organism and such being the case, it belongs with, and is part of, physiology. That . . . was the view held by a majority of the members of the American Physiological Society."[53]

Experimental physiology had growing relevance for fields that were traditionally viewed as morphologic as well. Founder William H. Welch, although primarily a pathologist and bacteriologist, had studied with Carl Ludwig in addition to several leaders of European pathology. He told Daniel Gilman in 1885, "Experimental physiology is the basis of experimental pathology."[54] Welch urged Franklin Mall to devote some time to physiology during his postgraduate training in Europe. "I do not believe that you will ever regret the time you give to experimental physi-

THE AMERICAN PHYSIOLOGICAL SOCIETY

ological work. It opens up quite a new perspective in medicine."[55] Welch believed that the advance of experimental physiology was directly linked to the reform of medical education. He claimed in 1916, "The physiological laboratory is traced, in this country, mainly to the work of Bowditch in Boston and Newell Martin at Johns Hopkins, but it cannot be said, I think, that physiology had taken the place which it should hold in medical education much before a quarter of a century ago. One of the great marks of progress in medical education is due to the recognition of the fundamental nature of physiological study for the training of the physician."[56] Welch became one of the strongest advocates of expanding the philosophy of the physiologists to all of the basic medical sciences, and, ultimately, to the clinical branches of medical education.

As with any social organization, certain members of the American Physiological Society had more influence on the group than did others. The elected officers were, as one would expect, in a position to shape the character of the society. During the first five years, Bowditch and Mitchell served as the society's president and Martin was secretary-treasurer. In addition to them, members of the council during these early years included John Curtis, Horatio Wood, and Russell Chittenden. Individuals who regularly attended the meetings undoubtedly played a more significant role in setting the agenda of the society than those who infrequently participated. There was a wide spectrum of participation by the twenty-eight original members in the annual meetings. The individuals who most consistently attended included the leading physiologists of the next generation. Founding members who attended 50 percent or more of the annual meetings between 1888 and 1899 included Henry Beyer, Henry Bowditch, Russell Chittenden, John Curtis, William Howell, Warren Lombard, Edward Reichert, and Joseph Warren. Before his return to England in 1893, Martin attended all but one of the meetings of the society. Mitchell's attendance dropped off in the middle of the 1890s as he became increasingly involved in other activities related to his interests in neurology, clinical medicine, and writing. Some of the founders attended few meetings or dropped out altogether as their interests changed or as their needs were better met by other organizations.

Several factors contributed to the pattern of attendance at the early meetings of the American Physiological Society. An average of 38 percent of the members attended the annual meetings between 1888 and 1899. The members held special triennial meetings, reflecting one of the original stimuli for founding the society, with the Congress of American

Physicians and Surgeons in September in addition to the regular annual December meetings. No consistent trend in attendance appears to depend on geographic location of the regular meeting with the exception of the 1897 meeting held in Ithaca, New York. Two factors help explain the low attendance at this meeting; held in December in conjunction with the American Society of Naturalists. It followed a special September meeting and Cornell University had no physiological laboratory.

The membership of the American Physiological Society steadily grew from twenty-eight to seventy-three between 1888 and 1899. A review of the attendance data at the nineteenth-century meetings of the society does not support the conclusion of one recent historian: "The chronic ill-health of the American Physiological Society . . . was symptomatic of the fragile condition of the discipline. Attendance at annual meetings dropped to a handful in the mid-1890s, and it was uncertain for some years whether the society would survive."[57] (See appendix 3.) The majority of the most active members in the society were once associated with Harvard or Johns Hopkins. Of the founding members who attended more than one-half of the annual meetings between 1888 and 1899, one-third had affiliations with Hopkins, one-third with Harvard, and the remaining one-third represented Yale, the College of Physicians and Surgeons of New York, and the University of Pennsylvania. In addition to the nine founders who attended more than one-half of the meetings between 1888 and 1899, several members elected in the earliest years of the American Physiological Society who frequently attended the regular meetings were Clifton Hodge, Frederic Lee, Graham Lusk, Samuel Meltzer, John Abel, and William Porter. This group of fifteen individuals were most active in the affairs of the society, both in terms of presenting papers and in determining its policies and agenda. Moreover, several were active participants in the reform movement to make American medicine more scientific.

The minutes of the early meetings of the American Physiological Society shed little light on the agenda of its members. Other manuscript sources provide some insight into their concerns, however. Curtis assumed the active role Dalton had played in the fight against the antivivisectionists and welcomed a group of allies. Communication and coordination among the experimental physiologists on the issue of vivisection were mandatory in Curtis's view. Shortly after the organization of the society, he claimed, "I have, unhappily, only too much familiarity with the law about 'vivisection' as I have in past years had repeatedly to waste my own time, & to see that of others wasted, in defending against its repeal. . . . All who are interested in experimental medicine should bear always in mind that the least indiscretion on the part of one will probably involve great injury & hardship to all the rest."[58]

Other members of the American Physiological Society were also active in the effort to limit the effectiveness of the antivivisectionists. In 1895, Mitchell, together with Curtis, Bowditch, and Martin's successor Howell, circulated a printed letter to America's leading biomedical scientists encouraging them to sign a formal statement in support of vivisection. Their letter also revealed the physiologists' goal of reforming medical education:

> The public should be informed concerning the relation between animal experimentation and the progress of general biology. They should be made to see that medical teaching is a university function, that the medical sciences are experimental and that they can be taught only by the experimental method. They should be told that to cut off research and demonstration on living animals would be as senseless as to cut off laboratory teaching in physics and chemistry and would bring medical teaching at a single blow to the level of the middle ages, to a blind reliance on authority instead of independent observation. It is in our opinion advisable to unite on a plan by which the scientific opinion of the community can be rapidly collected and effectively used.[59]

With Howell substituting for his departed mentor Martin, the signers of this letter represented the founders of the American Physiological Society.

These physiologists proposed that a coalition of representatives from six specialty societies be formed to combat the antivivisectionists. That group would then draft a document in support of animal experimentation that would be widely distributed after review by the constituent organizations. This effort was a success, and thirty-four individuals signed a document entitled " 'Vivisection' a Statement in Behalf of Science" that was circulated as a pamphlet and published in *Science* early in 1896. Half of the individuals who signed the document were members of the American Physiological Society. The version published in *Science* was supplemented by an introductory note signed by Charles W. Eliot, Francis A. Walker, president of the Massachusetts Institute of Technology, and Frank K. Paddock, president of the Massachusetts Medical Society. They claimed the statement "sets forth the importance of animal experimentation for the advancement of medicine, and may be accepted as an authoritative expression of expert opinion on this question."[60] This brief document bore witness to the emergence of a coalition of educators, full-time biomedical scientists, and representatives of the medical profession. Because of their dedication to the research ethic, the leaders of the American Physiological Society coordinated the efforts of those interested in reforming medical education in order to make medicine more scientific. Their response to the antivivisectionists now became a vehicle for encouraging a broader audience to support the ideals of the scientific reform movement. Only by expanding their coalition, and by encouraging the endowment of the expensive new scientific curriculum, could the physiologists and their fellow biomedical scientists hope to see their fields develop in the United States.

Curtis's laboratory at the College of Physicians and Surgeons of New York was equipped for physiological investigation, but inadequate funding and staffing kept it from becoming a major center of research in the nineteenth century. Curtis, who attended all but one of the regular society meetings between 1888 and 1898, found that the American Physiological Society satisfied certain of his needs. He hinted at his sense of intellectual isolation in a letter to Franklin Mall in 1891: "The longer I live the more I appreciate the 'touch of elbow' among the few men who are really interested in the things that you & I care for."[61] For Curtis, the society provided a forum for sharing concerns about the role of the basic medical sciences in the medical school curriculum, philanthropic support for research, the ongoing antivivisection debate, and related issues.

The society sought to expand the number of positions for its members as full-time basic medical scientists. Several members of the society expressed concern about the limited opportunities for scientific careers in medicine in this era. Writing to Franklin Mall in 1886, William Welch declared, "It is a great misfortune of our country that the opportunities are so few for man's engaging in scientific medical work."[62] Welch expressed the same concern two years later when Mall was considering a job offer at Clark University. The Hopkins pathologist asserted, "One thing ought to be considered that positions such as you are offered at Clark, in fact any kind of position where a man can carry on scientific work with a reasonable pecuniary support, are very scanty in this country."[63]

Although the American job market for scientists was gradually expanding in the late nineteenth century, positions were, as Welch claimed, still scarce. The American Physiological Society provided young biomedical scientists with a credential that could be used to make them more competitive in the scientific job market. Recurrent pulmonary problems, ultimately discovered to be due to tuberculosis, led Henry Sewall to request a year's leave of absence from the University of Michigan in the summer of 1888. Sewall nominated Joseph W. Warren, an instructor in Bowditch's physiology department at the Harvard Medical School, to serve in his absence. Sewall and Warren had both attended the founding meeting of the American Physiological Society in December 1887. Sewall informed the Michigan board of regents, "Dr. Warren is well known as a physiologist both in this country and abroad. He is one of the original members of the American Physiological Society, and has for several years been associated with the distinguished physiologist Prof. H. P. Bowditch. He has had considerable practical experience both in the work of the laboratory and in the lecture room. Dr. Warren is the author of numerous original papers."[64]

With the organization of the American Physiological Society, physiologists who belonged to the society were set apart from individuals who did not. Most members elected after the founding meeting joined the society when they held junior faculty appointments in medical school departments of physiology. Amateurs were not invited to join. One of the few medical practitioners among the founders was Isaac Ott who taught physiology part time but practiced medicine in Easton, Pennsylvania. Ott, who had previously worked with both Bowditch and Martin, was a prolific author and an American pioneer of pharmacology. Bowditch visited Ott's private laboratory in Easton, Pennsylvania, in the spring of 1889 and declared, "He is a most industrious little man. He manages to find time to do a great deal of excellent scientific work in the intervals of active practice. He must have an iron constitution."[65]

With the growing awareness of the distinction between amateur and professional scientists in this era, members of the American Physiological Society emphasized the incompatibility of successful physiological research and medical practice. Experimental physiology was now dominated by vivisection and instruments of precision, and it was difficult for practicing physicians to participate meaningfully in physiological research. William T. Porter, an 1885 graduate of St. Louis Medical College, whose interest in physiology was inspired by his German-born teacher of physiology Gustav Baumgarten and his recent exposure to German laboratories, informed his mentor in 1890:

> There can be no question that I can be more useful in St. Louis as
> a physiologist than as a practitioner. The making of a physiological
> institute in our community is worth living for. It is not possible
> to succeed in such an undertaking and to succeed in practice at
> the same time. To practice medicine and experimental physiology
> is to be an amateur in two things. I must make a choice. I must be
> one thing or the other. Physiology means absolute poverty for
> some years, comparative poverty during life. Practice means giv-

ing up the best thing in sight for the sake of material comforts.
These are the horns of the dilemma. I believe that I have chosen
wisely.

Porter's letter also reveals one of the reasons the job market for experimental physiologists was expanding. Medical schools that wanted to be
viewed as progressive could no longer ignore the trend toward full-time
basic medical science faculties and a curriculum that emphasized practical training in the laboratory and hospital. Porter explained, "The [St.
Louis Medical] College must very soon have a professional physiologist.
That such a thing pays is shown by the fact that Bellevue and Jefferson
find it to their interest. The schools with whom we wish to compete,
with whom we must compete, are already provided with professional
physiologists."[66]

The American Physiological Society made a modest but visible
commitment to scientific research with the establishment of a physiology prize in 1890. Mitchell, who was wealthy as a result of his successful
practice, sponsored the $200 prize. Designed "to encourage physiologi-
cal research," the prize would be awarded to the American who submitted the best paper based on research on the transmission of nerve im-
pulses or reflex action.[67] There were no papers submitted in response,
however. Perhaps this result is not surprising in view of the few Americans capable of undertaking experimental work of this nature and the
limited number of facilities adequately equipped for such a study. Unde-
terred, Mitchell, in the name of the society, offered a $250 prize the fol-
lowing year for the best paper on the regeneration of severed spinal
nerves. This prize was awarded to William Howell, Martin's former student, then at the University of Michigan, and Carl Huber, assistant professor of histology and embryology at Michigan. Mitchell urged the society to sponsor research and continued, anonymously, to subsidize these
efforts.

The enthusiasm for research voiced by several founders of the
American Physiological Society was rarely matched by opportunities at
America's medical schools in this era. William Howell changed institutions three times in six years in the hope that he would have more time
for research and less responsibility for elementary instruction. Following
the receipt of his doctorate from Johns Hopkins in 1884, Howell became
chief assistant in Martin's department with the title of assistant professor
of biology. Although Joseph Warren delivered the lectures at Michigan
in Sewall's absence during the 1888–89 term, his appointment was not
permanent. Sewall recommended Howell, his former colleague at Johns

Hopkins, as his successor in Ann Arbor. Writing from Baltimore, Howell explained to James B. Angell, president of the University of Michigan:

> The chief drawback to the pleasant position I hold at present is that the onerous duty of instructing thirty or more men in practical laboratory work—together with my lectures and executive duties leave me little or no time for original research. I understand that the Ann Arbor position offers opportunities for work of this kind and I therefore feel very anxious to obtain it, as I am prepared for and more than desirous of utilizing every chance to engage in good physiological work.[68]

Howell took the position at Ann Arbor but soon discovered he had not escaped the conflict between teaching and research.

The creation of the American Physiological Society formalized a network of scientists who sought to facilitate the careers of young physiologists. Although several of the founders had stable academic positions in the early 1890s, most of the younger members, like Howell, held poorly paid junior faculty positions that required them to devote much of their time to elementary teaching or simple demonstrations. Despite growing acceptance of the full-time concept for basic medical scientists, few positions were available to physiologists before the twentieth century. It was uncommon, even at leading medical schools, for there to be more than one, or at most two, full-time physiology positions. A second faculty post might be held by a poorly paid demonstrator. Eventually, however, junior faculty positions became available in response to the introduction of practical laboratory training for medical students.

Because the number of full-time positions for basic medical scientists and the pool of suitably trained individuals seeking to devote themselves to physiology were both small, career moves among the second generation of professional physiologists were often interdependent. This correlation is illustrated by a rather striking series of moves precipitated by the addition of a faculty position in physiology at the College of Physicians and Surgeons of New York in 1891. Following Dalton's death in 1889, James McLane assumed the presidency of the college. The following year he asked John Curtis to write a report on the status and needs of the physiology department. In his response, Curtis revealed the difficulties he confronted in attempting to introduce modern experimental physiology at the college.

Through his contacts with fellow members of the American Physiological Society, and his visit to European laboratories a few years earlier, Curtis was aware of the shortcomings of the college's physiology program. He argued that his department should perform three functions: provide basic instruction to medical students by lectures and demonstrations, train advanced workers for careers in physiology, and afford an opportunity for qualified individuals to undertake research. Now that the college had an adequate laboratory and modern apparatus, staffing was the major impediment to pursuing this agenda; Curtis was the only paid faculty member. Earlier, Curtis had paid Warren Lombard to serve as his assistant, but now his only helpers were medical student volunteers and the school's janitor when he was available. Curtis explained that much of his time was devoted to the preparation of routine demonstrations for elementary lectures, which precluded his attention to the "higher duties" of research and advanced teaching.

In order to expand the activities of the department, Curtis requested a full-time assistant who should,

> as the Professor now does, give his whole time to the College; and be of so high a class as to be regarded as the most promising candidate for the reversion of the Professorship. A physiologist has not, like a chemist, or an electrical expert, any opportunity to combine other remunerative work with his College duties; far less can he practice medicine. His work leads away from all so-called "practical" opportunities and depends wholly for its support upon the institution he serves. The Assistant's salary must therefore, suffice to attach an unmarried man to the College for a number of years.

Thus, he was now arguing that a full-time assistant was necessary to expand the goals of his department. This pattern would gradually appear at the leading medical schools throughout America. Curtis emphasized the central role of physiology in medical education and declared that it was also the foundation upon which experimental pathology and pharmacology were built. Noting the proposed union of the College of Physicians and Surgeons with Columbia College, he explained that his department should serve as the focal point for the scientific workers of both institutions. Physiology was no longer a subject of interest only to physicians. "Many eminent Physiologists today, are Doctors of Philosophy, and not of medicine." Curtis claimed, "Physiology holds a conspicuous place among the so-called Biological sciences, widely studied for their own sake, and not for medical purposes at all."[69]

When the merger between Columbia College and the College of Physicians and Surgeons became final in the spring of 1891, the medical faculty requested the board of trustees to enlarge the teaching staff in the basic medical sciences. A second paid position was created in the physi-

ology department: a demonstrator whose duties, in addition to the traditional responsibilities of preparing demonstrations for lectures, would
include an obligation "to carry on such original researches as the Professor shall approve [and] . . . to devote his entire working time to the
study, teaching and advancing of Physiology at Columbia College."[70]
The creation of this position initiated a series of interrelated career
moves among the second-generation physiologists.

The new position was filled by Frederic S. Lee, who had received a
doctorate in biology at Johns Hopkins in 1885 and subsequently spent a
year in Carl Ludwig's physiological institute. After his return to the
United States, Lee served as an instructor in Martin's laboratory at Johns
Hopkins until 1887 when he went to Bryn Mawr College to teach biology. Bryn Mawr had opened in 1885, and its character was strongly influenced by the Johns Hopkins University.[71] The biology department at
Bryn Mawr was patterned after Martin's in Baltimore. Edmund B. Wilson, the first professor of biology at Bryn Mawr, was one of Martin's first
pupils, although his interests were in morphology, and he had worked
mainly with William K. Brooks.[72] Lee was elected to membership in the
American Physiological Society in 1888 and, with Curtis, regularly attended the meetings of the society.

Joseph Warren, an assistant in Bowditch's department since 1881,
left Harvard in 1892 to fill the vacancy created at Bryn Mawr by Lee's
departure. When Warren left Harvard, Martin's former pupil Howell
was selected to take his place. Writing to Bowditch from Ann Arbor, less
than three years after his arrival at the University of Michigan, Howell
revealed:

> In many ways such a position as you describe would be more
> agreeable to me than the one I hold at present. Yet in some re-
> spects the reverse is true. The laboratory here is well provided
> with apparatus and the regents are generous in making appropria-
> tions for new instruments. The position is one of great freedom as
> far as the kind and the extent of work is concerned but heretofore
> the amount of teaching in the medical and literary departments
> has been so heavy that but little leisure time is left for research—
> though they have promised me relief in this regard. . . . My ambi-
> tion as a physiologist is to investigate.[73]

Reflecting the concerns raised by Martin and Curtis regarding the
need for adequate salaries for junior faculty members, Howell explained
to Bowditch, "If the conditions of the position are such that you could
offer me a larger salary I should feel as though I could accept the position cheerfully at once. . . . Certainly a man can not do his best work

for his College if he feels that he must always be looking for chances to augment his income from sources other than his regular salary."[74] Howell accepted Bowditch's offer and left Ann Arbor to become associate professor of physiology at the Harvard Medical School in 1892.

The interrelated career moves continued. The chair of physiology at the University of Michigan vacated by Howell was filled by Warren Lombard who had ties to Harvard University, Johns Hopkins, the College of Physicians and Surgeons, and Carl Ludwig's laboratory. Lombard, an original member of the American Physiological Society, and frequent participant in its early meetings, received his medical degree from Harvard in 1881. While a medical student, he worked briefly in Bowditch's laboratory.[75] Following his graduation from Harvard, Lombard traveled to Europe for postgraduate training in preparation for a career as a medical practitioner. Once abroad, Lombard decided to study with Carl Ludwig, and while working in Ludwig's laboratory in 1883, he met two recent Michigan graduates, John J. Abel and Franklin P. Mall. From them, Lombard learned about Sewall's laboratory and the scientific program at the University of Michigan. Upon his return to New York in 1885, Lombard found, as had Welch a few years earlier, that full-time basic medical science positions were scarce in America. He hoped to find an opening in Bowditch's laboratory but none was available. Lombard asked Bowditch whether John G. Curtis was "a man under whom I can work to advantage?"[76] Curtis hired Lombard as his assistant at the College of Physicians and Surgeons paying the recent German-trained physiologist's salary out of his own pocket, since the college had not yet approved a second paid position in physiology.

Mall had an opportunity to renew his friendship with Lombard when he visited Curtis at the college in 1886.[77] They also were together at Johns Hopkins in 1887 when Lombard was a graduate student in Martin's department, and Mall was a fellow in Welch's pathology department. Lombard's position at the College of Physicians and Surgeons did not offer the promise of a secure future as a physiologist. A better opportunity arose in 1889 when G. Stanley Hall, president of Clark University, offered Lombard the position of assistant professor of physiology at the new Worcester, Massachusetts, institution. Hall probably met Lombard at Johns Hopkins in 1887 when Hall was professor of psychology at the Baltimore university. They both attended the 1887 organizational meeting of the American Physiological Society.

Lombard accepted the Clark position and was joined by Mall who was appointed adjunct professor of anatomy. William Welch had taken an interest in Lombard's career when the young physiologist worked in

Martin's laboratory. Upon hearing of his appointment at Clark, Welch congratulated Lombard: "I believe that this position will open to you just the opportunity which you want and that you are just the man for the place. The work which lies before you seems to me more congenial and promising in results than a similar one in connection with any of our existing medical schools."[78] Welch and Martin were anxious to facilitate the careers of their scientific pupils. Harry Friedenwald, a student of both men, was told by his mother while he was studying in Berlin in 1886: "You must not break your connection with people like Martin and Welch, for they take an interest and really feel proud when any of their men achieve something."[79]

The promise of Clark University as an institution devoted to graduate education with emphasis on research went largely unfulfilled; anticipated funding for the support of faculty and facilities was not forthcoming. A mass resignation of the Clark faculty took place in January 1892, and several staff members, including Mall, were recruited to the newly founded University of Chicago.[80] When he joined in the mass resignation from Clark University, Lombard was left without a job. The dean of the University of Michigan, Victor Vaughan, was present at the 1890 meeting of the American Physiological Society, as was Lombard. When it became apparent that Howell was going to leave the University of Michigan, Vaughan wrote to Lombard to ask him if he would be interested in the physiology chair in Ann Arbor. Lombard accepted the offer and moved to Michigan in 1892.

Few would have guessed that one of the nation's most productive physiologists, Newell Martin, would suffer from alcoholism complicated by an intermittent painful neuropathy and resign at the age of forty-five from the premier physiology position in America in 1893. The impending opening of the Johns Hopkins Medical School made the appointment of a successor especially important to the Hopkins officials. Daniel Gilman, who had followed William Howell's career for nearly fifteen years, invited the Hopkins graduate to become professor of physiology in the medical school. Although he had been at Harvard for less than a year, Howell resigned from Bowditch's department to return to his alma mater. His resignation created an opening in the Harvard physiology department that was filled by William Porter, one of the few second-generation full-time physiologists who had not studied under either Bowditch or Martin.

Membership in the American Physiological Society, rather than previous institutional affiliation, provided the link that led to Porter's appointment at Harvard. Porter consistently attended the meetings of the society following his election to membership in 1891. While studying in Europe in 1890, Porter had declared his intention to devote himself to a career in physiology. Although Gustav Baumgarten and Porter persuaded the St. Louis Medical College to equip a physiological laboratory for Porter upon his return from Europe, the young physiologist did not receive consistent support from the officers or faculty of the school. He complained to Baumgarten in 1892, "I think you also understand that this continual, and necessary, struggle for money is distasteful to the extent of making me almost morbid."[81]

As was true of Bowditch, Porter was interested in the reform of medical education and recognized the interdependence of this movement and the further development of the basic medical sciences, especially experimental physiology. Competition for medical students and related financial considerations had recently led to a reorganization of the medical schools in St. Louis. Porter believed that competition for students would lead to new opportunities for physiologists. He applauded the recent decision of his institution to replace a teacher of chemistry who used old methods of instruction and was not committed to research with a "real scientist."[82] Porter stopped in Baltimore on his way to Europe in the spring of 1893 and learned from William Osler and William Welch that Martin had resigned. Porter was also informed that Howell would be leaving Boston to succeed Martin at Johns Hopkins. As he had planned, Porter departed for Europe to spend the summer working in the physiological institute of the University of Berlin. He would soon be offered a position in Bowditch's department at the Harvard Medical School, however.[83]

Porter had presented the results of his innovative experiments on the effects of ligation of the coronary arteries to the members of the American Physiological Society in December 1892. Howell and Bowditch were both present at that meeting, as was Reichert with whom Porter had worked briefly in Philadelphia. It is not surprising that, in view of Bowditch's own interest in cardiovascular physiology, he thought of Porter when Howell's departure created a vacancy in his department in 1893. By Christmas, Porter had moved to Boston and was at work in Bowditch's department.

The common denominator in all of these career moves was membership in, and regular attendance at the meetings of, the American Physiological Society. All of the second-generation physiologists whose job changes between 1889 and 1893 have just been described were active members of the society in its early years. Howell, Lombard, Sewall, and Warren were present at the organizational meeting in 1887. The leaders of the American Physiological Society considered the younger members when vacancies occurred in the physiology departments of America's best medical schools.

This brief flurry of hectic job hunting in the years immediately following the formation of the American Physiological Society was followed by a long period of stability for several of the second-generation professional physiologists. At Johns Hopkins, Howell was head of physiology for a quarter of a century. Porter remained at the Harvard Medical School for the duration of his career, although he failed to succeed Bowditch whose physiology chair was awarded to Walter B. Cannon in 1906. Curtis held the chair of physiology at the College of Physicians and Surgeons of New York until 1909, when he was succeeded by Frederic S. Lee who had been at the college since 1891. Lee remained at the college for the rest of his long career. Reichert was chairman of the University of Pennsylvania physiology program for more than three decades. Although Mitchell remained active in the affairs of the University of Pennsylvania and continued to dabble in venom research, his involvement in the affairs of the physiology department was minimal. After Howell's brief tenure in Ann Arbor, his successor Lombard held the chair at the University of Michigan for three decades. Although Henry Chapman of Jefferson Medical College was not an active member of the American Physiological Society, he did contribute to the literature of physiology and held the chair at Jefferson for thirty years.

Thus, the physiology departments at the leading medical schools of America attained a certain degree of stability in the early 1890s, as did several of the second-generation professional physiologists. The most prestigious and financially secure positions went to individuals who were active members of the American Physiological Society. The society served, in a sense, as a clearinghouse for pupils of Martin and Bowditch who wished to devote themselves to full-time careers in physiology. In the final decade of the nineteenth century, when better positions arose, the individuals who filled them were, in most cases, affiliated at some point during their training with the physiology programs at Harvard or Johns Hopkins.

As the number of physiologists increased and their opportunities for research improved, their productivity reached a level that suggested the need for a more specialized American journal for the publication of their results. Several medical and scientific specialties established their own American journals during the last quarter of the nineteenth century. With the inauguration of Foster's *Journal of Physiology* in England in 1878, Bowditch's desire for an American journal devoted to studies in anatomy and physiology was temporarily obviated. By the mid-1890s, however, the need for American journal devoted exclusively to physiology reappeared. The impetus came from William Porter, who joined Bowditch's department in 1893. Curricular changes and greater financial support of the basic sciences at the Harvard Medical School led to dramatic growth in Bowditch's physiology department. Porter informed his former teacher Gustav Baumgarten early in 1897:

> Next year the staff of the Department of Physiology in the Harvard Medical School will be raised from 6 to 10. The 4 newcomers will have the title of assistant. . . . They will give their entire time. The afternoons will be spent in instructing, or rather superintending, laboratory work in experimental physiology; the mornings in research. They are to receive $400.00, an M.A. degree (where eligible), and all the training in science which we can give them in a year. The idea is chiefly pedagological,—to train men in physiological science, to give them habits of thought which will be useful in whatever line of work they may take up. Applicants should have a good elementary training; they may or may not be physicians, but medical men are preferred.[84]

This revealing letter shows Porter's dedication to the research ethic and his belief that thinking physiologically had intrinsic merit.

The productivity of Bowditch's department and other physiology groups grew dramatically during the 1890s. Scientific editors recognized this trend and tried to adapt to it. Some consideration was given to expanding the scope of the *American Journal of Science* to include more physiological papers in 1894, and editor James B. Dana approached Bowditch to serve on the editorial board of the New Haven-based journal.[85] Bowditch's needs were served, to some degree, by the establishment of the *Journal of the Boston Society of Medical Sciences* in January 1896, but initially it was primarily a local publication with limited circulation. The Johns Hopkins University had had a commitment to establish journals for the publication of work by its faculty and other qualified individuals since its inception in 1876. Many of Martin's papers and those of his associates and pupils were published in the university's occasional *Studies from the Biological Laboratory*. Now Johns Hopkins set up two additional publications to provide the new medical faculty with an outlet for their scientific and clinical observations and research: the *Johns Hopkins Hospital Bulletin* and the *Johns Hopkins Hospital Reports*. Nevertheless, some biomedical scientists advocated an American journal devoted exclusively to their interests.

With the encouragement of his network of scientific friends, William Welch established the *Journal of Experimental Medicine* in 1896. This journal was a success but did not address the specific needs of the physiologists. The American Physiological Society had considered the establishment of a journal devoted exclusively to their science as early as 1894. The content of the early volumes of Welch's journal suggested there was enough research in physiology in American institutions to justify a journal devoted to this specialty. Welch informed fellow pathologist and bacteriologist Mitchell Prudden of Yale, "I am very glad that the physiologists will probably start a journal of their own, as this will relieve the pressure upon our pages which has become almost intolerable for a single annual volume. . . . We shall also be able to give a more homogeneous character to the Journal by the predominance of pathological and bacteriological papers, a change which the majority of our subscribers will probably appreciate."[86] A Boston writer explained, "The number of investigations in physiology and its allied sciences now made in this country is grown so large that the present means of publication are no longer sufficient. Physiologists can no longer print in foreign countries, often in foreign languages, or in general medical journals, without stunting a growth, which, unchecked, will come to be a gratification to every American, and a wholesome influence in American medicine."[87]

A critical mass of medical scientists now existed in the United States: they could form societies and establish journals upon disciplinary lines. The founding of the *American Journal of Physiology* signified the expansion and vigor of American physiology. Perhaps it overstated the case, since there were still few full-time physiologists. Nevertheless, the physiologists would gain visibility (and perhaps support) through their new journal. When the first issue of the *American Journal of Physiology* appeared in 1898, its editorial board consisted of Henry Bowditch, Russell Chittenden, William Howell, Frederic Lee, Jacques Loeb, Warren Lombard, and William Porter, who was primarily responsible for the establishment of the journal.[88]

American physiology also proclaimed its maturation to the world in 1896 when the William B. Saunders Company published the *American Text-Book of Physiology*. Edited by William Howell, this 1,052-page, six-pound volume contained contributions by ten of America's leading physiologists, all of whom were members of the American Physiological Society. In his preface, Howell observed:

> Many teachers of physiology in this country have not been altogether satisfied with the text-books at their disposal. Some of the more successful older books have not kept pace with the rapid

changes in modern physiology, while few, if any, of the newer books have been uniformly satisfactory in their treatment of all parts of this many-sided science. Indeed, the literature of experimental physiology is so great that it would seem to be almost impossible for any one teacher to keep thoroughly informed on all topics.[89]

This group of professional American physiologists could accomplish the task.

Before 1900, American physiologists had created their own society, their own journal, and an authoritative textbook. Their claims that the chairs in the basic sciences in the nations's medical schools must be held by full-time scientists imbued with the research ethic was gaining support. They managed to keep the antivivisection movement in check, although they were unable to eliminate it. The physiologists and those who shared their commitment to reforming American medical education and creating scientific careers were pleased with what they had accomplished after so many years of frustration. They were not complacent, however. With the beginning of a new century, the reformers were joined by powerful and well-financed allies from within and outside the medical profession. The result was a more influential coalition who set an even broader agenda in order to make American medicine scientific.

CHAPTER SIX

A Scientific Prescription for American Medicine

AMERICA'S PHYSIOLOGISTS became impatient by the turn of the century. They wanted more hours in the curriculum, more equipment, more assistants, and more time for research. From 1850, when Dalton and Mitchell studied with Claude Bernard, to 1887 when the American Physiological Society was formed, the gains of the physiologists were actually rather modest. By 1900, there were perhaps a dozen medical schools in America in which full-time physiologists taught and pursued research. Fewer institutions offered programs of advanced training in physiology. There were encouraging signs, however. Alumni and local citizens were beginning to contribute to medical schools so the curriculum could be improved and the faculty strengthened. By the early 1900s, the importance of the laboratory method of teaching the scientific branches was widely acknowledged.[1]

Contemporary laboratory manuals reveal the sophisticated exercises medical students performed in America's leading medical schools. In 1905, the committee on medical curricula of the Association of American Medical Colleges called for sixty hours of practical laboratory training in physiology in addition to ninety hours of lectures. These practical courses necessitated student apparatus, laboratory space, and instructors with training in experimental physiology.[2] Still more had to be done if American medicine was to become scientific, however, and the physiologists and their scientific colleagues could not do it all. They realized that a broader coalition was necessary if the reforms they had successfully introduced in America's leading medical schools were to become the standard.

Several of the most prominent and enthusiastic spokesmen for the medical education reform movement were active members of the American Physiological Society. This small band of full-time medical scientists worked hard to enlarge the scope and size of their network. They sought the support of scientifically oriented practitioners, educators, medical editors, and influential laymen. Encouraged by the introduction of practical laboratory teaching in physiology into several medical schools and the resultant increase in full-time positions, the reformers broadened their agenda.

Chicago physician, educator, and editor Nathan Smith Davis, who had urged improvements in medical education for nearly half a century, put the movement in perspective in 1891, when he claimed, those "who deny that medicine has any scientific character . . . betray the shallowness of their own attainments, and especially their ignorance of the real medicine of to-day. . . . Modern medicine is composed of facts and principles belonging to the wide domain of natural and physical sciences and their application to the relief of human suffering." In Davis's opinion, and that of the physiologists, the fundamental medical sciences formed the "basis of modern medicine."[3]

In 1893, the new medical school of the Johns Hopkins University embodied many features of the best continental institutions, including the full-time system for basic medical scientists and the research ethic. As was the case when the Johns Hopkins University opened nearly two decades earlier, the medical school set a new standard in this country. For the first time in an American medical school, all of the basic science teachers devoted their whole time to teaching and research. In 1886, seven years before instruction began, the Johns Hopkins trustees had decided their basic scientists would not be permitted to engage in medical practice. They believed "medical education in the United States now suffers from the fact that the chairs are almost always filled by practitioners and consequently the scientific work of the Schools of Medicine has been less efficient than it should be."[4] It was the rule, not the exception, that medical faculty members at Johns Hopkins, like the professors in the university's arts and sciences division, were hired, in part, on the basis of their commitment to, and accomplishments in, research.

John Shaw Billings, who, with Daniel Gilman and William Welch, selected the original faculty of the Johns Hopkins Medical School, argued that the highest priority in elevating American medical education was to hire competent teachers. This goal posed a problem, however. Ordinary medical lecturers were available, but they were not what Billings and his colleagues wanted. They sought a special class of individuals for Johns Hopkins, and few candidates were suitable. Billings asked, "How many anatomists, or physiologists, or pathologists, of the first class, thoroughly trained, authorities in their special fields, capable of increasing knowledge, and with the peculiar gift of ability to teach—do you suppose there are in this country? It is a liberal estimate to say that a dozen of each have thus far given evidence that they exist."[5]

Where could Gilman, Welch, and Billings turn to find specialists in the basic medical sciences imbued with the research ethic? They found them among the members of the American Physiological Society. All of the basic science professors hired to staff the Johns Hopkins Medical School were members of the society. The medical school's scientific chairs went to William H. Howell, professor of physiology; Franklin P. Mall, professor of anatomy; John J. Abel, professor of pharmacology; and William H. Welch, professor of pathology—all members of the American Physiological Society.

Mall, Abel, and Welch had studied under Carl Ludwig and, although they now identified themselves as specialists in their own scientific fields, they remained deeply committed to physiology as the basis of modern scientific medicine. The diversity of their interests demonstrates that these early members of the American Physiological Society shared a commitment to the full-time system, the experimental method, and the research ethic as much as (or even more than) they shared a single scientific focus. Now, in the Johns Hopkins Medical School, Americans had a native institution they held up as the ideal training ground for physicians and biomedical scientists. The new institution incorporated virtually all the reforms advocated for American medical education during the preceding half century. Matriculants were required to have a college degree, complete a four-year graded curriculum, participate in practical laboratory training in each of the basic medical sciences, and gain clinical experience at the bedside in the Johns Hopkins Hospital.

Encouraged by the organization of the Johns Hopkins Medical School and reforms at a few of the nation's leading medical schools, such as Harvard, the University of Pennsylvania, and the College of Physicians and Surgeons of New York, the physiologists and their biomedical colleagues continued their efforts to infuse the American medical profession and public with the research ideal. William Welch, among the strongest advocates of the full-time system and the research ethic, told members of the Harvard Medical School Association in 1892:

It would do much to advance medical education and to encourage original research in medicine in this country, if the way were more freely open for academic careers in the sense in which it is in the German universities; that is, if young men who do good scientific work, who publish valuable results of original investigation, and who acquire reputation among those who are competent to judge them, could look forward with some reasonable assurance to securing positions in our leading medical schools. The incentive of this reward acts as a powerful stimulus to original investigation in Germany.[6]

Welch was optimistic about the future of medical education in America and complimented the faculty and officers of the Harvard Medical School on their efforts to elevate its standards and encourage science. He applauded the creation of a new assistant professor position in the Harvard physiology department because it expanded the job opportunities for young Americans who wished to specialize in that scientific field.

Although he had chosen a career in pathology and bacteriology, Welch acknowledged the central role of physiology in medicine. Speaking two years later in Cleveland, he claimed that physiology

is of the first importance in medical education. It has attained a higher degree of precision in experimental methods than any other medical science. A good knowledge of physiology is the best corrective to irrational theories and practice in medicine. Physiology has become a highly specialized science, and should be represented in the medical school by a good physiological laboratory and a teacher who is thoroughly trained in physiological methods, and can devote his whole time to the subject.[7]

Within three years of joining the faculty at Johns Hopkins, Welch began delivering addresses throughout America on the importance of reforming medicine along scientific lines. He took his message to Yale in 1888, the University of Toronto in 1889, Harvard in 1892, Western Reserve University in 1894, the University of Pennsylvania in 1895, the University of Chicago in 1897, and back to Yale in 1901. Welch's missionary work on behalf of scientific medicine continued well into the twentieth century. He served as an effective and articulate spokesman on behalf of the scientific reform movement for nearly fifty years.

Hopkins anatomist Franklin Mall also acknowledged the central role of physiology in biology and medicine. In 1894, he claimed that the "greatest hope in biological investigation" lay with physiologists, and emphasized the relevance of physiological methods to all of the branches of medicine. Mall explicitly outlined the broader agenda of the scientific reformers in this address. The basic scientists should be encouraged and supported in their attempts to develop laboratories and adequately staffed departments. Eventually, Mall argued, "they could not only train students and investigators from many standpoints but also take charge of the first few years of medical education. This . . . will help materially to raise our standard of medicine to the dignified position it holds in Europe."[8] Thus, the type of medical teacher chosen to educate America's future physicians had important implications for the status of medicine in this country.

The reformers' appeals to the patriotism of Americans became increasingly persuasive and successful. This approach was even more effective once Europeans began to acknowledge the contributions made by America's biomedical scientists. Historian Thomas Bonner has reviewed the impressions of the leaders of German medicine and biomedical science who visited the United States in increasing numbers around the turn of the century "to observe, to criticize, to encourage, or to envy, as the case might be."[9] Indeed, Friedrich von Müller, a prominent Munich clinical teacher, was impressed by the extent of practical laboratory teaching in physiology in some American medical schools during a 1907 visit. The German universities still usually reserved practical laboratory exercises for graduate students, as Billings had informed Gilman some years earlier. Recognition by their European idols encouraged the reformers and heightened their enthusiasm for the cause of scientific medicine.

By the turn of the century, America's small but growing corps of full-time biomedical scientists contributed to the medical literature more frequently, and their papers were more significant. Europeans acknowledged the value of Newell Martin's isolated mammalian heart preparation and, along with American groups, refined it during the early years of the twentieth century. The important observations of William Porter and his colleagues at Harvard on the effects of ligation of the coronary arteries stimulated additional studies of this nature in Chicago and abroad during the early years of the century. Americans were no longer viewed simply as importers of scientific ideas and techniques. With the right training, adequate assistance, and the necessary apparatus, Americans, too, could make significant additions to biomedical knowledge.

Several years earlier, William Welch and William Osler had asserted that the lack of opportunities for young American medical graduates to devote themselves to investigation had retarded medical science in the United States.[10] In the early twentieth century, American productivity in medical research, measured by the output of scientific publications, grew in proportion to the increase in full-time scientists and the adoption of the research ethic among America's better medical schools. A sense of achievement and anticipation gradually replaced the complaint that Americans did not publish articles based on research, expressed so frequently by editors and reviewers during the middle of the nineteenth century.

The dawn of a new century was accompanied by a torrent of verbal and written assessments of the accomplishments of the nation during the preceding one hundred years. Medical reformers took advantage of this frenzy of retrospection and prediction. Billings attributed the dramatic advances in medicine during the nineteenth century to improvements in methods of investigation and diagnosis, "resulting from increase of knowledge in chemistry and physics; to better microscopes and new instruments of precision; to experimental work in laboratories; and to the application of scientific method and system in the observation and recording of cases of disease and of the results of different modes of treatment." He concluded his essay, published in the *New York Evening Post* and the *Reports of the Smithsonian Institution*, by urging the expansion of the scientific method in medicine. New methods of scientific investigation held great promise for the future, and, Billings argued, they must be applied more widely.[11]

Michael Foster, speaking before the British Association for the Advancement of Science in Toronto in 1897, commented on the development of physiology that had taken place in the fourteen years since the association had last met in the Western Hemisphere. He applauded the recent dramatic increase in the number of physiological laboratories, the "heart of physiology." He contrasted the teaching of physiology in 1884 with the situation in 1897, and in so doing, traced the evolution of the research ethic. No longer were teachers in the scientific branches of medicine content to deliver lectures augmented by an occasional demonstration. In the brief span of a decade and a half, Foster saw widespread adoption of the belief that medical students should be taught practically in the laboratory. The British physiologist applauded those schools that had adopted the research ethic for their basic science teachers: "Perhaps in no respect has the development during the past thirteen years been so marked as in this," exclaimed Foster.[12] He acknowledged the role his pupil Martin had played in the development of this enviable situation in America.

Americans increased their pleas for the endowment of institutions that had adopted the research ethic and the full-time faculty system.[13] Reformers sought new sources of philosophical and financial support. Weir Mitchell's longtime friend William W. Keen chose the endowment of medical colleges for the theme of his presidential address before the American Medical Association in 1900. The Philadelphia surgeon quoted Bowditch, Eliot, Welch, and other leaders of the scientific reform movement and proclaimed the value of practical laboratory training and individualized clinical instruction. Recounting the many discoveries in bacteriology and their implications for public health, he boasted, "What has not the laboratory done for us within the last few years?" Keen emphasized the necessity of expanding the research ethic: "No school is worthy of the name that does not provide for greater or less research work. . . . Twenty-five years ago there were practically few young men who were fitted for research work, especially laboratory work. Now every well-equipped school has attached to it one way or another a score or more of young men who are eager to work, longing for the opportunity for usefulness and distinction if they can only obtain a bare living." He encouraged the AMA to provide "scientific grants in aid of research" and predicted, "The results of such grants would be not only absolute additions to our knowledge, but the cultivation of a scientific spirit which would permeate the whole profession and elevate its objects and aims."[14] Thus, the expansion of the research ethic would benefit not only the laboratory workers, but, by elevating the prestige of the profession, all of America's physicians who subscribed to the philosophy of the new scientific medicine. Although others had made this point earlier, the audience of practitioners was never more receptive.

When the scientific reformers gained the support of the officers of the American Medical Association, they had a powerful ally in their goal of making American medicine scientific. The AMA came to play an important role in promoting scientific medicine early in the twentieth century. In 1895, the association had held its annual meeting in Baltimore, so its members had had an opportunity to see the unique structure and philosophy of the recently opened Johns Hopkins medical institutions. The following year the AMA conducted a survey of American medical schools.[15]

This 1896 AMA summary of the nation's medical schools was comprised of letters forwarded by the deans of the various institutions. Shortly thereafter the association actively investigated each American institution that claimed to provide medical training, rather than simply accepting the unverified reports of the schools' officials. Perhaps by coincidence, the published summary of nearly one hundred medical schools immediately followed an article entitled "The Value to the Medical Student of Physiologic Study" by John Benson, physiology professor at the College of Physicians and Surgeons of Chicago. In addition to advocating the full-time system for basic scientists and the adoption of the research ethic, Benson emphasized the importance of physiology to those who practiced medicine. The practitioner "must pay strict attention to this branch before he can hope to become a diagnostician, a pathologist or a therapeutist."[16] Members of the AMA heard such claims on behalf of medical science at their meetings and read the opinions of the reformers in their journal with increasing frequency over the next decade.

When the AMA established a committee on medical education in 1902, the reformers had a focal point within the organization. The committee had a broad agenda, but part of it addressed the specific goals of the biomedical scientists. Arthur Dean Bevan served as chairman of the committee and its descendant, the council on medical education, established by the AMA two years later. Bevan, born in Chicago in 1861, attended the Sheffield Scientific School at Yale where Daniel Gilman and his colleagues had established a pioneering premedical scientific course. At Sheffield, Bevan came into contact with Russell Chittenden and others deeply committed to the basic medical sciences and the advancement of medicine through research. Chittenden, a founder of the American Physiological Society, was, according to William Howell, "with Bowditch and Martin . . . instrumental in giving to American physiology an independent standing."[17]

From New Haven, Bevan returned to Chicago where he graduated from Rush Medical College in 1883. Subsequently, he studied in Leipzig, Vienna, and Berlin where he was exposed to the German university system with its emphasis on research and the full-time concept. Bevan was also influenced by his Chicago teachers Nicholas Senn and Christian Fenger. Senn, one of the earliest Americans to perform significant research in surgery, was a vocal advocate of the research ethic.[18] Fenger, a Danish immigrant who studied pathology under Karl Rokitansky before coming to America, successfully transmitted the ideals of European scientific medicine to the Midwest according to historian George Rosen.[19] In 1887, Bevan became professor of anatomy and surgery at Rush Medical College and spent his career at that institution. Although he was a practicing surgeon, not a full-time basic medical scientist, he was sympathetic to the goals of the physiologists and their fellow reformers.

As chairman of the AMA council on medical education, Bevan was in a position to facilitate the diffusion of the agenda of the reformers among America's practitioners. Other members of the council were Victor Vaughan of the University of Michigan, William Councilman of Harvard, Charles Frazier of the University of Pennsylvania, and John

Witherspoon of Vanderbilt University. Vaughan and Councilman were members of the American Physiological Society, and Frazier and Witherspoon, like Bevan, had a special interest in scientific medicine. Frazier had studied pathology under Rudolf Virchow as part of his preparation to become a surgeon, and Witherspoon was professor of physiology at the University of Tennessee in Nashville until 1894 when he was appointed to the chair of medicine at Vanderbilt. The council encouraged the development of the full-time faculty system for basic medical scientists and the adoption of the research ethic by America's medical schools. These themes recur throughout their annual reports, first published in 1905.

Victor Vaughan set the tone for the first annual conference when he claimed that modern medicine depended on the facts derived from scientific investigation that could be applied to the prevention, diagnosis, and treatment of disease. The Michigan physiological chemist and dean argued that "medicine can advance no faster than the sciences on which it is founded advance. Discovery of facts must precede their application. Therefore, medical men must encourage research work, and it is a duty imposed on every medical school to advance the bounds of scientific knowledge."[20]

By the third meeting of 1907, some member of the council or its secretary had visited 160 American medical schools in an ambitious attempt to evaluate the quality of medical training in these institutions. As would be the case with Abraham Flexner's more widely known survey published three years later, the visitors from the AMA "found schools which are absolutely worthless, without any equipment for laboratory teaching, without any dispensaries, without any hospital facilities; some which are no better equipped to teach medicine than is a Turkish-bath establishment or a barber-shop." Adopting the solution long advocated by the scientific reformers, the AMA council proposed endowments as the only hope of improving the low state of medical education in many of America's medical schools: "The public must be taught the necessities and the possibilities of modern medicine, and philanthropists shown that medicine well deserves the same support that has been given to theology, to colleges of liberal arts, to libraries, etc."[21] The committee recognized that only limited funds would become available and sought to direct those funds to elite institutions. They suggested that only schools that included extensive laboratory work and possessed well-equipped facilities, staffed by full-time basic medical scientists, should be supported; the others should adopt these reforms or discontinue instruction.

Charles Eliot compared the present circumstances at the Harvard

Medical School with those in 1870 in his address to the AMA council in 1908. The Harvard president credited Bowditch and his reform-minded scientific colleagues for the dramatic changes at Harvard:

> The whole laboratory method, for instance, has come in during these forty years. The medical school as I first knew it, had but one laboratory and that was a perfectly disgraceful, dirty and abominable dissecting room, but it was infinitely precious since the only laboratory instruction given was in the horrible dissecting room. Now, nineteen-twentieths of the instruction in the medical school is either laboratory work or clinical work which in a sense is also laboratory work.[22]

During this same meeting, William Councilman, Welch's first assistant in pathology at Johns Hopkins, and now professor of pathology at Harvard, also emphasized the dramatic changes in medical education, science, and practice that had occurred during his thirty-year career as a medical scientist.

With the organization of the Carnegie Foundation for the Advancement of Teaching in 1905, a new opportunity arose for the AMA council to enlist a formidable and well-financed ally in their attempt to reform American medical education. Andrew Carnegie, an industrialist, and one of the wealthiest men in the nation, had been persuaded by Henry S. Pritchett, president of the Massachusetts Institute of Technology, to establish a foundation to improve the status of teaching in America. Those interested in the reform of medical education turned to the Carnegie Foundation for assistance. Pritchett served as president of the foundation, and Charles Eliot, long interested in the establishment of scientific medicine in America, served as chairman of the board of trustees of the foundation from 1905 to 1909. Pritchett recruited Abraham Flexner to undertake a thorough investigation of the medical schools of the United States, Canada, and Europe.

Flexner was a logical choice for the job of surveying America's medical schools. Like Charles Eliot and Daniel Gilman, he was an educator who had visited European universities and was interested in improving America's institutions of higher learning. Flexner's recent assessment of the status and needs of America's colleges demonstrated his concern for educational reform.[23] Although he was not a physician, Flexner had reason to be interested in the advance of medical education and the support of medical research. He was an 1884 graduate of the Johns Hopkins University, and his brother Simon had been a graduate student in pathology at Johns Hopkins in 1890, following the receipt of his medical degree from the University of Louisville.

Simon Flexner was profoundly influenced by William Welch, owing much of his philosophy of medical science and education to him. Indeed, Simon also owed his job, director of the new Rockefeller Institute for Medical Research, to Welch. John D. Rockefeller established this well-endowed institute in New York City in 1901. Welch served as the chairman of the advisory board of the new foundation to support medical research. In this capacity, he had a great deal to do with the organization of the institute and was responsible for many of the appointments to its original staff.[24] Abraham Flexner watched his brother's career with interest and heard of the new opportunities for medical research available at Johns Hopkins and the Rockefeller Institute, models for the expansion of the full-time system and the research ethic.

Abraham Flexner revealed the results of his Carnegie-sponsored survey of North American medical schools in 1910. His widely circulated report held up the Johns Hopkins Medical School as the ideal American institution for the training of physicians and the advance of medical knowledge. This selection was not motivated by simple institutional loyalty. Johns Hopkins had the highest standard of admission for its pupils, the most comprehensive curriculum that emphasized practical training in the laboratory and at the bedside, and was staffed by a talented group of biomedical scientists and clinicians imbued with the research ethic.

Henry Pritchett's lengthy introduction outlined the significance of Flexner's report and its implications for society. Pritchett described the changes in medical schools that had taken place during the prior two decades. He argued that medical education was not simply a problem for the profession; it had implications for society as a whole. He pointed out the need "to educate the public" that most patients did not receive the best possible care because most medical graduates were unsophisticated in the sciences fundamental to medicine and lacked clinical experience. Pritchett concluded, "A right education of public opinion is one of the problems of future medical education."[25]

In his detailed and candid report, Flexner described the transition of medicine from an age of empiricism to the modern era of science. He attributed this development to the advance of physics, chemistry, and biology and "the elaboration out of them of a method just as applicable to practice as to research. The essential dependence of modern medicine on the physical and biological sciences, already adverted to, will hereafter become increasingly obvious in the wealth of the curricula based upon them, and no less in the poverty of those constructed without them." Flexner outlined his interpretation of the ideal arrangement for the basic science courses in positive terms that demanded, rather than recommended, the acceptance of his suggestions: "The medical laboratories *must* be manned, equipped, and organized like university laboratories devoted to non-medical subjects. The laboratory staff consists *necessarily* of a chief—the professor in charge—with a corps of paid assistants, cooperating with him in the work of teaching, busy at other times with their problems, as he is with his." (Emphasis added.) Only professional scientists were suitable to teach the basic medical sciences and research was "*required* of the medical faculty because only research will keep the teachers in condition." (Emphasis added.) In a repudiation of the part-time teacher in the scientific branches, Flexner exclaimed, "The one person for whom there is no place in the medical school, the university, or the college, is precisely he who has hitherto generally usurped the medical field,—the scientifically dead practitioner, whose knowledge has long since come to a standstill and whose lectures, composed when he first took the chair, like pebbles rolling in a brook get smoother and smoother as the stream of time washes over them."[26] This situation was most likely to be found in the proprietary medical schools in which the research ethic was virtually nonexistent and the teachers were practitioners with little or no experience or interest in the scientific approach to medical education.

Flexner's descriptions of the nation's medical schools, based on personal visits, were purposely provocative. Although he declared a few institutions outstanding, and Johns Hopkins the ultimate model, he judged many schools unfit for survival. Those medical schools that had adopted the research ethic and the full-time faculty system in the basic sciences generally fared well in the report. He described laboratory facilities at Johns Hopkins and Harvard as unexcelled for teaching and research. The University of Michigan, the College of Physicians and Surgeons of New York, and the University of Pennsylvania also got high marks for their support of the basic sciences, and, as mentioned earlier, most members of the American Physiological Society came from these institutions during its first quarter century. The institutions that produced and sustained physiologists also best served Flexner's purpose (and that of the reformers): the training of scientific physicians. Flexner's comprehensive and candid report catalyzed the reform movement and hastened the closing or consolidation of many marginal medical schools. On the occasion of Flexner's ninetieth birthday, physiologist and medical historian John Fulton emphasized the value of his contributions to medical education and to "the cause of scientific medicine."[27]

Reformers had advocated medical research for nearly half a century as well as the development of a system whereby biomedical scientists were paid a salary that would enable them to devote their whole time to teaching and investigation. By 1910, this system existed in a few of America's leading medical institutions. Nevertheless, the majority of medical schools did not have sufficient endowment or income to adopt the full-time faculty system or encourage research, even if they had wanted to do so. The efforts of the AMA and the Carnegie Foundation sped up the medical schools' adoption of the full-time faculty system for the basic medical sciences and the research ethic. It was made possible, not by simple rhetoric, but by massive and unprecedented economic aid to medical schools willing to adopt the philosophy and structure of the new scientific medical education outlined by Flexner and the AMA council on medical education, whose views owed much to the physiologists and their biomedical colleagues. Most of the funding came from the Rockefeller-endowed General Education Board, strongly influenced by Welch and Flexner.[28]

The reform movement came to fruition in an era of progressivism in which the efforts of individuals and organizations touched all segments of society to achieve a better standard of living for Americans. The reform of medical education and the endowment of research were increasingly viewed (and portrayed) as part of the larger movement to advance society. In 1910, Henry Pritchett heard Arthur Bevan declare at the sixth annual conference of the AMA council on medical education: "To-day medicine is a science, and it is the most important of all sciences both from the standpoint of the welfare of the individual and the welfare of the community." Now, according to Bevan, the patient should be able to distinguish the scientific from the unscientific practitioner: "The individual citizen, if he is wise, can secure for himself and his family the benefits and the protection of modern scientific medicine by securing the services of a well-trained scientific physician. He is foolish and unfortunate who selects for his medical adviser the poorly trained medical man, the pathist, the pretender, or the charlatan, who cannot give him the benefits of modern medical knowledge."

Bevan's approach was not new. Others had attempted to undermine the homeopaths and other sectarians by claiming they were unscientific. His solution—endowment—had repeatedly been advocated for more than a quarter of a century. But now, there were palpable examples of substantial gifts to support medical education and research; and these had paid dividends. Bevan declared, "Certainly one of the best investments John D. Rockefeller ever made was the money given to the Rockefeller Institute, which resulted in finding a cure for cerebrospinal meningitis, and the most far-reaching and beneficial investment the state or a rich philanthropist could make would be in money given to medical research and medical education."[29]

The AMA could not have found a more ardent supporter of the full-time system and the research ethic than William Welch who served as its president in 1910. In his presidential address, Welch surveyed the recent activities of the AMA which he considered a "scientific association." He pointed out that the character of the AMA had changed in 1901 in response to the decision to base membership and the right of representation on participation in the state medical societies. In Welch's mind this change had led to unprecedented cooperation between practitioners and biomedical scientists who now shared many of the same goals for the profession and for society. He complimented the pioneering efforts of the AMA council on medical education and claimed that their impressions of America's medical schools were confirmed by Abraham Flexner's recent report.

In Welch's view, the facts collected by the AMA council and the Carnegie Foundation

> while confirmatory of general impressions, acquire impressive
> significance when marshaled in concrete, statistical form and are
> of enormous consequences to the medical profession and the com-
> munity. The attitude of physicians should be clear in this matter,
> for the strength and credit of the profession, the great interests of
> public health, municipal, state and national, and the welfare of
> the individual all depend on the quality of training given in our
> medical schools.

Already, there was the promise of aid to those schools willing to adopt the full-time system in the basic medical sciences and the research ethic. Welch enthusiastically described the reforms just beginning at Washington University in St. Louis made possible "by splendid gifts of enlightened benefactors."[30]

The AMA was now an active participant in the scientific reform movement which was no longer limited to several dozen physiologists and their scientific colleagues, a handful of institutional presidents, and a few medical editors. Officers and influential members of the AMA encouraged the thousands of practitioners that belonged to that organization to join the call for the reform of medical education. Members were repeatedly told, and they came to believe, that their image in society would benefit from their association with the leaders of medical science. The reformers now had influence within the AMA, the same organization whose politics had led to the schism between the elite scientifically oriented physicians and the ordinary practitioners only a quarter of a century earlier. Other benefits to the scientific reformers, and the physiologists in particular, also resulted from this new coalition with the AMA.

Through various committees and with resolutions, the AMA had long supported Dalton and other physiologists in their efforts to suppress the antivivisection movement. Many members of the American Physiological Society contributed their time and energy to thwart the ongoing attempts of the antivivisectionists to halt animal experimentation. Although a pathologist, William Welch "had the highest opinion of the value of the [American Physiological] Society as a means for the promotion of scientific medicine in this country," and participated in its meetings.[31] He was deeply committed to experimental medicine and became one of his generation's leaders in the fight against the antivivisection movement. He valued the experimental method above all other approaches and recognized the central role vivisection must play in the advance of medical knowledge. As president of the AMA, Welch encouraged physicians to continue to support animal experimentation. Action, not simple rhetoric, was necessary, and the AMA began to serve as a clearinghouse for published responses to the attacks of the antivivisectionists through its council on defense of medical research established in 1908.

Welch, more confident of success in the fight against the antivivisectionists than some physiologists, asserted that all physicians now acknowledged the benefits of animal experimentation and boasted, "One is almost inclined to welcome an agitation which has afforded us the opportunity to present to the public conclusive evidence on this question in the admirable papers already published and in the course of preparation under the supervision of the Council on Defense of Medical Research."[32] The AMA published more than twenty pamphlets explaining the value of animal experimentation early in the twentieth century.[33] Although American physiologists wrote many articles defending vivisection, several clinicians, and even Charles Eliot, contributed to the series. The physiologists and others interested in experimental medicine now had the philosophical and financial support of the AMA. The enormous organization whose annual meetings were attended by more than three thousand individuals was a powerful influence once it adopted the support of scientific medical education as part of its agenda. In addition to

Welch, other AMA leaders of the scientific reform movement included Victor Vaughan, president in 1914, and Arthur Bevan, president in 1918.

The expansion of the full-time system from the basic medical scientists to the clinical faculty of America's medical schools was, in Abraham Flexner's opinion, "a perfectly natural evolution."[34] During the first two decades of the twentieth century, most of America's medical schools adopted the full-time system for the basic medical sciences, and many encouraged their medical teachers to perform research. Having finally succeeded in achieving the goals set nearly half a century earlier by such individuals as Daniel Gilman and Henry Bowditch, several of the scientific reformers turned their attention to the clinical branches of medical education. Physiologists and their disciples played a significant role in this new and expanded effort to reform medical teaching in America. Once again, the model was derivative: the German medical schools had employed full-time teachers in the clinical branches for several decades. Carl Ludwig, the mentor of many of America's leading experimental physiologists and other basic medical scientists, was responsible for suggesting that the full-time concept should ultimately be extended to the clinical faculty in medical schools in the United States. The German physiologist discussed this subject with his American pupil Franklin Mall in 1885 when the recent Michigan medical graduate was working in the Leipzig Physiological Institute.

Mall met William Welch when they were both studying in Europe in 1885. After returning to America, Mall went to Baltimore where he worked as a fellow in Welch's new pathology department at Johns Hopkins. Thereafter, he briefly held chairs at Clark University and the University of Chicago. A new opportunity arose in 1893, when he was invited to become the first professor of anatomy at the medical school of Johns Hopkins University. He informed William Harper, president of the University of Chicago, that though he was pleased with his prospects at the midwestern university he had decided to accept the Hopkins offer because "a desire to better medical education in this country" outweighed other considerations.[35] Mall believed, as did Bowditch and Martin, that basic medical scientists had a special opportunity and a responsibility to encourage reforms in medical education. At Johns Hopkins, he met several other individuals who shared his interest in scientific medicine. Among his colleagues was Lewellys Barker, who became an associate in Mall's anatomy department in 1894 following a fellowship with Welch in pathology. At Mall's suggestion, Barker went abroad for postgraduate study in Leipzig where he worked in the physiological institute and in other laboratories. Soon, Mall, Barker, and Welch were working together to encourage the expansion of the full-time system to clinical teachers in America's medical schools.

Mall encouraged Barker to accept an invitation to chair the anatomy department at the University of Chicago in 1900. Two years later, in an address to the western alumni of Johns Hopkins, Barker outlined the basic philosophy of the full-time system as it might be applied to clinical teachers. He advanced the same arguments that had long been used in support of the full-time concept for the basic medical sciences and concluded, "There is no reason why internal medicine, surgery, obstetrics and certain other branches should not be similarly elevated; on the contrary, for the sake of people who need help in time of illness, for the sake of the medical profession, on account of our universities and for the prestige of the science of the nation, there is every reason for that elevation." Barker's suggestion for inaugurating this reform was also familiar: endowments were necessary to expand the full-time plan to the clinical teachers. In rhetoric reminiscent of Daniel Gilman, he explained that endowed professorships in the clinical branches should be given only to individuals who gave their entire time to teaching and research in the medical schools and hospitals; they should not engage in private practice.

The extension of the research ethic to the clinical faculty and to medicine as a whole was mandatory in Barker's view. He recounted several recent advances in practical medicine that resulted from scientific research in laboratories, and argued:

> Experimentation ought not to be confined to those physiologists and pathologists who are not clinicians. What we need above all at this time are physicians and surgeons trained in physiology and pathology who will spend a part of their time in careful observation in the wards and over the operating table; who will there collect facts which will give them ideas to be submitted to experimental test, and who, during the rest of their time, will go down into the laboratories adjacent to the wards and actually make these experiments. The men who do this should give their whole time to the university.[36]

Barker was optimistic that philanthropists would support this extension of the full-time system, because they had been convinced of the value of medical research to mankind. The Rockefeller Institute for Medical Research had just been established, and he was familiar with the details of its development through his friends Welch and Simon Flexner. Barker's paper generated much interest and controversy among those concerned with the reform of medical education, and some individuals lent their support to the plan.[37]

The second-generation professional American physiologists and their scientific colleagues participated in the movement to encourage the expansion of the full-time system and the research ethic to the clinical subjects in the medical school. In 1909, Charles Minot, Bowditch's first postdoctoral student, a founding member of the American Physiological Society, and now chairman of the department of histology and embryology at the Harvard Medical School, told the new medical graduates of Washington University that the skill of exact observation was the most important quality of a medical practitioner. It could be learned, Minot argued, only through practical training in the laboratory and on the ward. He complained, "Have we not to deplore the fact that very few physicians think physiologically? . . . I deem the opinion sound which regards physiology as the central discipline of medicine, and maintains that a generous development of clinical physiology is the improvement needed above all others in our medical curriculum."[38]

Joseph H. Pratt, a Harvard faculty member with strong ties to Johns Hopkins, shared Minot's views. Pratt, who was elected to membership in the American Physiological Society in 1910, developed his philosophy of medical education while a student at some of the leading institutions in the reform movement. A pupil of Russell Chittenden at the Sheffield Scientific School, of Franklin Mall, Lewellys Barker, William Welch, and Wiliam Osler at the Johns Hopkins Medical School, Pratt was also influenced by the basic scientists at the Harvard Medical School where he accepted an appointment in pathology in 1898. There, William Porter, Henry Bowditch, and William Councilman further stimulated his interest in scientific medicine.[39]

In a 1912 address, Pratt applauded recent developments in the basic medical sciences in America and paid tribute to his teacher Bowditch. He quoted another admirer of Bowditch who had said, "'He stood for the highest ideals of progress and maintained always that the old-fashioned "practical" physicians must be replaced by men scientifically trained and animated by the scientific spirit.'" Pratt went on to advocate the development of the clinical full-time system, because

> even in our best schools the teachers of the clinical subjects are
> practitioners of medicine dependent upon private work for their
> bread and butter. Many of them, impelled by financial consider-
> ations, think first of their private practice, secondly of their hospi-
> tal, and lastly of their school. Many of the clinical teachers lack

the scientific spirit. That is not their fault in most instances, for they were trained by men of the same stamp, and the scientific spirit must be instilled into a man when he is young if it is to live and grow.[40]

The solution, in Pratt's opinion, was to provide adequate salaries so that clinical teachers could give up, or at least nearly give up, private practice and devote themselves to teaching, research, and hospital work on behalf of the medical school. Only by exposing medical students to teachers imbued with the ideals and methods of science could American medicine become scientific.

Physiologists and other basic medical scientists advocated the establishment of new types of positions in medical schools for clinical scientists who could "bridge the gap between the practicing physician and the laboratory-based scientist."[41] In a 1904 review entitled "Problems of Physiology at the Present Time," William Howell noted the growing separation of physiology from clinical medicine. As an experimental science based on physics and chemistry, and now "an independent science, with specific problems of its own, physiology has naturally loosened its connections with the art of medicine." He emphasized that experimental physiologists must not dwell solely on applied research. The pathologist and the clinician could use the methods of the physiologist, however, to pursue the "practical problems of medicine." Although he did not explicitly describe the functions of the clinical scientist, Howell advocated an "outlying division of workers who will keep the subject [physiology] in touch with practical medicine."[42]

Two leading second-generation professional physiologists, Frederic S. Lee and Walter B. Cannon, served on the AMA committee on medical research shortly after the publication of Flexner's 1910 report. Lee was a former student of Martin and Ludwig, and succeeded John Curtis as Dalton Professor of Physiology at the College of Physicians and Surgeons of New York in 1904. Cannon, Bowditch's former pupil, had succeeded his teacher as Higginson Professor and chairman of the Harvard physiology department in 1906. Lee served as an officer of the American Physiological Society almost continuously from 1895 to 1919, as did Cannon from 1905 to 1920. Both were leading spokesmen in the unending fight against the antivivisectionists. In their 1917 report to the AMA, written with Richard Pearce, these physiologists reiterated themes central to the scientific reform movement initiated by their teachers several decades earlier, and they extended the traditional agenda. Lee and Cannon emphasized the importance of medical training in shaping the physician's attitude toward medicine as a science, and proclaimed the crucial role of the medical school teacher in this process. They applauded the widespread acceptance of the research ethic for basic scientists in medical schools and advocated full-time clinical chairs in recognition of the importance of science in clinical medicine and to help free the schools from any hint of "commercialism."[43]

The third author of this AMA report, Richard Pearce, had been a medical student at Harvard in the 1890s where he studied under Bowditch. After accepting a position in pathology at the University of Pennsylvania, he studied in Leipzig, where he witnessed the German emphasis on science in both the preclinical and clinical years of the medical curriculum. Pearce, who held the recently founded chair of research medicine at the University of Pennsylvania, became a leader in the movement to establish the research ethic in clinical medicine. Several of his essays were reprinted with those of other basic medical scientists and scientifically oriented clinicians in a volume entitled *Medical Research and Education* in 1913.[44] Of the twenty contributors to this volume, more than two-thirds were members of the American Physiological Society. Those who were not members of that organization were anatomists, pathologists, or practitioners with a special interest in experimental physiology and medicine.

James McKeen Cattell, an energetic popularizer of American science, published this volume. With ties to two founders of the American Physiological Society, he was elected to membership in 1895. As a fellow at Johns Hopkins University in the early 1880s, Cattell was strongly influenced by Newell Martin. Subsequently, he was exposed to the British and German university systems as a postgraduate student. As was true of several of the early American physiologists, Cattell had difficulty finding a suitable position after returning from Europe. Weir Mitchell and others helped him establish himself as a physiological (experimental) psychologist. These experiences contributed to his enthusiasm for encouraging the development of scientific careers in America.[45] The reformers whose articles were reprinted in his volume shared his publishing goal. In a letter to Henry Bowditch's widow he stated, "I trust that the book, of which I enclose the table of contents, will be of some use in advancing medical research and education in this country."[46]

This collection of essays was introduced by an extensive historical review of medical research from antiquity to the twentieth century in which Richard Pearce described four eras and aspects of medical research: "1. The epoch-marking labors of isolated individuals working independently. 2. The application of the exact methods of physics, chemistry and biology to medicine. 3. The development of laboratories for the organized and intensive investigation of the various problems of medicine. 4. The idea of diminishing suffering and ameliorating social conditions." This scheme was simple and clearly linked the medical reform movement to larger issues in society. Moreover, Pearce's outline was familiar to many of those interested in medical reform: all of his stages had existed in American physiology during the preceding half century.

Pearce traced the recent development of the full-time system in the basic medical sciences and advocated the extension of the research ethic to the clinical branches because "it is the duty of the university so to organize its laboratories and hospital that this advance of medicine by research may continue, side by side with teaching, as a university function of benefit to student and faculty, as well as to the state and the general public welfare, and thus as an aid to the advancement of civilization." Calling attention to the social aspects of the movement to make medicine more scientific, Pearce quoted Charles Eliot's recent address at the opening of the Rockefeller Institute for Medical Research: "Medical research habitually strives to arrive at something beyond abstract truth. It seeks to promote public and private safety and happiness, and the material welfare of society."[47]

As the reform movement matured, and additional full-time basic science positions were established, it became necessary to address the issue of the proper balance between basic research and investigations designed to answer practical medical questions. Indeed, as physiology became professionalized, and many physiologists sought to uncover fundamental mechanisms, scientists considered defining a new class of workers who would pursue clinical investigation using the principles of experimentation devised or refined by the physiologists.

The professionalization of physiology and the other basic medical sciences had some negative implications for the quality of clinical teaching in America's medical schools in the opinion of Samuel Meltzer. A European immigrant trained in physiology by Hugo Kronecker at the University of Berlin, Meltzer combined the life of a busy practitioner and a productive investigator before becoming the head of physiology at the Rockefeller Institute in 1904. Meltzer was elected to membership in the American Physiological Society at the first regular meeting in 1888. Active in the society, he believed it was important "as a means of promoting the advance of physiological science," in the words of William Howell.[48]

Meltzer regretted that most clinical medicine in America's medical schools was taught by busy practitioners. Moreover, he believed that the quality of clinical teaching had suffered as a result of the loss "of the brainy men who now devote their energies to the pure sciences of medicine."[49] William Welch recalled that Meltzer often emphasized, especially to young physicians, "that the field of clinical research is just as interesting, as rewarding, as important and just as capable of scientific advancement by research as that of physiology or the other branches of medicine to which the term 'science' is sometimes, although erroneously, limited."[50]

The expansion of the full-time system and the research ethic to the clinical faculty became possible because of massive financial support by the Rockefeller-sponsored General Education Board. Although he gave credit to Franklin Mall and Lewellys Barker for suggesting the expansion of the full-time system to the clinical faculty, Abraham Flexner outlined the way in which this innovation might be accomplished. In a confidential report prepared for the Rockefeller Foundation in 1911, Flexner emphasized that the original plan of full-time faculty members imbued with the research ethic had succeeded in its goal of producing teacher-investigators "who would lead in the rehabilitation and modernization of medical science and education."

Turning to the clinical branches, Flexner criticized the tendency of the physician staff of Johns Hopkins to be distracted from research by the promise of a higher income from consultations. This situation was intolerable, in his view, because "the increasing complexity and promise of clinical study in the wards and laboratories attached to them will not be satisfied with devotion and interest any less complete than that of the physiologist."[51] The solution advocated by Flexner was to extend the full-time system to the clinical chairs, and the General Education Board was ready to finance this new venture. Although the proposal to extend the full-time system to the clinical faculty brought forth criticism from a wide variety of observers including scientifically oriented physicians like William Osler and Arthur Bevan, it was soon inaugurated at Johns Hopkins and gradually spread to other progressive schools supported by the General Education Board.

The reformers whose goal was to make medicine scientific had finally found a patron. The physiologists and their colleagues in other basic medical sciences had not done it alone; they could not. They were part, a critical part, of a larger movement that eventually reshaped the ideals and structure of American medical education. As the medical profession and the American people acknowledged the value of research, medicine in the United States did, indeed, become scientific. No longer was it necessary for medical scientists to support their research by seeing patients. Science in the laboratory and science at the bedside were worthy of support, first by philanthropists and later by the federal government.

During the late nineteenth century it was necessary for the reformers to use the European model to support their claims that endowment would lead to better doctors and meaningful discoveries. A combination of idealism and nationalism inspired their patrons to support them without demanding immediate proof that their investment was yielding dividends. Few could question the success of European workers in discovering new facts with implications for the prevention, diagnosis, and ultimate cure of disease. Unless they were intellectually inferior, and no one was willing to concede this, Americans should be able to join in the production of new knowledge if they had the opportunity. Productivity in research was not quantified at the turn of the century. Nevertheless, all interested observers had to acknowledge the extraordinary growth in the number of scientific publications coming from the new American laboratories of physiology, physiological chemistry, anatomy, pharmacology, experimental pathology, and bacteriology.

New journals devoted to medical science joined the *American Journal of Physiology* and the *Journal of Experimental Medicine* showing that Americans were producing knowledge. Among those that appeared in the United States during the first quarter of the twentieth century were the *American Journal of Anatomy* (1901), *Journal of Medical Research* (1901), *Journal of Biological Chemistry* (1905), *Anatomical Record* (1906), *Journal of Pharmacology and Experimental Therapeutics* (1909), *Physiological Reviews* (1921), and the *American Journal of Pathology* (1925). By the twentieth century the names of Americans appeared with increasing frequency in the scientific sections of the *Index Medicus*, inaugurated by John Shaw Billings in 1879. This growing visibility in the world of medical science reassured interested observers that American medical investigators could indeed be productive once they had the time and facilities necessary to devote themselves to research.

It is not my purpose to chronicle the discoveries made by America's physiologists and their scientific colleagues. Nevertheless, it is important to show that accomplishment followed their rhetoric once they obtained the support they sought. Several approaches may be used to demonstrate the increasing frequency of discoveries in medical science attributed to Americans during the period under study. Joseph Ben-David has shown, in a series of publications, the factors that led to an increase in scientific productivity among American physicians and biomedical scientists during the nineteenth century. He derived quantitative data from a chrono-

228 THE DEVELOPMENT OF AMERICAN PHYSIOLOGY

logical summary of important medical discoveries published by medical historian Fielding Garrison in 1929. Although these data include discoveries that cover a broad range of subjects in clinical medicine as well as the basic medical sciences and related life sciences, the trends are dramatic. Ben-David showed that Americans were taking over the German predominance of scientific discoveries by the turn of the century: "The American share [of medical discoveries] was rapidly increasing from the 1880s and became the largest by 1910–1919."[52]

In 1911 Fielding Garrison had undertaken the study that Ben-David used. During the next year, he had compiled a list of "important milestones and landmarks of progress" of works in medicine and the collateral sciences. An American, Garrison can be criticized for placing undue emphasis on contributions from physicians and biomedical scientists in the United States. Nevertheless, his 1912 list has been revised continuously, and since 1943 Leslie T. Morton, a British medical librarian, has edited the work and retained most of the American physiology citations in the original edition.[53] Garrison's 1912 list appeared at the time the physiologists were entering their second quarter century as a profession defined by the establishment of the American Physiological Society. His original compilation included several contributions by members of the society and was the result of contemporary rather than retrospective evaluation of the significance of their publications.

Garrison's list was arranged chronologically and by topic. As I have shown, several founding and early members of the American Physiological Society actually worked and published in a broad range of related scientific disciplines. Their names appear in his sections devoted to biology, anatomy, embryology, histology, morphology, physiological chemistry, pathology, and bacteriology, in addition to physiology. It was the collective activity of these workers that demonstrated the productivity of America's nascent full-time medical scientists to interested observers in the medical profession and in society at large when Garrison's list appeared. The physiologists made no effort to isolate themselves from other basic medical scientists who shared their agenda. For this reason it is appropriate to consider the contributions of members of the American Physiological Society to scientific fields outside traditional physiology in evaluating their productivity before 1912.

The sections of Garrison's list dealing with the medical sciences noted above were reviewed. Members of the American Physiological Society who published books (number of books indicated in parentheses) cited in Garrison's 1912 list included Jacques Loeb (4), Charles S. Minot (1), Franklin P. Mall (1), Wilbur O. Atwater (2), Russell H. Chittenden

(1), Francis G. Benedict (2), Herbert H. Donaldson (1), Harvey C. Cushing (1), George F. Nuttall (1), Christian A. Herter (1), S. Weir Mitchell (2), and Edward T. Reichert (1). Members of the American Physiological Society who wrote articles listed by Garrison were Franklin P. Mall (5), Charles S. Minot (2), Jacques Loeb (3), Ross G. Harrison (2), William Osler (1), Alexis Carrel (2), H. Newell Martin (3), William H. Howell (4), William T. Porter (3), George F. Nuttall (3), Henry P. Bowditch (2), John C. Dalton (1), S. Weir Mitchell (2), Isaac Ott (1), Archibald B. Macallum (1), William G. MacCallum (3), G. Stanley Hall (1), William H. Welch (5), Simon Flexner (4), George Sternberg (1), Victor C. Vaughan (1), William T. Councilman (2), and Eugene Opie (1).

America's biomedical scientists were productive, and their work was significant, at least in the opinion of Garrison (and Morton). The physiologists and their scientific colleagues could point to accomplishments in their chosen fields when asked to justify the support they received from their institutions and from philanthropists who wanted to see that their gifts were not leading to "intellectual atrophy and degradation," as Henry Chapman had claimed patronage often did in an 1876 essay.[54]

The biomedical scientists could point to another palpable result of the endowment of research in 1912 when Alexis Carrel won the Nobel Prize in Physiology or Medicine. Carrel had emigrated from France in 1904 after completing medical training in Paris. He had been interested in experimental medicine in France and sought a job in America so that he could pursue his studies on blood vessel surgery. Carrel accepted a position in the physiology department of the University of Chicago where he worked with Charles C. Guthrie. This pair published several papers on experimental vascular surgery, and their efforts attracted the attention of surgeon Harvey Cushing, then at Johns Hopkins. Cushing invited Carrel to lecture on his experiments at Johns Hopkins in 1905, where the young investigator met "the most eminent American scholars."[55] At this time, Carrel also visited the Rockefeller Institute which was being constructed in New York and met its director Simon Flexner. Soon, Flexner offered him a position at the institute which the Frenchman promptly accepted because it offered the promise of consistent funding for his research.

Carrel's receipt of the Nobel Prize for his work on vascular surgery and the transplantation of tissues and organs brought international recognition to the Rockefeller Institute. President William Howard Taft classed Carrel's contributions with those of William Harvey, Louis Pasteur, Robert Koch, and Walter Reed, and the popular and medical press celebrated the receipt of the prestigious prize by an American researcher. The cause of the scientific reformers was served as well. Carrel closed his Nobel Lecture with the assertion that it is only "through a more fundamental study of the biological relationships existing between living tissues that the problems involved [in organ transplantation] will come to be solved and thereby render possible the benefits to humanity which we hope to see accomplished in the future."[56]

A community of productive biomedical scientists had been established in the United States by World War I. European models had finally been adapted to the American context. Dalton, Mitchell, Bowditch, and Martin each contributed something different to the movement that ultimately saw widespread acceptance of the full-time medical faculty system and adoption of the research ethic by America's medical schools. Bowditch and Mitchell both survived beyond 1910 to see their efforts at elevating medical education to the status of a science gain support from many segments of American society. Physiology, the profession to which Bowditch devoted his career, and to which Mitchell remained loyal despite his failure to win an academic chair, grew steadily during the early twentieth century.

Charles Greene, a physiologist and historian of the American Physiological Society, claimed in 1938:

> The second quarter century of the American Physiological Society opened under most auspicious circumstances. At this time, 1913, in the United States we were in the midst of a profound wave of accelerated education progress. There were new universities like Chicago and Stanford recently established with unbelievably great financial resources. There were scientific laboratories erected under a new wave of idealism. . . . Under such circumstances the enormous growth in membership, scientific researches, and publications in the field of physiological, biochemical, and general biological sciences ceases to be an occasion of wonder.[57]

It has been my aim in this book to demonstrate how the "circumstances," as Greene called them, came to exist that allowed the physiologists and their colleagues in the medical education reform movement to establish themselves as the spokesmen for scientific medicine and to attract the endowments necessary to achieve their goals of making medicine scientific. It took half a century and the efforts of a broad coalition of scientists, educators, medical writers, and physicians to achieve this situation, but they succeeded.

Original Members of the
American Physiological Society

Name	Birthdate/ Birthplace	College	Medical School	Postgrad. Study	Institution in 1887
Henry G. Beyer	1850 Germany	Germany	Bellevue	JHU	U.S. Navy
Henry P. Bowditch	1840 Mass.	Harvard	Harvard	Europe	Harvard
Henry C. Chapman	1845 Pa.	Penn	Penn	Europe	Jefferson
Russell Chittenden	1856 Conn.	Yale		Yale	Yale
John G. Curtis	1844 N.Y.	Harvard	P&S	Harvard	P&S
John C. Dalton, Jr.	1825 Mass.	Harvard	Harvard	Europe	P&S
Henry H. Donaldson	1857 N.Y.	Yale		JHU	JHU
Frederick W. Ellis	1857 Mass.		Harvard	Harvard	Practice/ Monson, Mass.
George L. Goodale	1839 Maine	Amherst	Harvard		Harvard
G. Stanley Hall	1846 Mass.	Williams		Harvard, Europe	JHU
Hobart A. Hare	1862 Pa.	Penn	Penn	Europe	Penn
William H. Howell	1860 Md.	JHU		JHU	JHU
Joseph Jastrow	1863 Poland	Penn		JHU	JHU
Warren P. Lombard	1855 Mass.	Harvard	Harvard	Europe, JHU, P&S	P&S
H. Newell Martin	1848 Ireland	Trinity, Dublin	London	Europe	JHU
T. Wesley Mills	1847 Canada	Toronto	McGill	Europe	McGill

Name	Birthdate/ Birthplace	College	Medical School	Postgrad. Study	Institution in 1887
Charles S. Minot	1852 Mass.	MIT		Harvard, Europe	Harvard
S. Weir Mitchell	1829 Pa.	Penn	Jefferson	Europe	Practice/ Philadelphia
William Osler	1849 Canada	Trinity, Ontario	McGill	Europe	JHU
Isaac Ott	1847 Pa.	Lafayette	Penn	JHU, Penn, Harvard	Practice/ Easton, Pa.
Edward T. Reichert	1855 Pa.		Penn	Europe	Penn
William T. Sedgwick	1855 Conn.	Yale		JHU	MIT
Henry Sewall	1855 Va.	Wesleyan		JHU, Europe	Michigan
Robert M. Smith	1854 Pa.	Penn	Penn	Europe	Penn
Victor C. Vaughan	1851 Va.	Mt. Pleas., Mo.	Michigan	Michigan	Europe
Joseph W. Warren	1848 Mass.	Harvard	Europe	Europe	Harvard
William H. Welch	1850 Conn.	Yale	P&S	JHU, Europe	JHU
Horatio C. Wood, Jr.	1841 Pa.		Penn		Penn

Sources: The data in this appendix have been derived from William H. Howell, "The American Physiological Society"; J. McKeen Cattell, ed., *American Men of Science*, 1906; and other standard biographical sources listed in the bibliography.

Note: Abbreviations: JHU = Johns Hopkins; MIT = Massachusetts Institute of Technology; P&S = College of Physicians and Surgeons of New York; Penn = University of Pennsylvania. The generic term "Europe" has been used for postgraduate study abroad. Individuals often studied in several institutions and in different countries.

Institutional Affiliation of Members of the American Physiological Society at the Time of Their Election to the Society

	Original Members (1887)		Members Elected 1888–1899		Total Elected 1887–1899	
	No.	%	No.	%	No.	%
Johns Hopkins	6	21	9	18	15	19
Harvard	4	14	8	16	12	15
Pennsylvania	5	18	5	10	10	13
Yale	1	4	5	10	6	8
P&S N.Y.	3	11	2	4	5	6
Michigan	2	7	3	6	5	6
Jefferson	1	4	1	2	2	3
MIT	1	4	1	2	2	3
McGill	1	4	1	2	2	3
Washington Univ.	0		2	4	2	3
Chicago	0		2	4	2	3
Clark	0		1	2	1	1
Toronto	0		1	2	1	1
Bryn Mawr	0		1	2	1	1
Columbia	0		1	2	1	1
Syracuse	0		1	2	1	1
Northwestern	0		1	2	1	1
Weslyan	0		1	2	1	1
Manitoba	0		1	2	1	1
Army/Navy	1		1	2	2	3
Practice	3		3	6	6	8

Source: Adapted from William H. Howell, "The American Physiological Society."

Attendance at the Regular (December) Meetings of the American Physiological Society, 1887–1899

Year	Location	Number of Members Attending	Total Members	Percentage Attending
1887	New York	17	28	61
1888*	Philadelphia	14	28	50
1889	New York	11	32	34
1890	Boston	16	35	46
1891*	Philadelphia	10	39	26
1892	Princeton	12	41	29
1893	New Haven	15	43	35
1894*	Baltimore	21	47	45
1895	Philadelphia	22	51	43
1896	Boston	28	59	47
1897*	Ithaca	11	62	18
1898	New York	33	62	53
1899	New Haven	25	73	34

Source: The data have been derived from the American Physiological Society Minutes, Vol. 1, 1887–1919, APS Archives.

*A special meeting was held in September of these years in conjunction with the Congress of American Physicians and Surgeons.

Journal Abbreviations

Am. J. Educ.	American Journal of Education
Am. J. Med. Sci.	American Journal of the Medical Sciences
Am. Med. Times	American Medical Times
Am. Nat.	American Naturalist
Anat. Rec.	Anatomical Record
Ann. Med. Hist.	Annals of Medical History
Ann. Rep. Smithsonian	Annual Report of the Board of Reagents of the Smithsonian Institution
Atlantic Mon.	Atlantic Monthly
BAAS Rep.	British Association for the Advancement of Science Reports
Biog. Mem. Nat. Acad. Sci.	Biographical Memoirs. National Academy of Sciences
Boston Med. Surg. J.	Boston Medical and Surgical Journal
Brit. For. Med. Chir. Rev.	British and Foreign Medico-Chirurgical Review
Brit. Med. J.	British Medical Journal
Bull. Hist. Med.	Bulletin of the History of Medicine
Bull. N. Y. Acad. Med.	Bulletin of the New York Academy of Medicine
Canada Med. Surg. J.	Canada Medical and Surgical Journal
Coll. Clin. Rec.	College and Clinical Record
Hist. Sci.	History of Science
JAMA	Journal of the American Medical Association
J. Hist. Biol.	Journal of the History of Biology
J. Hist. Med.	Journal of the History of Medicine and Allied Sciences

J. Med. Educ.	*Journal of Medical Education*
J. Physiol.	*Journal of Physiology*
Johns Hopkins Circ.	*Johns Hopkins University Circulars*
Johns Hopkins Hosp. Bull.	*Johns Hopkins Hospital Bulletin*
Johns Hopkins Med. J.	*Johns Hopkins Medical Journal*
Med. Exam.	*The Medical Examiner and Monthly Record of Medical Science*
Med. Hist.	*Medical History*
Med. News	*Medical News*
Med. Rec.	*Medical Record*
Med. Surg. Rep.	*Medical and Surgical Reporter*
Med. Times Gaz.	*Medical Times and Gazette*
N. Am. Med. Chir. Rev.	*North American Medico-Chirurgical Review*
N. Am. Rev.	*North American Review*
N. Y. Med. J.	*New York Medical Journal*
Phila. Med. Times	*Philadelphia Medical Times*
Pop. Sci. Mon.	*Popular Science Monthly*
Proc. AAAS	*Proceedings of the American Association for Advancement of Science*
Proc. Acad. Nat. Sci. Phila.	*Proceedings of the Academy of Natural Science of Philadelphia*
Proc. Am. Philo. Soc.	*Proceedings of the American Philosophical Society*
Proc. Bost. Soc. Nat. Hist.	*Proceedings of the Boston Society of Natural History*
Trans. AMA	*Transactions of the American Medical Association*
Trans. Am. Philo. Soc.	*Transactions of the American Philosophical Society*
Trans. Coll. Phys. Phila.	*Transactions of the College of Physicians of Philadelphia*
Trans. Med. Chi. Md.	*Transactions of the Medical and Chirurgical Faculty of Maryland*
Trans. Med. Soc. N. Y.	*Transactions of the Medical Society of the State of New York*
Trans. Med. Soc. Penn.	*Transactions of the Medical Society of Pennsylvania*
Trans. N. Y. Acad. Med.	*Transactions of the New York Academy of Medicine*
Trans. Stud. Coll. Phys. Phila.	*Transactions and Studies of the College of Physicians of Philadelphia*
Univ. Penn. Med. Bull.	*University of Pennsylvania Medical Bulletin*
Yale J. Biol. Med.	*Yale Journal of Biology and Medicine*

Notes

See the Bibliography (pp. 279–80) for full citations of archival sources.

Introduction

1. Abraham Flexner, *Medical Education in the United States and Canada*, 63.

2. Claude Bernard, *An Introduction to the Study of Experimental Medicine*, 205; Thomas H. Huxley, "On the Educational Value of the Natural History Sciences" (1854), in *Science and Education*, 50 (Huxley's emphasis); and Owsei Temkin, "Basic Science, Medicine, and the Romantic Era," *Bull. Hist. Med.* 37 (1963): 123.

3. See Joseph Ben-David, "Scientific Productivity and Academic Organization in Nineteenth-Century Medicine," in *The Sociology of Science*, ed. Bernard Barber and Walter Hirsch (New York: Free Press of Glencoe, 1962), 305–28.

4. *Proceedings of the National Medical Conventions, Held in New York, May 1846, and in Philadelphia, May 1847* (Philadelphia: Collins, 1847), 63–77.

5. Anne E. Crowley, Sylvia I. Etzel, and Edward S. Petersen, "Undergraduate Medical Education," *JAMA* 254 (1985): 1565–72.

6. Daniel C. Gilman, "Present Aspects of College Training," *N. Am. Rev.* 136 (1883): 526–40.

7. D. Webster Cathell, *The Physician Himself: And What He Should Add to His Scientific Acquirement*, 2d ed. (Baltimore: Cushings & Bailey, 1882), 18.

8. William Osler, "Medicine," in *The Progress of the Century* (New York: Harper & Brothers, 1901): 176–77.

9. Joseph Ben-David, "Roles and Innovations in Medicine," *American Journal of Sociology* 65 (1960): 557.

Chapter 1: John Call Dalton, Jr.

1. S. Weir Mitchell, "Memoir of John Call Dalton, 1825-1889," *Biog. Mem. Nat. Acad. Sci.* 3 (1890): 179. See also "John Call Dalton," in Thomas Francis Harrington, *The Harvard Medical School*, 2:886-901 (includes Dalton's bibliography); and Alonzo Brayton Ball ("Minutes of Special Trustees Meeting on Appreciation for the Work of J. C. Dalton after his Death"), 26 February 1889, Columbia Archives. See also Sidney H. Sobel, "John Call Dalton, Jr., M.D. (1825-1889), Scientist and Teacher: A Scientific Biography" (B.A. thesis, Harvard University, 1957). The author thanks John V. Taggert for forwarding a copy of the Sobel essay.

2. Mitchell, "John Call Dalton," 184.

3. See John O. Green, *A Memorial of John C. Dalton, M.D.* (Cambridge: [Harvard] University Press, 1864); Morrill Wyman, Jr., *A Brief Record of the Lives and Writings of Dr. Rufus Wyman (1778-1842) and His Son Dr. Morrill Wyman (1812-1903)* (Cambridge, 1913); and Oliver Wendell Holmes, "Memoir of Professor Jeffries Wyman," *Massachusetts Historical Society Proceedings* 14 (1875): 4-24.

4. John C. Dalton [Sr.] to Jeffries Wyman, 28 December 1836, Wyman Papers.

5. Diary of Rufus Wyman, 30 November 1837, published in Wyman, *A Brief Record*, 49.

6. Jeffries Wyman to Morrill Wyman, 17 December 1843, Wyman Papers.

7. Ibid., 9 January 1847, Wyman Papers.

8. John C. Dalton [Sr.] to Jeffries Wyman, 13 April 1848, Wyman Papers.

9. Elisha Bartlett, *Sketches of the Character and Writings of Eminent Living Surgeons and Physicians of Paris* (Boston: Carter, Hendee & Babcock, 1831). See also William Osler, "Elisha Bartlett: A Rhode Island Philosopher," in *An Alabama Student and Other Biographical Essays* (Oxford and New York: Oxford University Press, 1908), 108-58.

10. Elisha Bartlett, *An Essay on the Philosophy of Medical Science* (Philadelphia: Lea & Blanchard, 1844), 85-86. Bartlett's emphasis.

11. Holmes to his parents, 13 August 1833, published in John T. Morse, Jr., *Life and Letters of Oliver Wendell Holmes*, 2 vols. (Cambridge: Riverside Press, 1896), 1:108-9. See also Thomas Dwight, "Reminiscences of Dr. Holmes as Professor of Anatomy," *Scribner's Magazine* 17 (1895): 121-28, and David Cheever, "Oliver Wendell Holmes: The Anatomist," *Harvard Graduates Magazine* 3 (1894): 154-59.

12. See "New York Academy of Medicine. Report of the Meeting of December 21, 1859," *Med. Surg. Rep.* 3 (1859): 304-9.

13. Bruce Sinclair, "Americans Abroad: Science and Cultural Nationalism in the Early Nineteenth Century," in *The Sciences in the American Context: New Perspectives* ed. Nathan Reingold (Washington: Smithsonian Institution Press, 1979), 36.

14. *Report of the Committee of Internal Health on the Asiatic Cholera, Together with a Report of the City Physician on the Cholera Hospital* (Boston, 1849).

15. Frederick Clayton Waite, *The Story of a Country Medical College: A History of the Clinical School of Medicine and the Vermont Medical College, Woodstock, Vermont, 1827-1856* (Montpelier: Vermont Historical Society, 1945).

16. "Vermont Medical College," *Boston Med. Surg. J.* 52 (1855): 447.

17. John C. Dalton, Jr., "On the Gastric Juice, and Its Office in Digestion," *Am. J. Med. Sci.* n.s. 28 (1854): 313.

18. See John C. Dalton [Jr.], *History of the College of Physicians and Surgeons in the City of New York*, and John Shrady, ed., *The College of Physicians and Surgeons of New York*.

19. Board of Trustees of the College of Physicians and Surgeons to the Regents of the University (1847), quoted in Dalton, *History of the College of Physicians and Surgeons*, 91.

20. Alonzo Clark, *The Claims of the Medical Profession*, rev. ed. (Albany: New York State Medical Society, 1853).

21. Dalton, *History of the College of Physicians and Surgeons*, 93.

22. Brown-Séquard to Wyman, 12 October 1852, Wyman Papers. See also James M. D. Olmsted, *Charles-Edouard Brown-Séquard*.

23. John W. Draper, *The Indebtedness of the City of New York to Its University* (New York: Alumni Association of the University of the City of New York, 1853). See also Donald Fleming, *John William Draper and the Religion of Science* (Philadelphia: University of Pennsylvania Press, 1950).

24. Francis Donaldson, "Bernard's Recent Discoveries in Physiology," *Am. J. Med. Sci.* n.s. 22 (1851): 363.

25. Benjamin Silliman, Jr., to William Brewer, 1 February 1854, published in Lewis I. Kuslan, "Benjamin Silliman, Jr.: The Second Silliman," in *Benjamin Silliman and His Circle*, ed. Leonard G. Wilson, 163. Silliman's emphasis.

26. William M. Cornell, "Comparative Anatomy and Physiology," *Boston Med. Surg. J.* 50 (1854): 216. Cornell's emphasis.

27. Brown-Séquard to Wyman, 12 October 1852, Wyman Papers.

28. James L. Cabell, "Report of the Committee on Medical Education," *Trans. AMA* 7 (1854): 81.

29. John C. Dalton, Jr., *Introductory Address, Delivered at the College of Physicians and Surgeons, New York, October 16, 1855* (New York: John J. Schroeder, 1855), 11, 17-19. Dalton's emphasis.

30. Du Bois-Reymond to Ludwig, 9 April 1850, published in Paul F. Cranefield, ed., *Two Great Physiologists of the Nineteenth Century*, 57-58.

31. Dalton, *Introductory Address*, 28. Dalton's emphasis.

32. J[ohn] C. D[alton], Review. "Leçons de Physiologie expérimentale . . . [and] Mémoire sur le Pancréas . . . Par M. Claude Bernard," *Am. J. Med. Sci.* n.s. 33 (1857): 402.

33. J[ohn] C[all] B[artlett], "The Profession in New York: Impressions of a Visitor," *Boston Med. Surg. J.* 58 (1858): 301.

34. Samuel D. Gross, "Reports on the Causes Which Impede the Progress of American Medical Literature," *Trans. AMA* 9 (1856): 337-62.

35. Mitchell, "John Call Dalton," 185.

36. "The Present Aspect of the Profession of Medicine," *Boston Med. Surg. J.* 59 (1858): 104.

37. Henry Jacob Bigelow, *Science and Success* (Boston: David Clapp, 1859).

38. John C. Dalton, Jr., *A Treatise on Human Physiology: Designed for the Use of Students and Practitioners of Medicine* (Philadelphia: Blanchard and Lea, 1859).

39. [? Oliver W. Holmes], "Bibliographical Notices. A Treatise on Human Physiology . . . by John C. Dalton," *Boston Med. Surg. J.* 60 (1859): 80.

40. O[liver] W. H[olmes], "Bibliographical Notices. The Physiological Anatomy and Physiology of Man . . . by Robert B. Todd and William Bowman," *Boston Med. Surg. J.* 56 (1857): 302. See also "American Subserviency to Foreign Original Research," *Med. Surg. Rep.* 3 (1859): 292–93. Joseph Leidy was a prominent Philadelphia anatomist.

41. W[illiam] A. H[ammond], "Bibliographical Notices: A Treatise on Human Physiology . . . by John C. Dalton, Jr.," *Am. J. Med. Sci.* n.s. 41 (1861): 515–16.

42. See John C. Cardwell, "A History of the Department of Physiology of the Long Island College of Medicine," *Long Island Medical Bulletin* 9 (1932): 3–4; 10 (1933): 1–5, 5–7, 10–12, and Joseph Howard Raymond, *History of the Long Island College Hospital and Its Graduates: Together with the Hoagland Laboratory and the Polhemus Memorial Clinic* (Brooklyn: Alumni Association of the Long Island College Hospital, 1899).

43. D[aniel] F. Wright, Oliver W. Holmes, S. G. Armor, and W. H. Byford, "Report of the Committee on Medical Literature," *Trans AMA* 13 (1860): 773.

44. [George Shrady], "American vs. European Science," *Med. Rec.* 4 (1869): 133–34.

45. [George Shrady], "The Practice in Medicine in a Pecuniary Point of View," *Med. Rec.* 3 (1868): 373–75.

46. *John Call Dalton, M.D., U.S.V.* (Cambridge: H. O. Houghton & Co., 1892). See also John C. Dalton, Jr., to Charles Dalton, 14 September [1862], and 5 August [1863], published in *Massachusetts Historical Society Proceedings* 56 (1923): 444, 462–63.

47. See Austin Flint [Jr.] *Collected Essays and Articles on Physiology and Medicine*, 2 vols. (New York: D. Appleton & Co., 1903), and Austin Flint, Jr., *The Physiology of Man: Designed to Represent the Existing State of Physiological Science, as Applied to the Functions of the Human Body*, 5 vols. (New York: D. Appleton & Co., 1865–1874).

48. Robley Dunglison, *Introductory Lecture to the Course on the Institutes of Medicine* (Philadelphia: Joseph M. Wilson, 1860), 7.

49. See Samuel Chew, *Lectures on Medical Education, or on the Proper Method of Studying Medicine* (Philadelphia: Lindsay & Blakiston, 1864).

50. Claude Bernard, *Rapport sur les Progrès et la Marche de la Physiologie générale en France* (Paris: L. Hachette, 1867). See also [William James], "Rap-

port sur le [*sic*] Progrès et la Marche de la Physiologie générale en France. . . . Par M. Claude Bernard," *N. Am. Rev.* 107 (1868): 322–28.

51. Claude Bernard, *Lectures on the Phenomena of Life Common to Animals and Plants*, trans. Hebbel E. Hoff, Roger Guillemin, and Lucienne Guillemin (Springfield, Ill.: Charles C. Thomas, 1974), 10.

52. Pasteur quoted in Ashley Miles, "Reports by Louis Pasteur and Claude Bernard on the Organization of Scientific Teaching and Research," *Notes and Records of the Royal Society of London* 37 (1982): 116.

53. Claude Bernard, *Introduction à l'Étude de la Médecine expérimentale* (Paris: Baillière, 1865); in English: Claude Bernard, *An Introduction to the Study of Experimental Medicine*, trans. Henry Copley Greene.

54. Henry to Agassiz, 13 August 1864, published in A. Hunter Dupree, "The Founding of the National Academy of Sciences: A Reinterpretation," *Proc. Am. Philo. Soc.* 101 (1957): 339–40.

55. See Sydney H. Coleman, *Humane Society Leaders in America*.

56. "Poisoning as a Science," *Nation* 1 (1865): 242–43.

57. F[rancis] Donaldson, *Physiology the True Basis of Rational Medicine: An Introductory Lecture Delivered at the University of Maryland, October 17, 1866* (Baltimore: Kelly & Piet, 1866).

58. [George Shrady], "Medical Journalism," *Med. Rec.* 1 (1866): 453–55.

59. Dalton to Delafield, 8 November 1866, published in "Vivisection," *Boston Med. Surg. J.* 75 (1866): 371.

60. John C. Dalton, *Vivisection* (New York: Baillière, 1867), 13. Dalton's emphasis; idem, "Vivisection: What It Is, and What It Has Accomplished," *Bull. N. Y. Acad. Med.* 3 (1866): 159–98.

61. "Vivisection," *Boston Med. Surg. J.* 75 (1866): 369.

62. "Experimental Physiology," *Med. Surg. Rep.* 15 (1866): 524. See also "Experimental Physiology," *Med. Surg. Rep.* 5 (1860): 40–42.

63. John C. Dalton [Jr.], "Vivisection," *Trans. Med. Soc. N.Y.* (1867) (Albany: Van Benthuysen & Sons, 1867), 30.

64. [Henry Bergh], "Scientific Barbarity," excerpts published in Dalton, "Vivisection" (1867), 31.

65. Dalton to Wyman, 18 February (1867), Wyman Papers.

66. Quoted by Saul Benison, "In Defense of Medical Research," *Harvard Medical Alumni Bulletin*, 44 (1970): 17. See also "Mr. Bergh and the Doctors," *N. Y. Med. J.* 5 (1867): 71–80; and "The Society for the Prevention of Cruelty to Animals," *Med. Rec.* 2 (1867): 86.

67. John C. Dalton [Jr.], "Sugar Formation in the Liver," *Trans. N. Y. Acad. Med.* (1871): 28–58.

68. William H. Welch, "Some of the Conditions Which Have Influenced the Development of American Medicine, Especially during the Last Century," *Johns Hopkins Hosp. Bull.* 19 (1908): 34.

69. George Shrady, "Editorial," *Med. Rec.* 6 (1871): 398. See also Henry S. Hewitt, *The Relations and Reciprocal Obligations between the Medical Profession and the Educated and Cultivated Classes* (New York, 1869), and Edward S. Dunster, "The Relations of the Medical Profession to Medical Education," *N.Y. Med. J.* 12 (1870): 481–503.

70. C[ornelius] R. Agnew, "Some of the Relations of the Medical Profession to Education," *Trans. Med. Soc. N. Y.* (1874): 73–74.

71. Welch to Dennis, 5 September 1877, Welch Papers. For an assessment of the state of science and medicine in New York City in this era, see Douglas Sloan, "Science in New York City, 1867–1907," *Isis* 71 (1980): 35–76, and Charles Rosenberg, "The Practice of Medicine in New York a Century Ago," *Bull. Hist. Med.* 41 (1967): 233–53.

72. "Speech of Prof. Tyndall" in *Proceedings at the Farewell Banquet to Professor Tyndall* (New York: D. Appleton & Co., 1873), 48.

73. Simon Newcomb, "Exact Science in America," *N. Am. Rev.* 119 (1874): 286–308.

74. See Howard S. Miller, *Dollars for Research.*

75. Daniel B. St. John Roosa, "Anniversary Address," in *A Doctor's Suggestions to the Community* (New York: G. P. Putnam's Sons, 1880), 45.

76. George C. Freeborn, *History of the Association of the Alumni of the College of Physicians and Surgeons, New York* (Lancaster, Pa.: New Era Printing Co., 1909).

77. Dalton, *History of the College of Physicians and Surgeons*, 112.

78. Charles Heitzman, *Microscopical Morphology of the Animal Body in Health and Disease* (New York: J. H. Vail & Co., 1883), [v.] See also S. Oakley Vanderpole, "Pathological Anatomy: The Necessity for Its Study, and Its Influence upon Medicine as a Positive Science," *Trans. Med. Soc. N. Y.* (1872): 81–103.

79. John C. Dalton, Jr., "Objects Proposed in Raising a Fund for Improving the Means of Medical Education in New York" (1876), Columbia Archives. Dalton's corrections. See also "Expensiveness of Scientific Education," *Pop. Sci. Mon.* 7 (1875): 746–48; F. W. Clarke, "Laboratory Endowment," *Pop. Sci. Mon.* 10 (1877): 729–36; and "The Endowment of Medical Colleges," *Med. Rec.* 12 (1877): 152–53.

80. "Scientific Cruelty," *New York Times*, 13 December 1875, Curtis Papers. See also Frederic S. Lee, "John Green Curtis," *Columbia University Quarterly* 16 (1913): 54–57.

81. John C. Dalton [Jr.], *Experimentation on Animals, as a Means of Knowledge in Physiology, Pathology, and Practical Medicine* (New York: F. W. Christern, 1875).

82. Clarke to Dalton, 4 October 1874, published in Dalton, *Experimentation on Animals*, 69.

83. Austin Flint [Sr.] to Dalton, 9 November 1874, published in Dalton, *Experimentation on Animals*, 70.

84. "Vivisection," *Med. Rec.* 10 (1875): 88.

85. "A Memorial from Various Medical Societies and Associations," *Med. Rec.* 17 (1880): 246–47. See also "Whether Vivisection Pays," *Med. Rec.* 18 (1880): 42–43. The extent of the use of vivisection in research and teaching in New York is described in Burt G. Wilder, "Vivisection in the State of New York," *Pop. Sci. Mon.* 23 (1883): 169–80.

86. Dalton to Billings, 31 January 1881 and 1 February 1881, Billings Pa-

pers. The latter letter contains a brief historical sketch of the committee on experimental medicine as well as a list of the original members.

87. Harriet V. Bills, "Paris as a Medical Center," *Physician and Surgeon* 5 (1883): 404–5. See also Henry Hun, *A Guide to American Medical Students in Europe.*

88. See Albert Leffingwell, *An Ethical Problem: Or Sidelights upon Scientific Experimentation on Man and Animals* (New York: C. P. Farrell, 1914), and idem, "Does Vivisection Pay?" in *The Vivisection Question* (New Haven: Tuttle, Morehouse & Taylor Co., 1901), 1–19.

89. John C. Dalton [Jr.], *The Experimental Method in Medical Science,* 108.

90. For background on the American response to the germ theory see Howard D. Cramer, "The Germ Theory and the Early Public Health Program in the United States," *Bull. Hist. Med.* 22 (1948): 233–47, Phyllis Allen Richmond, "American Attitudes towards the Germ Theory," *J. Hist. Med.* 9 (1954): 428–54, and Gert H. Brieger, "American Surgery and the Germ Theory of Disease," *Bull. Hist. Med.* 40 (1966): 135–45.

91. See John C. Dalton [Jr.], *The Origin and Propagation of Disease* (New York: D. Appleton & Co., 1874); idem, "Spontaneous Generation," *N. Y. Med. J.* 15 (1872): 113–52; and idem, "Microscopic Fungi," *Med. Rec.* 8 (1873): 385–88.

92. Lister's development of the antiseptic system can be traced through many papers he wrote on the subject during the closing decades of the nineteenth century. These are reprinted in *The Collected Papers of Joseph Baron Lister,* 2 vols. (Oxford and New York: Oxford University Press, 1909). See also Charles Illingsworth, "On the Interdependence of Science and the Healing Art as Illustrated by Lister's Discovery of the Nature of Wound Sepsis," *Annals of the Royal College of Surgeons of England* 35 (1964): 1–14.

93. J[ohn] C. Dalton [Jr.], *Topographical Anatomy of the Brain,* 3 vols. (Philadelphia: Lea Brothers & Co., 1885).

94. "The Faith of Professors of Medical Colleges as Shown by Their Works," *Detroit Lancet* 5 (1882): 490–91.

95. Vanderbilt to the Trustees of the College of Physicians and Surgeons, 17 October 1884, published in Shrady, *College of Physicians and Surgeons,* 1:162.

96. Michael Mulhall, "The Increase of Wealth," *N. Am. Rev.* 140 (1885): 78.

97. William Gilman Thompson, "The Present Aspect of Medical Education," *Pop. Sci. Mon.* 27 (1885): 591, 592.

98. Henry D. Noyes, "Pathfinding in Medicine," *Med. Rec.* 28 (1885): 589.

99. See "Gift to Bellevue Hospital Medical College," *Med. News* 44 (1884): 520; Arnold H. Eggerth, *The History of the Hoagland Laboratory;* and "The Loomis Laboratory," *Med. News* 52 (1888): 244.

100. "Medical College Endowments," *JAMA* 3 (1884): 493.

101. Horace W. Davenport, "Physiology, 1850–1923: The View from Michigan," see esp. 50–67.

102. Lombard to Velyien E. Henderson, 25 May 1932, APS Archives.
103. Lee, "John Green Curtis," 56.
104. Draper to James W. McLane, 2 March 1889, Rare book room, New York Academy of Medicine, New York, N.Y.
105. John C. Dalton, "Magendie as a Physiologist," *International Review* 8 (1880): 120–25.
106. Mitchell, "John Call Dalton," 179.

Chapter 2: S. Weir Mitchell

1. Anna R. Burr, *Weir Mitchell: His Life and Letters;* Richard D. Walter, *S. Weir Mitchell, M.D.: Neurologist: A Medical Biography* (Springfield, Ill.: Charles C. Thomas, 1970); Ernest Earnest, *S. Weir Mitchell: Novelist and Physician* (Philadelphia: University of Pennsylvania Press, 1950); *S. Weir Mitchell, M.D., LL.D., F.R.S., 1829–1914: Memorial Addresses and Resolutions* (Philadelphia, 1914); and W. Bruce Fye, "S. Weir Mitchell, Philadelphia's 'Lost' Physiologist," *Bull. Hist. Med.* 57 (1983): 188–202. Mitchell prepared an autobiography late in his life, "Autobiography of S. Weir Mitchell," Historical Society of Pennsylvania Library, Philadelphia, Pa. Another version of this autobiography was available to Burr in the preparation of her biography.
2. S. Weir Mitchell, "Memoir of John Call Dalton, 1825–1889," *Biog. Mem. Nat. Acad. Sci.* 3 (1890): 179.
3. George W. Corner, *Two Centuries of Medicine*, 21. See also John Morgan, *A Discourse upon the Institution of Medical Schools in America* (1765; reprint ed., Philadelphia: University of Pennsylvania Press, 1965).
4. John Fulton, *Physiology*. For background on the European influence on medical education, medical science, and medical practice in the United States before the Civil War, see Francis R. Packard, "Foreign Influences on American Medicine," in *History of Medicine in the United States*, 2 vols. (New York: Paul B. Hoeber, 1931), 2:951, and Whitfield J. Bell, Jr., *The Colonial Physician & Other Essays* (New York: Science History Publications, 1975).
5. Henry Fairfield Osborn, "Biographical Memoir of Joseph Leidy: 1823–1891," *Biog. Mem. Nat. Acad. Sci.* 7 (1913): 335–96; William S. Middleton, "Joseph Leidy, Scientist," *Ann. Med. Hist.* 5 (1923): 100–112; and "The Joseph Leidy Commemorative Meeting Held in Philadelphia, December 6, 1923," *Proc. Acad. Nat. Sci. Phila.* 75 (1923): 1–87.
6. Samuel Jackson, *Address to the Medical Graduates of the University of Pennsylvania* (Philadelphia: Collins, 1840), 13, 13–14. See also William S. Middleton, "Samuel Jackson," *Ann. Med. Hist.* n.s. 7 (1935): 538–49 and Joseph Carson, *A Discourse Commemorative of the Life and Character of Samuel Jackson, M.D.* (Philadelphia: Collins, 1872).
7. Alexis de Tocqueville, *Democracy in America*, ed. J. Mayer and Max Lerner (New York: Harper & Row, 1966). The original French edition appeared in 1835. See also George H. Daniels, *American Science in the Age of Jackson* (New York: Columbia University Press, 1968).

8. Samuel Henry Dickson, *The Late Prof. J. K. Mitchell, M.D.* (Philadelphia: Joseph M. Wilson, 1858).

9. The experiments are described in Robley Dunglison, *Human Physiology*, 7th ed. (Philadelphia: Blanchard & Lea, 1850), 150. See also Samuel X. Radbill, ed., "The Autobiographical Ana of Robley Dunglison, M.D.," and Jerome J. Bylebyl, "William Beaumont, Robley Dunglison, and the 'Philadelphia Physiologists,'" *J. Hist. Med.* 27 (1970): 1-21.

10. Mitchell to Elizabeth Mitchell, 2 February 1851, published in Burr, *Weir Mitchell*, 67.

11. "Autobiography of Mitchell," 41.

12. Brown-Séquard's Philadelphia lectures were published: [Charles-] E. Brown-Séquard, "Experimental Researches Applied to Physiology and Pathology," *Med. Exam.* 16 (1852): 481-504, 549-69, 698-709.

13. William W. Keen, "The History of the Philadelphia School of Anatomy and Its Relation to Medical Teaching," in *Addresses and Other Papers* (Philadelphia: W. B. Saunders Co., 1905): 60.

14. S. Weir Mitchell, "The Relations of the Pulse to Certain States of Respiration," *Am. J. Med. Sci.* n.s. 27 (1854): 387-98. See also S. Weir Mitchell to Alexander Henry, 30 September 1853, American Philosophical Society Library, Philadelphia, Pa. See also S. Weir Mitchell, "A Case of Curious Cutaneous Disease," *Med. Exam.* 16 (1852): 74-76; and idem, "Observations on the Generation of Uric Acid, and Its Crystalline Forms," *Am. J. Med. Sci.* n.s. 24 (1852): 121-25.

15. S. W[eir] M[itchell], Book Review of Joseph Jones, "Investigations, Chemical and Physiological, Relative to Certain American Vertebrata," *N. Am. Med. Chir. Rev.* 1 (1857): 697-99. See also James O. Breeden, *Joseph Jones, M.D.: Scientist of the Old South* (Lexington: University of Kentucky Press, 1975), and S. Weir Mitchell, "Report on the Progress of Physiology and Anatomy," *N. Am. Med. Chir. Rev.* 2 (1858): 105-19.

16. Mitchell, "Report on Physiology," 119.

17. Joseph Leidy, *Lecture Introductory to the Course on Anatomy, in the University of Pennsylvania* (Philadelphia: Collins, 1853), 19. Other contemporary writers also pointed out the low productivity of Americans in medical research. See Samuel D. Gross, "Reports on the Causes Which Impede the Progress of American Medical Literature," *Trans. AMA* 9 (1856): 337-62; Edward B. Hunt, "Views and Suggestions on the Practice and Theory of Scientific Publications," *Proc. AAAS* 11th meeting (Cambridge: Joseph Lovering, 1858), 158-64; and "American Subserviency to Foreign Original Research," *Med. Surg. Rep.* 3 (1859): 293-95.

18. John K. Mitchell, *Impediments to the Study of Medicine* (Philadelphia: Collins, 1850), 19-20.

19. Bonnie Ellen Blustein, "The Philadelphia Biological Society, 1857-61: A Failed Experiment?" *J. Hist. Med.* 35 (1980): 188-202. See also David Riesman, "Men and Events in the History of the Philadelphia Pathological Society," *Ann. Med. Hist.* n.s. 6 (1934): 359-75.

20. See Bonnie Ellen Blustein, "A New York Medical Man: William Alex-

ander Hammond, M.D., 1828–1900, Neurologist" (Ph.D. diss., University of Pennsylvania, 1979); Jack D. Key, *William Alexander Hammond, M.D. (1828–1900)* (Rochester, Minn.: Davies, 1979); and Jack D. Key and Bonnie Ellen Blustein, *William A. Hammond, M.D. (1828–1900): The Publications of an American Neurologist* (Rochester, Minn.: Davies, 1983).

21. William A. Hammond, "Experiments with Bibron's Antidote to the Poison of the Rattlesnake," *Am. J. Med. Sci.* n.s. 35 (1858): 94–96. For Mitchell's recollections of his early interest in snakes and their venom, see S. Weir Mitchell, "The Poison of Serpents," *Century Magazine* 37 (1889): 503–14.

22. W[illiam] A. H[ammond], "Book Review. John C. Dalton, A Treatise on Human Physiology," *Am. J. Med. Sci.* n.s. 37 (1859): 446–58.

23. William A. Hammond and S. Weir Mitchell, "Experimental Researches Relative to Corroval and Vao: Two New Varieties of Woorara, the South American Arrow Poison," *Am. J. Med. Sci.* n.s. 38 (1859): 13–60.

24. William Hammond to Joseph Leidy, 19 September 1859, Leidy Papers.

25. See S. Weir Mitchell, "Researches upon the Venom of the Rattlesnake: With an Investigation on the Anatomy and Physiology of the Organs Concerned," *Smithsonian Contributions to Knowledge* 12 (1860): 1–145; and idem, "On the Treatment of Rattle-snake Bites, with Experimental Criticism upon the Various Remedies Now in Use," *N. Am. Med. Chir. Rev.* 5 (1861): 269–310.

26. Holmes to Mitchell, [May 1860], Mitchell Papers, Trent Collection. See also Holmes to Mitchell, 28 December 1858, Mitchell Papers, Trent Collection; Claude Bernard, "Lectures upon Experimental Pathology and Operative Physiology, Delivered at the College of France during the Winter Session, 1859–1860," *Med. Times Gaz.* 2 (1860): 295–97; and W. A. Hammond and S. Mitchell, "Recherches expérimentales sur le Corroval et la Vao," *Journal de la Physiologie de l'Homme et des Animaux* 2 (1859): 707–9.

27. S. Weir Mitchell, "Speech on the Two Hundred and Fiftieth Anniversary of the Founding of Harvard College," in *A Record of the Commemoration . . . of the Founding of Harvard College* (Cambridge: John Wilson & Son, 1887), 318.

28. John C. Dalton [Jr.], "Vivisection: What It Is and What It Has Accomplished," *Bull. N. Y. Acad. Med.* 3 (1866): 159–98.

29. S. Weir Mitchell, "The Annual Oration," *Trans. Med. Chi. Md.* (1877): 51–68. Elsewhere, Mitchell claimed Jackson told him, "You will lose a patient for every experiment you make in the laboratory." Mitchell, "John Call Dalton," 181.

30. Robley Dunglison [1852] quoted in Radbill, "Robley Dunglison," 151–52. Dunglison's emphasis.

31. Brown-Séquard to Mitchell, 20 July 1861, Mitchell Papers, Trent Collection.

32. Mitchell to Wyman, 26 February 1863, Wyman Papers. Mitchell's emphasis.

33. See George W. Adams, *Doctors in Blue: The Medical History of the Union Army in the Civil War* (New York: Henry Schuman, 1952), and Richard

H. Shryock, "A Medical Perspective on the Civil War," *American Quarterly* 14 (1962): 161–73.

34. S. Weir Mitchell, "Some Personal Recollections of the Civil War," *Trans. Coll. Phys. Phila.* 4th ser., 27 (1905): 87–94.

35. Mitchell to Elizabeth Mitchell, 10 August 1861 [1862], published in Burr, *Weir Mitchell*, 109–10. Mitchell later recalled, "The years from 1862 to 1865 left a busy Army surgeon small leisure for laboratory work." [S. Weir Mitchell], *A Catalogue of the Scientific and Literary Work of S. Weir Mitchell* (Philadelphia, 1894).

36. Allen to Leidy, 3 February 1862, Leidy Papers.

37. Hammond to Leidy, 1 March 1863, Leidy Papers.

38. Mitchell to Leidy, 2 March 1863, Leidy Papers. Mitchell's emphasis. Mitchell refers to Jacob Mendez DaCosta with whom he taught at the Summer Association and who was his colleague at Turner's Lane Hospital. See M. A. Clark, "Memoir of J. M. DaCosta," *Am. J. Med. Sci.* 125 (1903): 318–29.

39. Mitchell to Wyman, 4 February [March] 1863, Wyman Papers. Mitchell's emphasis. The content of this letter and that of 26 February 1863 from Mitchell to Wyman and other contemporary correspondence virtually prove that Mitchell misdated this letter, erroneously substituting February, the month just ended, for March.

40. Henry to Leidy, 11 March 1863, Reynolds Collection.

41. Henry to Tyndall, 22 October 1872, published in Charles Weiner, "Science and Higher Education," in *Science and Society in the United States,* ed. David D. Van Tassel and Michael G. Hall, (Homewood, Ill.: Dorsey Press, 1966), 177.

42. See Charles Nancrede, "Francis Gurney Smith [Jr.], M.D. 1818–1878," *Trans. Med. Soc. Penn.* n.s. 12 (1878): 404–8; and Joseph M. Toner, "Francis Gurney Smith [Jr.] M.D.," *Trans. AMA* 29 (1878): 762–63.

43. William B. Carpenter, *Principles of Human Physiology,* ed. with additions, by Francis Gurney Smith (Philadelphia: Lea & Blanchard, 1848). Smith contributed a highly regarded supplement on the clinical application of the microscope to Carpenter's work on this same subject; see William B. Carpenter, *The Microscope and Its Revelations,* ed. Francis Gurney Smith (Philadelphia: Blanchard & Lea, 1856).

44. Oliver Wendell Holmes et al., "Report of the Committee on Medical Literature," *Trans. AMA* 1 (1848): 249–86, see esp. 286.

45. Francis G. Smith, "Experiments on Digestion," *Med. Exam.* n.s. 12 (1856): 385–94, 513–18.

46. "Minutes of the Board of Trustees, University of Pennsylvania," 5 May 1863, Pennsylvania Archives. In addition to Mitchell and Smith, four other individuals submitted their names as candidates for the vacant chair: Henry Hartshorne, I. Chester Norris, James Aitken Meigs, and Charles-E. Brown-Séquard. The last two candidates were ineligible because they were nominated too late. For background on the University of Pennsylvania board of trustees see Joseph Carson, *A History of the Medical Department of the University of Pennsylvania, from Its Foundation in 1765* (Philadelphia: Lindsay & Blakiston, 1869), 53,

and *University of Pennsylvania: Biographical Catalogue of the Matriculants of the College, 1749-1893* (Philadelphia, 1894), xv-xvi.

47. Mitchell to Henry, 6 May 1863, Henry Papers. Background on Philadelphia society in this era is provided by E. Digby Baltzell, *Philadelphia Gentlemen: The Making of a National Upper Class* (1971; reprint ed., Philadelphia: University of Pennsylvania Press, 1979). Joseph Leidy recently described the attacks and insinuations, motivated by envy and competition, that could be expected from one's medical colleagues. See Joseph Leidy, *Valedictory Address to the Class of Medical Graduates of the University of Pennsylvania* (Philadelphia: Collins, 1858).

48. [George Shrady], "Medical Appointments," *Med. Rec.* 1 (1866): 477-78.

49. Alfred Stillé, *Address before the Philadelphia County Medical Society* (Philadelphia: Collins, 1863).

50. Henry to Mitchell, 7 May 1863, Reynolds Collection.

51. Holmes to Mitchell, [? June 1863], Mitchell Papers, Trent Collection. See also letters from William Hammond to Mitchell, 10 May 1863, published, in part, in Burr, *Weir Mitchell*, 118, and John Call Dalton [Jr.] to Mitchell, 17 May 1863, Mitchell Papers, Trent Collection.

52. S. Weir Mitchell, "Paralysis from Peripheral Irritation: With Reports of Cases," *N. Y. Med. J.* 2 (1866): 321-55, 401-23.

53. William Frederick Norwood, "Medical Education in the United States before 1900," in *The History of Medical Education*, ed. Charles D. O'Malley, 463-99.

54. S. Weir Mitchell, "The Object and Duties of a Neurological Society," *Journal of Nervous and Mental Diseases* 11 (1884): 262-66.

55. Mitchell to Wyman, 14 April 1868, Wyman Papers.

56. Wyman to Mitchell, 18 April 1868, Mitchell Papers, Trent Collection.

57. The relevant correspondence is in the Mitchell Papers, Trent Collection. The letters are acknowledged in the "Minutes of the Board of Trustees of the Jefferson Medical College," 23 April 1868, Jefferson Archives.

58. Agassiz to Mitchell, 28 May 1868, quoted in Burr, *Weir Mitchell*, 119-20.

59. See Henry C. Chapman, "Memoir of James Aitken Meigs," *Trans. Coll. Phys. Phila.* 3d ser., 5 (1880): cxvii-cxxxiii; George Hamilton, "Biographical Sketch of James Aitken Meigs, M.D.," *Trans. Med. Soc. Penn.* 13 (1880): 385-400; and Lawrence Turnbull, *Memoir of James Aitken Meigs, A.M., M.D.* (Philadelphia: Pugh Madeira, 1881).

60. Meigs to Isaac Hays, 12 July 1856, Gratz Collection. Historical Society of Pennsylvania, Philadelphia, Pa.

61. J[ames] A. M[eigs], "Book Review: E. Brown-Séquard. 'Journal de la Physiologie.'" *Am. J. Med. Sci.* n.s. 36 (1858): 505-8.

62. James A. Meigs, *Some Remarks on the Methods of Studying and Teaching Physiology* (Philadelphia: J. B. Lippincott Co., 1859).

63. "The Special Courses in the Jefferson Medical College," *Med. Surg. Rep.* 14 (1866): 175.

64. A list of letters in support of Meigs appears in Hamilton, "James Aitken Meigs," 5. See also Henry to Meigs, 2 May 1868; Henry to the Trustees of the Jefferson Medical College, 8 May 1868; and Meigs to Henry, 5 May 1868, in which Meigs outlines the positions he had held and the contributions he had made to physiology and anthropology. All in the Henry Papers. See also Curtis M. Hinsley, Jr., *Savages and Scientists: The Smithsonian Institution and the Development of American Anthropology, 1846–1910* (Washington: Smithsonian Institution, 1981).

65. Henry to the Trustees of the Jefferson Medical College, 25 May 1868, Reynolds Collection.

66. Henry to Mitchell, ?10 May 1868, and Mitchell to Henry, May 1868 and 16 May 1868, Henry Papers. For insight into the intense hostility between Democrats and Republicans in this period, in which George Woodward played a significant role, see Joel H. Silbey, *A Respectable Minority: The Democratic Party in the Civil War Era, 1860–1868* (New York: W. W. Norton, 1977).

67. Mitchell to "My Dear Sir," 28 May 1868, Gratz Collection, Historical Society of Pennsylvania, Philadelphia, Pa.

68. Turnbull, "James Aitken Meigs," 16.

69. Samuel G. Snowden to [James Ross Snowden], 15 May 1868, Historical Society of Pennsylvania, Philadelphia, Pa.

70. "Minutes of the Board of Trustees of the Jefferson Medical College," 2 June 1868, Jefferson Archives. See also Meigs to Henry, 8 June 1868, Henry Papers. A list of members of the Jefferson board of trustees is in Edward Louis Bauer, *Doctors Made in America* (Philadelphia: J. B. Lippincott Co., 1963), 354–55.

71. "Election of Dr. J. Aitken Meigs," *Med. Surg. Rep.* 18 (1868): 501; see also *Medical News & Library* 26 (1868): 106 which described the appointment as "an excellent one."

72. Wyman to Mitchell, 8 June 1868, Mitchell Papers, Trent Collection.

73. Mitchell to Wyman, 10 June [1868], Wyman Papers. Mitchell's emphasis. Other contemporary elections also hinged on social, political, and religious factors in the minds of some observers. See "The Chair of Anatomy in the Jefferson Medical College," *Med. Surg. Rep.* 28 (1873): 485–86; "The Contest at Jefferson College Concours," *Med. Surg. Rep.* 29 (1873): 32–33; "Hospital Appointments in Philadelphia," *Med. Rec.* 7 (1872): 376; and Leo James O'Hara, "An Emerging Profession: Philadelphia Medicine, 1860–1900" (Ph.D. diss., University of Pennsylvania, 1976), see esp. 37.

74. Mitchell to Wyman, 10 June [1868], Wyman Papers. The elite clientele of urban physicians of this era often left the cities during the summer months. Consequently, reduced practice demands provided more time for research and writing. See, for example, "The Summer Exodus from the City," *Boston Med. Surg. J.* 58 (1858): 482–83.

75. Mitchell to Henry, 3 June 1868, Henry Papers.

76. Henry to Mitchell, 5 June 1868, Henry Papers.

77. Mitchell to [James J. Putnam], 24 September [?1874], Putnam Papers, Countway.

78. [George Shrady], "American vs. European Medical Science," *Med. Rec.* 4 (1869): 133–34. See also Samuel D. Gross, "American vs. European Medical Science," *Med. Rec.* 4 (1869): 189–91; and [George Shrady], "American vs. European Medical Science Again," *Med. Rec.* 4 (1869): 181–86.

79. Frank Woodbury, "James Aitken Meigs," *Trans. AMA* 31 (1880): 1072.

80. James Aitken Meigs, *Valedictory Address to the Graduating Class of Jefferson Medical College* (Philadelphia: Collins, 1870), 20–21, 22. Meigs's emphasis.

81. Aleš Hrdlička, *Physical Anthropology: Its Scope and Aim: Its History and Present Status in America* (Philadelphia: Wistar Institute, 1919), 28–77. See also Frank Spencer, "The Rise of Academic Physical Anthropology in the United States, 1880–1980: A Historical Overview," *American Journal of Physical Anthropology* 56 (1981): 353–64; and "The Science of Anthropology," *Med. Surg. Rep.* 18 (1868): 223–24.

82. Edward J. Nolan, "A Biographical Notice of Henry Cadwalader Chapman, M.D., Sc.D.," *Proc. Acad. Nat. Sci. Phila.* (April 1910): 255–70. See also Leonard M. Rosenfeld, "Physiology at Jefferson Medical College (1842–1982)," *Physiologist* 27 (1984): 113–27.

83. Henry C. Chapman, *On Medical Education* (Philadelphia: Collins, 1876), 12–13.

84. Henry C. Chapman, "Lecture Introductory to the Course of Jefferson Medical College for the Session of 1880–81," *Coll. Clin. Rec.* 1 (1880): 181.

85. [Horatio C. Wood, Jr.], "The Value of Vivisection," *Scribner's Magazine* (September 1880): 770. See also George B. Roth, "An Early American Pharmacologist: Horatio C. Wood (1841–1920)," *Isis* 30 (1939): 38–45, and Horatio C. Wood, "Reminiscences of an American Pioneer in Experimental Medicine," *Trans. Coll. Phys. Phila.* 3d ser., 42 (1920): 175–86.

86. Wood, "Vivisection," 770. Outside of Philadelphia, the individuals Wood is probably referring to are H. Newell Martin at Johns Hopkins; Henry P. Bowditch at Harvard; Austin Flint, Jr., at the Bellevue Hospital Medical College; and John C. Dalton at the College of Physicians and Surgeons of New York. Isaac Ott, a practitioner who studied under Bowditch and Martin, and once used the facilities at the University of Pennsylvania, worked in his own private physiological laboratory in Easton, Pennsylvania.

87. "A Society for the Suppression of Vivisection," *Med. News* 42 (1883): 162. See also "Does Vivisection Pay?" *Med. News* 43 (1883): 383–84.

88. A list of this equipment is in "College News and Miscellany," *Coll. Clin. Rec.* 4 (1884): 165–66. See also "The Chair of Physiology at the College," *Coll. Clin. Rec.* 1 (1880): 10–11 and "College News," *Coll. Clin. Rec.* 1 (1880): 143.

89. William H. Howell, "The American Physiological Society during Its First Twenty-Five Years."

90. Holmes to Mitchell, 16 April 1872, Mitchell Papers, Trent Collection. The book Holmes refers to is S. Weir Mitchell, *Injuries of Nerves and Their Consequences* (Philadelphia: J. B. Lippincott Co., 1872).

91. See George B. Wood, *Introductory Lectures and Addresses, on Medical Subjects, Delivered Chiefly before the Medical Classes of the University of Pennsylvania* (Philadelphia: J. B. Lippincott Co., 1859).

92. "Medical Teaching in Philadelphia," *Phila. Med. Times* (March 15, 1871): 218–20.

93. Alfred Stillé, *Medical Education: What It Is and What It Might Be Made* (Philadelphia: Collins, 1873). See also William Osler, "Alfred Stillé," *Univ. Penn. Med. Bull.* 15 (1902): 126–32.

94. Wood to Billings, 1 December 1875, Billings Papers.

95. Ibid. See also Francis Newton Thorpe, *William Pepper, M.D., LL.D.* (Philadelphia: J. B. Lippincott Co., 1904).

96. Chapman to Leidy, 7 June 1875, Leidy Papers. Joseph Carson had been professor of materia medica and therapeutics at the University of Pennsylvania since 1850 and was an influential faculty member.

97. Rogers to the Committee of the Board of Trustees on the Medical Department, December 1875. A copy of this printed letter is in "Minute Book of the Medical Faculty of the University of Pennsylvania," vol. 6, Pennsylvania Archives.

98. *Catalogue and Announcement of the Medical Department of the University of Pennsylvania for the One Hundred and Twelfth Session, 1877–78* (Philadelphia: Collins, 1877), 16.

99. Nancrede, "Francis Gurney Smith."

100. George Strawbridge, William Pepper, H. C. Wood, Jr., "Report of Committee of the Hospital Professors of the University of Pennsylvania to the Medical Committee of the Board of Trustees on the Subject of Elevating the Standard of Medical Education," 22 November 1875, Pennsylvania Archives.

101. Tyson to [Calvin Ellis], 27 December 1874, Letters to the Dean, Countway. See also James Tyson, *Selected Addresses: On Subjects Relating to Education, Biography, Travel, Etc.* (Philadelphia: P. Blakiston's Son & Co., 1914); and Kenneth M. Ludmerer, "Reform at Harvard Medical School, 1869–1909," 343–70.

102. Horatio C. Wood, Jr., "Medical Education in the United States," *Lippincott's Magazina* (December 1875): 707. Wood's emphasis. The significant differences in the medical curriculum at Harvard compared with the University of Pennsylvania, Jefferson Medical College, and the College of Physicians and Surgeons of New York are graphically displayed in "The Order of Lectures in Some of the Principal Eastern Medical Schools, during the Session of 1875–76." *Med. Rec.* 10 (1875): 637–40. Only Harvard had laboratory work and a graded curriculum.

103. Wood, "Medical Education," 711.

104. Smith to the Board of Trustees of the University of Pennsylvania, 23 April 1877, "Minute Book of the Medical Faculty of the University of Pennsylvania," vol. 6, Pennsylvania Archives.

105. Ott to Bowditch, 25 April 1875, Bowditch Papers.

106. "A Step Forward in Medical Education," *Med. Surg. Rep.* 26 (1877): 16–17.

107. S. Weir Mitchell, "The Annual Oration before the Medical and Chirurgical Faculty of Maryland," *Trans. Med. Chi. Md.* (1877): 67-68.

108. A[lonzo] B. Palmer, "The Fallacies of Homeopathy," *N. Am. Rev.* 134 (1882): 314. See also William G. Rothstein, *American Physicians in the Nineteenth Century.*

109. William Pepper, Jr., Manuscript autobiographical notes, Pepper Collection. See also Fred B. Rogers, "William Pepper, 1843-1898: Physician, Educator, Philanthropist," *J. Med. Educ.* 34 (1959): 885-89, and Thorpe, *William Pepper.*

110. William Pepper, *Higher Medical Education: The True Interest of the Public and of the Profession* (Philadelphia: Collins, 1877).

111. Corner, *Two Centuries of Medicine,* 159.

112. S. Weir Mitchell, *Address Dedicatory of the New Buildings Erected by the University of Pennsylvania for Its Dental School and Medical Laboratories* (Philadelphia: J. B. Lippincott Co., 1878), 1-2, 15-16.

113. "Speech Delivered by Dr. William Pepper of Philadelphia, at the Opening of the New Laboratory of McGill University, Montreal, Canada, October 22/85," Pepper Papers.

114. "Endowment of Research," *Med. Surg. Rep.* 46 (1882): 658. See also "Endowments," *Med. Surg. Rep.* 48 (1883): 106; "Memorial Chairs in Our Medical Colleges," *Med. News* 41 (1882): 11-12; and "Aid for Original Scientific Research," *American* 3 (1881): 70-71.

115. "Nitro-Glycerin," *Med. News* 40 (1882): 408. Author's emphasis. See also W. Bruce Fye, "Nitroglycerin: A Homeopathic Remedy," *Circulation* 73 (1986): 21-29, and idem, "T. Lauder Brunton and Amyl Nitrite: A Victorian Vasodilator," *Circulation* 74 (1986): 222-29.

116. Brown-Séquard to Francis Gurney Smith, Jr., 5 April 1878, and 9 April 1878, Trent Collection.

117. Biographical material on Dupuy is contained in James M. D. Olmsted, *Charles-Edouard Brown-Séquard.* See also Eugene Dupuy, "Researches," and translations of several letters of recommendation for Dupuy in the Pennsylvania Archives.

118. Agnew to Tyson, 13 May 1878, "Minute Book of the Medical Faculty of the University of Pennsylvania," vol. 6, Pennsylvania Archives.

119. Horatio C. Wood [Jr.], "Memoir of Harrison Allen, M.D.," *Trans. Coll. Phys. Phila.* 3d ser., 20 (1898): xliii. See also "Harrison Allen," *Proc. Acad. Nat. Sci. Phila.* 49 (1897): 510-18.

120. Allen to Leidy, 12 February 1870, College of Physicians of Philadelphia, Philadelphia, Pa. See also Allen to Leidy, 21 December 1874, College of Physicians of Philadelphia.

121. "Aid for Original Scientific Research," 70.

122. William Bacon Stevens et al., "Printed Letter," 1 May 1882, Pennsylvania Archives.

123. S. Weir Mitchell quoted in Corner, *Two Centuries of Medicine,* 179.

124. Edward T. Reichert, "On the Physiological Action of Potassium Nitrite . . . With a Note on the Physiological Action on Man, by S. Weir Mitchell," *Am. J. Med. Sci.* 80 (1880): 158-80.

125. S. Weir Mitchell, "Remarks upon Some Recent Investigations on the Venom of Serpents," *Lancet* 2 (1883): 94.

126. S. Weir Mitchell and Edward T. Reichert, "Researches upon the Venoms of Poisonous Serpents," *Smithsonian Contributions to Knowledge* 26 (1886): 1–186. Mitchell encouraged the study of snake venom into the twentieth century when he partially subsidized Hideyo Noguchi's study of this subject. See Hideyo Noguchi, *Snake Venoms* (Washington: Carnegie Institute, 1909), iii, and S. Weir Mitchell, "The Poison of Serpents," *Proceedings of the Pathological Society of Philadelphia* n.s. 6 (1903): 81–84.

127. Bowditch to the Trustees of the University of Pennsylvania, 3 March 1885, in *To the Trustees of the University of Pennsylvania (1885)*, Pennsylvania Archives. This printed pamphlet includes several letters of support for Smith as well as his bibliography of thirty-three publications and a list of his appointments. Other letters of support came from Michael Foster, C-E. Brown-Séquard, John Burdon-Sanderson, and Alfred Stillé.

128. S. Weir Mitchell quoted in Corner, *Two Centuries of Medicine*, 179.

129. Wood and Tyson to the Board of Trustees, 20 October 1886, in "Minute Book of the Medical Faculty of the University of Pennsylvania," vol. 7, Pennsylvania Archives.

130. Ibid. For a listing of the physiological apparatus available at the university's chief competitor, Jefferson Medical College, see *Coll. Clin. Rec.* 4 (1884): 165–66.

131. Bowditch to Pepper, 31 March, 1895, Pepper Collection.

132. Flexner to Welch, [Spring 1902], quoted in Corner, *Two Centuries of Medicine*, 205–6.

133. William Osler, "Weir Mitchell," *Johns Hopkins Hosp. Bull.* 1 (1890): 64.

134. S. Weir Mitchell, "Lectures on the Conduct of the Medical Life," *University Medical Magazine* 5 (1893): 651–74.

Chapter 3: Henry P. Bowditch

1. S. Weir Mitchell, Russell H. Chittenden, William H. Howell, and Walter B. Cannon, "In Memory of Henry P. Bowditch, M.D." *Boston Med. Surg. J.* 164 (1911): 629. See also Walter B. Cannon, "Henry Pickering Bowditch," *Biog. Mem. Nat. Acad. Sci.* 17 (1922): 181–96; Frederick W. Ellis, "Henry Pickering Bowditch and the Development of the Harvard Laboratory of Physiology," *New England Journal of Medicine* 219 (1938): 819–28; W. Bruce Fye, "Why a Physiologist? The Case of Henry P. Bowditch," *Bull. Hist. Med.* 56 (1982): 19–29; idem, "Henry Pickering Bowditch: A Case Study of the Harvard Physiologist and His Impact on the Professionalization of Physiology in America" (Master's essay, Johns Hopkins University, 1978); Charles S. Minot, "Henry Pickering Bowditch," *Science* N.S. 33 (1911): 598–601; Harold Bowditch, *The Bowditch Family of Salem*, Massachusetts ([Boston], 1936); and Thomas Francis Harrington, *Harvard Medical School*. An unpublished chronology of Bowditch's life including excerpts from his correspondence was prepared by his son,

Harold Bowditch. See [Harold Bowditch], "Henry Pickering Bowditch, M.D.,"
Bowditch Papers; hereafter "Harold Bowditch Notes."

2. *Report of the Committee of the Overseers of Harvard College Appointed to Visit the Lawrence Scientific School during the Year 1860: Together
with the Reports Submitted by the Professors* (Boston, 1861). See also
"Lawrence Scientific School," *Am J. Educ.* 1 (1856): 205–24, and Edward
Lurie, *Louis Agassiz.*

3. "Report of the Committee on Medical Education," *Trans. AMA* 4
(1851): 409–46; see esp. 443–46. See also Margaret W. Rossiter, *The Emergence
of Agricultural Science,*and Rolf King, "E. N. Horsford's Contribution to the
Advancement of Science in America," *New York History* 36 (1955): 307–19.

4. See Wyman to H. P. Bowditch, 29 December 1869, Bowditch Papers,
and Jeffries Wyman, "Experiments with Vibrating Cilia," *Am. Nat.* 5 (1871):
611–16.

5. "Dr. Brown-Séquard's Lectures," *Boston Med. Surg. J.* 47 (1853): 452.
His 1852 lectures were published; see "Dr. Brown-Séquard's Experimental Re-
searches," *Boston Med. Surg. J.* 49 (1854): 249, and [Charles]-E. Brown-
Séquard, *Experimental Researches Applied to Physiology and Pathology*
(New York: Baillière, 1853). See also H. Richard Tyler and Kenneth L. Tyler,
"Charles-Edouard Brown-Séquard: Professor of Physiology and Pathology of
the Nervous System at Harvard Medical School," *Neurology* 34 (1984):
1231–36.

6. Brown-Séquard to George Cheyne Shattuck, 17 March 1865, Shattuck
Papers, Countway.

7. C[harles]-E. Brown-Séquard, *Advice to Students: An Address Delivered at the Opening of the Medical Lectures of Harvard University, Nov. 7,
1866* (Cambridge: John Wilson & Son, 1867), 32. Brown-Séquard emphasized
the practical utility of a thorough knowledge of physiology in an address delivered in Ireland the previous year. C[harles]-E. Brown-Séquard, "On the Importance of Application of Physiology to the Practice of Medicine and Surgery,"
Dublin Quarterly Journal of Medicine 39 (1865): 421–36.

8. [Henry P. Bowditch and William T. Porter], "The Department of Physiology," in *The Harvard Medical School* (Boston, 1906), 87. In an obituary of
Brown-Séquard, Bowditch listed his important discoveries, but asserted: "One
of his strongest claims to remembrance rests upon the stimulus to research which
flowed from his activity in the various medical communities in which he resided
and on the enthusiasm for pure science which he imparted to all who came into
personal relations with him." Henry P. Bowditch, "Memoir of Charles-Edouard
Brown-Séquard, 1817–1894," *Biog. Mem. Nat. Acad. Sci.* 4 (1902): 97.

9. See David Cheever, "Oliver Wendell Holmes, the Anatomist," *Harvard
Graduates Magazine* 3 (1894): 154–59, and Thomas Dwight, "Reminiscences of
Dr. Holmes as Professor of Anatomy," *Scribner's Magazine* 17 (1895): 121–28.

10. Oliver W. Holmes, *Teaching from the Chair and at the Bedside* (Boston: David Clapp & Son, 1867), 5.

11. William James to H. P. Bowditch, 5 April 1868, Bowditch Papers.

12. Holmes to his parents, 13 January 1834, published in John T. Morse,

Jr., *Life and Letters of Oliver Wendell Holmes*, 2 vols. (Cambridge: Riverside Press, 1896), 1:125–26. See also Walter R. Steiner, "Some Distinguished American Medical Students of Pierre-Charles-Alexander Louis of Paris," *Bull. Hist. Med.* 7 (1939): 783–93, and Henry I. Bowditch, *Brief Memories of Louis and Some of His Contemporaries in the Parisian School of Medicine of Forty Years Ago* (Boston: John Wilson & Son, 1872).

13. Henry I. Bowditch to Olivia Bowditch, 25 August 1866, published in Vincent Y. Bowditch, *Life and Correspondence of Henry Ingersoll Bowditch*, 2:70.

14. William G. Rothstein, *American Physicians in the Nineteenth Century*.

15. James to Bowditch, 12 December 1867, published in Henry James, ed., *The Letters of William James*, 2 vols. (Boston: Atlantic Monthly Press, 1920), 1:120–24. See also Ralph Barton Perry, *The Thought and Character of William James* (Cambridge: Harvard University Press, 1948); Gay Wilson Allen, *William James;* and [William James], "Rapport sur le [*sic*] Progrès et la Marche de la Physiologie générale en France. Par M. Claude Bernard," *N. Am. Rev.* 107 (1868): 322–28.

16. Bowditch to Wyman, 14 January 1869, Wyman Papers.

17. Wyman to Bowditch, 9 February 1869, Bowditch Papers.

18. H. P. Bowditch to J. I. Bowditch, 12 February 1869, Bowditch Papers.

19. Benjamin A. Gould, "Address," *Proc. AAAS* 18th meeting, (Cambridge: Joseph Lovering, 1870): 1–37.

20. Wyman to Bowditch, 9 February 1869, Bowditch Papers.

21. "How to Study Medicine—No. VI," *Boston Med. Surg. J.* 79 (1868): 317.

22. "The Progress of Medical Science," *Boston Med. Surg. J.* 79 (1868): 284.

23. See Robert V. Bruce, "A Statistical Profile of American Scientists, 1836–1876," in George H. Daniels, ed., *Nineteenth-Century American Science*, 63–94; Clark A. Elliott, "The American Scientist, 1800–1863: His Origins, Career, and Interests"; and Stephen Sargent Vischer, *Scientists Starred, 1903–1943 in American Men of Science*.

24. J. I. Bowditch to H. P. Bowditch, 1 March 1869, Bowditch Papers.

25. H. P. Bowditch to J. I. Bowditch, 18 March 1869, published in Cannon, "Henry Pickering Bowditch."

26. William James to Mary Walsh James, [c. September 1863], published in James, *Letters of William James*, 1:45–46.

27. Wyman to Bowditch, 9 February 1869, Bowditch Papers.

28. Wyman to H. I. Bowditch, 10 February 1869, Bowditch Papers.

29. J. I. Bowditch to H. P. Bowditch, 15 February 1869, appended to Wyman to H. I. Bowditch, 10 February 1869, Bowditch Papers.

30. Ibid.

31. Edward Lloyd Howard and Christopher Johnston, "Report of the Committee on Specialties, and on the Propriety of Specialists Advertising," *Trans. AMA* 20 (1869): 111–13.

32. See Henry James, *Charles W. Eliot, President of Harvard University, 1869–1909;* Hugh Hawkins, *Between Harvard and America;* and William Allen

Neilson, *Charles W. Eliot: The Man and His Beliefs*, 2 vols. (New York: Harper & Brothers, 1926).

33. Rogers to Eliot, 6 June 1865, published in Emma Rogers and William T. Sedgwick, eds., *Life and Letters of William Barton Rogers*, 2 vols. (Boston: Houghton, Mifflin, 1896), 2:239. See also Samuel C. Prescott, *When M.I.T. was "Boston Tech": 1861–1916* (Cambridge: Technology Press, 1954).

34. [Charles W. Eliot], "The New Education: Its Organization," *Atlantic Monthly* 23 (1869): 216.

35. Eliot to Rogers, 20 June 1865, published in Rogers and Sedgwick, *William Barton Rogers*, 2:243.

36. "The Presidency of Harvard College," *Nation*, 7 (1868): 547–48.

37. Jeffries Wyman to Morrill Wyman, 15 April 1869, Wyman Papers.

38. J. I. Bowditch to H. P. Bowditch, 15 June 1869, Bowditch Papers.

39. Charles W. Eliot, "Inaugural Address as President of Harvard College," in *Educational Reform: Essays and Addresses* (New York: Century Co., 1901): 6, 35. See also "The New Regime at Harvard," *Nation* 9 (1869): 408–9.

40. H. P. Bowditch to H. I. Bowditch, 12 April 1869, Bowditch Papers.

41. Johannes Müller, *Handbuch der Physiologie des Menschen*, 2 vols. (Coblenz: J. Hölscher, 1834–1840).

42. Clement Smith to Mrs. Henry Rood, 24 January 1866, Smith Collection, Harvard University Archives, Cambridge, Mass.

43. James to Bowditch, 15 June 1868, Bowditch Papers. See also W. Bruce Fye, "Carl Ludwig and the Leipzig Physiological Institute: 'A Factory of New Knowledge,'" *Circulation* 74 (1986): 920–28.

44. Bowditch to Wyman, 31 October 1869, Wyman Papers.

45. H. P. Bowditch to H. I. Bowditch, 5 December 1869, Bowditch Papers.

46. Henry P. Bowditch, "Letter to the Editor," *Boston Med. Surg. J.* 82 (1870): 307. See also idem, "The Physiological Laboratory at Leipzig," *Nature* 3 (1870): 142–43.

47. Henry P. Bowditch, Über die Eigenthümlichkeiten der Reizbarkeit, welche die Muskelfasern des Herzens zeigen," *Berichte über die Verhandlungen der Königlichen Sächsischen Gesellschaft der Wissenschaften zu Leipzig. Math. Phy. Klasse* 23 (1871): 652–89. See also Wilfried F.H.M. Mommaerts, "Heart Muscle," in *Circulation of the Blood: Men and Ideas*, ed. Alfred P. Fishman and Dickinson W. Richards (New York: Oxford University Press, 1964), 127–98. Ludwig's students often mentioned his practice of assisting them but accepting no credit.

48. Eliot to H. P. Bowditch, 14 December 1869, transcribed in a letter from H. P. Bowditch to J. I. Bowditch, 9 January 1870. See also J. I. Bowditch to H. P. Bowditch, 9 December 1869, Bowditch Papers.

49. H. P. Bowditch to Eliot, 9 January 1870, transcribed in a letter from H. P. Bowditch to J. I. Bowditch, 9 January 1870, Bowditch Papers.

50. Bowditch to Lucy Bowditch, 27 February 1870, Bowditch Papers.

51. Ibid., [1869], published in Walter B. Cannon, "Henry Pickering Bowditch," 185. See also Edward D. Churchill, ed., *To Work in the Vineyard of*

Surgery: The Reminiscences of J. Collins Warren (1842-1927) (Cambridge: Harvard University Press, 1958).

52. See James Clark White, *Sketches from My Life: 1833-1913* (Cambridge: Riverside Press, 1914), and Abner Post, "James Clark White, M.D.," *Boston Med. Surg. J.* 175 (1916): 79–83.

53. White to Eliot, 17 August 1869, Eliot Papers. See also White to Eliot, 21 October 1869, Eliot Papers.

54. Ibid., 28 September 1870, Eliot Papers. The address to which White is referring is Oliver Wendell Holmes, *Teaching from the Chair and at the Bedside* (Boston: David Clapp & Son, 1867).

55. James C. White, "An Introductory Lecture Delivered before the Medical Class of Harvard University," *Boston Med. Surg. J.* 83 (1870): 279, 289.

56. James to Bowditch, 22 May 1869, Bowditch Papers.

57. Holmes to Motley, 3 April 1870, published in Morse, *Life and Letters of Oliver Wendell Holmes*, 2:186–89.

58. Eliot to G. J. Brush, 26 June 1863, published in Hawkins, *Between Harvard and America*, 28.

59. Eliot, "Inaugural Address," 27. See also Seymour Harris, *Economics of Harvard* (New York: McGraw-Hill, 1972). As Harvard's financial situation improved, Eliot became a strong advocate of research. See Charles W. Eliot, "Character of the Scientific Investigator," *Educational Review* 32 (1906): 157–64.

60. *A Memoir of Henry Jacob Bigelow* (Boston: Little, Brown & Co., 1900).

61. Bigelow to Eliot, 15 April 1871, Eliot Papers. Bigelow's emphasis.

62. Henry J. Bigelow, *Medical Education in America* (Cambridge: Welch, Bigelow & Co., 1871), 3, 39, 42, 45, 75, 49.

63. Holmes, quoted in James, *Charles W. Eliot*, 1:282.

64. Holmes to John L. Motley, 22 December 1871, published in Morse, *Life and Letters of Oliver Wendell Holmes*, 2:190.

65. J. I. Bowditch to H. P. Bowditch, 27 March 1870. See also J. I. Bowditch to H. P. Bowditch, 15 March 1870, Bowditch Papers, and Jeffries Wyman to Morrill Wyman, 5 April 1870, Wyman Papers.

66. [Graham Lusk], "Physiology at the Harvard Medical School: 1870–1871: A Part of the Introductory Lecture and Synopsis of the Experimental Demonstrations Given by William T. Lusk," *Boston Med. Surg. J.* 166 (1912): 921–22. Biographical sketches of Lusk are included in [William Chittenden Lusk], *War Letters of William Thompson Lusk* (New York, 1911).

67. James J. Putnam to Charles G. Putnam, 10 July 1870. Putnam Papers, Countway.

68. Jeffries Wyman to Morrill Wyman, 26 June 1870, Wyman Papers.

69. B. Joy Jeffries, "Letter to the Editor," *Boston Med. Surg. J.* 82 (1870): 421.

70. Bowditch to Eliot, 21 April 1871, Eliot Papers.

71. H. P. Bowditch to J. I. Bowditch, 21 April 1871, Bowditch Papers.

72. J. I. Bowditch to H. P. Bowditch, 22 March 1871, Bowditch Papers.

73. H. P. Bowditch to J. I. Bowditch, 21 April 1871, Bowditch Papers.

74. J. I. Bowditch to H. P. Bowditch, 10 May 1871, Bowditch Papers.

75. "Harvard University Medical Faculty. Minutes of the Meetings," vol. 3, 16 June 1871, Countway.

76. Harrington, *Harvard Medical School*, 3:1047–48. See also "Dr. George Swett," *Boston Med. Surg. J.* 81 (1869): 15.

77. *A Catalogue of the Officers and Students of Harvard University for the Academic Year 1871–1872*, 2d ed. (Cambridge: Riverside Press, 1872), 85.

78. David Cheever, "An Introductory Lecture Delivered before the Medical Class of Harvard University, Oct. 2, 1871," *Boston Med. Surg. J.* 85 (1871): 213. Cheever's emphasis.

79. "Recent Advances in Physiology," *Brit. For. Med. Chir. Rev.* (April 1874): 270. Author's emphasis.

80. "The Time Has Come," *Phila. Med. Times* (April 1, 1872): 251–53. This author observed that the circumstances in Great Britain were different from those in America.

81. Lankester to Bowditch, 1 August [1873?], Bowditch Papers.

82. *The Harvard University Catalogue, 1872–1873* (Cambridge, Mass.: Charles W. Sever, 1873).

83. Forceps, "Changes in the Harvard Medical College: How the Various Branches Are Taught," *N. Y. Med. J.* 20 (1874): 190–91.

84. James to Bowditch, 12 December 1867, Bowditch Papers. See also William James to Henry James, 24 August 1872 and 24 November 1872, published in James, *Letters of William James*, 1:165–67, and [William James], "Vivisection," *Nation* 20 (1875): 128–29.

85. H[enry] P. B[owditch], "Vivisection," *Boston Med. Surg. J.* 88 (1873): 94.

86. Robert S. Harper, "The First Psychological Laboratory," *Isis* 41 (1950): 158–61.

87. A list of publications from Bowditch's laboratory between 1873 and 1887 is in Fye, "Henry Pickering Bowditch," (1978): 187–90.

88. H[enry] P. B[owditch], "Report on Physiology," *Boston Med. Surg. J.* 90 (1874): 89.

89. H[enry] P. B[owditch], "Bibliographical Notice of Handbook for the Physiological Laboratory." *Boston Med. Surg. J.* 89 (1873): 360–61. See also Edward Klein, John Burdon-Sanderson, Michael Foster, and T. Lauder Brunton, *Handbook for the Physiological Laboratory*, 2 vols., ed. J. Burdon-Sanderson (Philadelphia: Lindsay & Blakiston, 1873).

90. See Martin to H. P. Bowditch, 14 January 1877, and E. Ray Lankester to H. P. Bowditch, 5 August [1875], Bowditch Papers.

91. See Martin to H. P. Bowditch, 14 January 1877, and Michael Foster to H. P. Bowditch, 3 July 1877, Bowditch Papers. Foster's letter is transcribed in "Harold Bowditch Notes." For an overview of the literature of medicine in America in this era see John S. Billings, "A Century of American Medicine: Literature and Institutions," *Am. J. Med. Sci.* 72 (1876): 439–80.

92. Minot to Bowditch, 14 January 1873, transcribed in "Harold Bowditch Notes." See also Frederick T. Lewis, "Charles Sedgwick Minot," *Anat. Rec.* 10

(1916): 113–64, and Henry H. Donaldson, "Charles Sedgwick Minot," *Proc. Bost. Soc. Nat. Hist.* 35 (1915): 79–93.

93. William Osler, "Harvard School of Medicine," *Canadian Journal of Medical Science* 2 (1877): 274–76. See also William Osler, "Brief Description of the New Physiological Laboratory, McGill College," *Canada Med. Surg. J.* 9 (1880): 198–201, and Harvey Cushing, *Life of Sir William Osler*, 2:142.

94. *Catalogue of Harvard University . . . 1876–1877* (Cambridge, 1876), 116.

95. Charles Eliot, [Remarks at a] "Meeting to Promote the Erection of a New Building," 22 October 1874, quoted in Harrington, *Harvard Medical School*, 3:1105–6.

96. Oliver Wendell Holmes, [Remarks at a] "Meeting to Promote the Erection of a New Building," 22 October 1874, quoted in Harrington, *Harvard Medical School*, 3:1107.

97. "Expensiveness of Scientific Education." *Pop. Sci. Mon.* 7 (1875): 746–48.

98. Josiah P. Cooke, Jr., *Scientific Culture* ([Boston], 1875), 7, 10. See also Richard Proctor, "The Endowment of Scientific Research," *Pop. Sci. Mon.* 7 (1875): 354–63, and Frank W. Clark, "American Colleges *versus* American Science," *Pop. Sci. Mon.* 9 (1876): 467–69.

99. Frederick W. Ellis, "Henry Pickering Bowditch," 822.

100. Palmer to Angell, 7 May 1877, Angell Papers. See also [Henry S. Frieze], *Memorial of Alonzo Benjamin Palmer* (Cambridge: Riverside Press, 1890); *The Reminiscences of James Burrill Angell* (New York: Longmans, Green & Co., 1911); and Horace W. Davenport, "Physiology, 1850–1923: The View from Michigan."

101. Cheever to Angell, March 1876, Angell Papers.

102. E[lias] W. Gray, "The Relation of Physiology to the Practice of Medicine," *Trans AMA* 25 (1874): 153.

103. M. Wall to Calvin Ellis, 10 June 1873, "Harvard Medical School Deans Office File, c. 1838–1900. Incoming Correspondence, November 1871–1892," Countway.

104. "Medical Science," *Phila. Med. Times* 7 (1877): 154–55. William H. Welch who recently returned to America from postgraduate medical training in Europe shared this view. See William Welch to Emeline Welch, 21 April 1878, quoted in Simon Flexner and James Thomas Flexner, *Henry Welch and the Heroic Age of American Medicine*, 112–13.

105. J.R.W. Hitchcock, "Recent Original Work at Harvard," *Pop. Sci. Mon.* 17 (1880): 483.

106. "The Harvard Medical School, 1880–81: Plans for the Future," *Boston Med. Surg. J.* 106 (1882): 66. See also "The Medical Teaching of the Future in Boston and at the Harvard Medical School," *Boston Med. Surg. J.* 109 (1883): 426–27.

107. [Joseph W. Warren], "Description of the Physiological Laboratory of the Harvard Medical School," *Science* 4 (1884): 130.

108. "The Biological Laboratory of the Johns Hopkins University," *Science* 3 (1884): 350–54.

109. Osler to Schäfer, 12 March 1884, Sharpey-Schafer Collection.

110. Hall quoted in a letter from H. Newell Martin to Daniel C. Gilman, 11 July 1883, Gilman Papers.

111. H. P. Bowditch to Selma Bowditch, 10 April [1884], Bowditch Papers.

112. Ellis, "Henry Pickering Bowditch," 825.

113. Oliver Wendell Holmes, "The Address Delivered in Huntington Hall," in *The New Century and the New Building of the Harvard Medical School, 1783-1883: Addresses and Exercises at the One Hundredth Anniversary of the Foundation of the Medical School of Harvard University* (Cambridge: John Wilson & Son, 1884), 24-25.

114. Oliver Wendell Holmes, "Endowment of the Harvard Medical School," in *The New Century*, 52.

115. Minot to Eliot, 16 May 1883, Eliot Papers. Other members of the Harvard faculty shared Minot's view that Bowditch was "most fit" for the job. See also Minot to Eliot, 18 May 1883, Eliot Papers.

116. James, *Charles W. Eliot*, 2:63.

117. See Fielding Garrison, *John Shaw Billings: A Memoir.*

118. Billings to Bowditch, 12 December 1884, "Harold Bowditch Notes," Bowditch Papers.

119. George B. Shattuck, "The President's Address," *Bulletin of the Harvard Medical Alumni Association*, no. 7 (1894): 18-19.

120. Ludwig to H. P. Bowditch, 2 March 1888, (original in German), "Harold Bowditch Notes." See also Brown-Séquard to H. P. Bowditch, 19 September 1888, Bowditch Papers.

121. Henry P. Bowditch, "The Advancement of Medicine by Research," *Science* n.s. 4 (1896): 100.

122. Ibid., "Reform in Medical Education," *Boston Med. Surg. J.* 139 (1898): 643-46; and idem, "The Medical School of the Future," *Philadelphia Medical Journal* 5 (1900): 1011-22.

123. See Harrington, *Harvard Medical School*, 3:1173, and Charles S. Minot to H. P. Bowditch, 27 June 1901, Bowditch Papers.

124. "Henry Pickering Bowditch: Obituary," *Lancet* 1 (1911): 975.

125. Osler to Selma Bowditch, [1911], "Harold Bowditch Notes," Bowditch Papers.

Chapter 4: H. Newell Martin, Johns Hopkins, and the Research Ethic

1. Background on the Johns Hopkins University is provided by Hugh Hawkins, *Pioneer;* John C. French, *A History of the University Founded by Johns Hopkins;* Alan M. Chesney, *The Johns Hopkins Hospital and the Johns Hopkins University School of Medicine: A Chronicle. Vol. 1. Early Years, 1867-1893;* and Richard H. Shryock, *The Unique Influence of the Johns Hopkins University on American Medicine.*

2. "Self-Made Men as Public Benefactors," *Nation* 9 (1869): 406-7.

3. Daniel Coit Gilman, "Johns Hopkins and the Trustees of His Choice,"

in *The Launching of a University and Other Papers*, 36. See also Mark B. Beach, "Professors, Presidents and Trustees."

4. [Daniel Coit Gilman] "Death of Hon. George W. Dobbin," *Johns Hopkins Circ.* no. 91 (July 1891): 148–49.

5. See Glenn C. Altschuler, *Andrew D. White: Educator, Historian, Diplomat* (Ithaca: Cornell University Press, 1979); *Autobiography of Andrew Dickson White: With Portraits*, 2 vols. (New York: Century Co., 1905); and Hugh Hawkins, "Three University Presidents Testify," *American Quarterly* 11 (1959): 99–111.

6. Andrew D. White, "Remarks," in *Proceedings at the Farewell Banquet to Professor Tyndall* (New York: D. Appleton & Co., 1873): 80. See also Katherine Sopka, "An Apostle of Science Visits America: John Tyndall's Journey of 1872–1873," *Physics Teacher* 10 (1972): 369–75.

7. White to James Carey Thomas, 13 March 1874, typescript in J.H.U. Collection, JHUSC. The Cornell president also encouraged the trustees to review his recent paper on scientific education. See White to Reverdy Johnson, Jr., 1 May 1874, J.H.U. Collection, JHUSC, and Andrew D. White, "Scientific and Industrial Education in the United States," *Pop. Sci. Mon.* 5 (1874): 170–91.

8. "Remarks of President Eliot of Harvard College Before the Trustees of the Johns Hopkins University, 4 June 1874," J.H.U. Collection, JHUSC. See also Reverdy Johnson, Jr., to Eliot, 13 May 1874, Eliot Papers.

9. "Remarks of James B. Angell of the University of Michigan before the Trustees of the Johns Hopkins University," J.H.U. Collection, JHUSC.

10. See Hawkins, *Pioneer*; Franklin, *Life of Daniel Coit Gilman*, and Francesco Cordasco, *The Shaping of American Graduate Education*.

11. Daniel C. Gilman, "Scientific Schools in Europe," *Am. J. Educ.* 1 (1856): 315, 327. See also Richard Emmons Thursfield, *Henry Barnard's "American Journal of Education"* Johns Hopkins Studies in Historial and Political Science, ser. 63, no. 1 (Baltimore: Johns Hopkins Press, 1945).

12. Gilman, "Scientific Schools," 327–28.

13. See [Theodore Dwight Woolsey], *Appeal in Behalf of the Yale Scientific School. With an Appendix* [Scientific Schools in Europe by Daniel C. Gilman] (New Haven, 1856); James D. Dana, *Science and Scientific Schools* (New Haven: S. Babcock, 1856); and Russell H. Chittenden, *History of the Sheffield Scientific School of Yale University, 1846–1922*.

14. [Daniel C. Gilman], "Our National Schools of Science," *N. Am. Rev.* 105 (1867): 516–17.

15. See Gilman to Porter, 12 September 1872, published in Franklin, *Daniel Coit Gilman*, 106–7, and George Wilson Pearson, *Yale College: An Educational History, 1871–1921* (New Haven: Yale University Press, 1952), see esp. 57–65.

16. Daniel C. Gilman, "The University of California in Its Infancy," in *University Problems in the United States* (New York: Century Co., 1896), 168. See also Gert H. Brieger, "The California Origins of the Johns Hopkins Medical School," *Bull. Hist. Med.* 51 (1977): 339–52.

17. Gilman to White, 5 April 1874, published in Franklin, *Daniel Coit Gilman*, 155–57.

18. See Robert Morris Ogden, ed. *The Diaries of Andrew D. White* (Ithaca: Cornell University Library, 1959), entry dated 15 August 1874, 183, and Gilman to White, 30 September 1874 and 18 October 1874, published in part in Franklin, *Daniel Coit Gilman*, 169–70.

19. Eliot to Gilman, 1 July 1874, Gilman Papers.

20. Gilman to White, 4 November 1874, published in Franklin, *Daniel Coit Gilman*, 171.

21. [Daniel C. Gilman], manuscript fragments, [April 1875], published in Franklin, *Daniel Coit Gilman*, 179.

22. Gilman's interview, published in the *Nation* 28 (January 1875), is reprinted in Franklin, *Daniel Coit Gilman*, 188–89.

23. Henry to the Committee of Arrangements of the Tyndall Banquet, 3 February 1873, in *Proceedings at the Farewell Banquet to Professor Tyndall* (New York: D. Appleton & Co., 1873), 11–24.

24. Henry to Gilman, 25 August 1875, Gilman Papers.

25. Henry to Reverdy Johnson, Jr., 19 February 1876, Gilman Papers.

26. Gilman to Eliot, 14 May 1875, Eliot Papers. Gilman's emphasis. See also Gilman to Eliot, 1 December 1876, Eliot Papers.

27. See Fielding H. Garrison, *John Shaw Billings*, and Jean A. Curran, "John Shaw Billings: Contributions to the Advancement of Medical Education," in *John Shaw Billings Centennial* (Bethesda: National Library of Medicine, 1975), 29–41.

28. John S. Billings, "The Medical College of Ohio before the War," *Cincinnati Lancet-Clinic* n.s. 20 (1888): 297–305.

29. John S. Billings, *A Report on Barracks and Hospitals: With Descriptions of Military Posts* (Washington: Surgeon General's Office, 1870). See also "Alfred Alexander Woodhull, John Shaw Billings, and the Johns Hopkins Hospital, 8 June 1871," *J. Hist. Med.* 13 (1958): 531–37, and letters of Woodhull to Billings, 3 June 1874 and 18 June 1874, Billings Papers.

30. John S. Billings, "Hospital Construction and Organization," in *Hospital Plans. Five Essays Relating to the Construction, Organization & Management of Hospitals, Contributed by Their Authors for the Use of the Johns Hopkins Hospital of Baltimore* (New York: William Wood & Co., 1875), 4, 5. See also Gert H. Brieger, "The Original Plans for the Johns Hopkins Hospital and Their Historical Significance," *Bull. Hist. Med.* 39 (1965): 518–28.

31. John S. Billings, *Johns Hopkins Hospital, Reports and Papers Relating to Construction and Organization*, no. 1 (Washington, 1876), 7.

32. "A New University," *Boston Med. Surg. J.* 92 (1875): 266–67.

33. See Cyril Bibby, *T. H. Huxley: Scientist, Humanist, and Educator;* Mário A. di Gregorio, *T. H. Huxley's Place in Natural Science;* and Leonard Huxley, ed., *Life and Letters of Thomas Henry Huxley.*

34. Gilman to the Johns Hopkins Trustees, 13 September 1875, published in Franklin, *Daniel Coit Gilman*, 206. See also Daniel C. Gilman, "The Launching of the University," in *The Launching of a University*, 3–38, and Roy

M. MacLeod, "The X-club, a Social Network of Science in Late Victorian England," *Notes and Records of the Royal Society of London* 24 (1970): 305–22.

35. Thomas H. Huxley, "Universities: Actual and Ideal" (1874), in *Science and Education*, 219.

36. Ibid., "On the Educational Value of the Natural History Sciences" (1854), in *Science and Education*, 50. Huxley's emphasis.

37. [Daniel C. Gilman], "On the Selection of Professors, Read to the Trustees" [December 1875], J.H.U. Collection, JHUSC. See also Minutes of the Board of Trustees of the Johns Hopkins University, 6 December 1875, Hamburger Archives; Gilman to James B. Angell, 10 December 1875, Angell Papers; and "Remarks of Professor D. C. Gilman," *Proceedings of the Agassiz Memorial Meeting. California Academy of Sciences* (San Francisco: California Academy of Sciences, 1874), 8–13.

38. Welch to Dennis, 7 November 1875, Welch Papers.

39. Eliot to Gilman, 23 March 1876, Gilman Papers.

40. See C. S. Breathnach, "Henry Newell Martin (1848–1893) [*sic*]: A Pioneer Physiologist," *Med Hist.* 13 (1969): 271–79; W. Bruce Fye, "H. Newell Martin: A Remarkable Career Destroyed by Neurasthenia and Alcoholism," *J. Hist. Med.* 40 (1985): 133–66; A. McGehee Harvey, "Fountainhead of American Physiology: H. Newell Martin and His Pupil William Henry Howell," *Johns Hopkins Med. J.* 136 (1975): 38–46; Henry Sewall, "Henry Newell Martin," *Johns Hopkins Hosp. Bull.* 22 (1911): 327–33; William H. Howell, "Early Days in the Biological Laboratory," Howell Papers; and Carl P. Swanson, "A History of Biology at the Johns Hopkins University," *Bios* 22 (1951): 223–62.

41. Gerald L. Geison, *Michael Foster and the Cambridge School of Physiology*.

42. Thomas H. Huxley and Henry N. Martin, *A Course of Elementary Instruction in Practical Biology* (London: Macmillan Co., 1875).

43. Huxley to Gilman, 20 February 1876, Gilman Papers.

44. Gilman to Huxley, 14 March 1876, Huxley Papers, American Philosophical Society Library, Philadelphia, Pa. (a microfilm set of the Huxley Papers). The original collection is deposited in the Archives, Imperial College, London, and is described in Warren R. Dawson, *The Huxley Papers: A Descriptive Catalogue of the Correspondence, Manuscripts and Miscellaneous Papers of the Rt. Hon. Thomas Henry Huxley* (London: Macmillan Co., 1946).

45. Martin to Gilman, 5 April 1876, Gilman Papers.

46. Huxley to Gilman, 27 June 1876, Gilman Papers.

47. "Notes," *Nature* 14 (1876): 79.

48. Daniel C. Gilman, "The Johns Hopkins University in Its Beginning: An Inaugural Address, Baltimore 1876," in *University Problems*, 23–24.

49. Huxley to Gilman, 23 April 1876, Gilman Papers.

50. John Grey McKendrick, "The Future of Physiological Research," *BAAS Rep.* 46 (1876): 132–33.

51. "Partial Arrangements for Instruction, 1876–77," *Johns Hopkins University, Official Circulars*, no. 4 (Baltimore, August 1876), 5–6.

52. Thomas H. Huxley, "Address on University Education," in *American*

Addresses: With a Lecture on the Study of Biology (New York: D. Appleton & Co., 1877), 99–127. See also William Pierce Randall, "Huxley in America," *Proc. Am. Philo. Soc.* 114 (1970): 73–99.

53. H. Newell Martin, "The Study and Teaching of Biology," *Pop. Sci. Mon.* 10 (1877): 299–300, 301, 303.

54. "Professor Martin on Scientific Education," *Pop. Sci. Mon.* 10 (1876): 369.

55. Gilman to Martin, 3 January 1877, Gilman Papers.

56. The paper is William Lee, "On the Effect of Stimulation on an Excised Nerve," *Med. Rec.* 12 (1877): 548–50. Lee was an 1865 medical graduate of the University of Maryland. See Martin to Bowditch, 9 January 1892, Bowditch Papers.

57. Martin to Schäfer, 18 February 1877, Sharpey-Schafer Collection.

58. See Richard C. French, *Antivivisection and Medical Science in Victorian Society.* See also Michael Foster, "Vivisection," *Pop. Sci. Mon.* 4 (1874): 672–85.

59. Billings to Gilman, 11 November 1876, Chesney Archives.

60. Ibid., 14 April 1876, Gilman Papers. See also Gilman to Billings, 7 April 1876, Billings Papers; "Bestowal of Fellowships," *Johns Hopkins University, Official Circulars,* no. 3 (Baltimore, 1876); and Hawkins, *Pioneer,* 79–93.

61. The relevant correspondence is Gilman to Martin, 9 April 1877 and 18 March 1878, and Martin to Gilman, 9 April 1877 and 18 March 1878, Gilman Papers. See also George L. Smith to Gilman, 20 March 1878, Gilman Papers, and French, *A History of the University,* 91–92.

62. Foster to Henry P. Bowditch, 3 July 1877, in "Harold Bowditch Notes," Bowditch Papers.

63. Martin to Gilman, 1 April, 1878, Gilman Papers.

64. See Remsen to Gilman, 25 August 1876, Gilman Papers.

65. John S. Billings, *Medical Education* (Baltimore: William K. Boyle, 1878), 3.

66. See Chesney, *Johns Hopkins Hospital,* 1:33–34, and Garrison, *John Shaw Billings,* 191–98.

67. Relevant letters from these individuals are preserved in the Billings Papers.

68. Billings, *Medical Education,* 5.

69. Billings to Gilman, 28 March 1878, Gilman Papers. I have been unable to find evidence that Billings's comments were circulated as he had hoped.

70. Hays to Billings, 8 January 1877, Billings Papers.

71. J[ohn] S. B[illings], "Higher Medical Education," *Am. J. Med. Sci.* n.s. 76 (1878): 189.

72. "Johns Hopkins University," *Phila. Med. Times* 9 (1878): 10–12. See also James Chadwick to Billings, 31 August [1878], Billings papers; Horatio Wood to Billings, 28 January 1879, Billings Papers; *Johns Hopkins University, Official Circulars,* no. 11 (Baltimore, June 1877); and Gilman, "The Launching of the University," 123.

73. H. Newell Martin, "To the Editor of the Philadelphia Medical Times," *Phila. Med. Times* 9 (1878): 95–96.

74. [George Shrady], "The Preliminary Medical Course at Johns Hopkins," *Med. Rec.* 14 (1878): 151–52.

75. [Ibid.], "The International Congress of Medical Science," *Med. Rec.* 16 (1879): 397.

76. Daniel Gilman, "A Report to the Trustees of the Johns Hopkins University [1878], published in Alan M. Chesney, "Two Documents Relating to Medical Education at the Johns Hopkins University," *Bull. Hist. Med.* 4 (1936): 483, 491. See also "The Johns Hopkins University," *Boston Med. Surg. J.* 99 (1878): 605–9.

77. *Fourth Annual Report of the Johns Hopkins University* (Baltimore, 1879), 53.

78. Eugene F. Cordell, *The Medical Annals of Maryland, 1799–1899*, 836.

79. H. Newell Martin, "The Physiology of Secretion," *Trans. Med. Chi. Md.* (1879): 74.

80. Hall to Henry P. Bowditch, 24 February 1880, Bowditch Papers. Hall's emphasis.

81. Sewall to Sharpey-Schafer, 14 July 1934, Sharpey-Schafer Collection. See also Henry Sewall, *Henry Newell Martin*, and Gerald B. Webb and Desmond Powell, *Henry Sewall*.

82. See W. Bruce Fye, "Heparin: The Contributions of William Henry Howell," *Circulation* 69 (1984): 1198–1203, and E. O. Jordan, George C. Whipple, and C.-D. A. Winslow, *A Pioneer of Public Health: William Thompson Sedgwick* (New Haven: Yale University Press, 1924). For a list of the physiological apparatus available in Martin's department at this time, see *Fourth Annual Report of the Johns Hopkins University* (Baltimore, 1879), 62–63.

83. Sedgwick to Gilman, 19 May 1880, Gilman Papers. Another of Martin's fellows, Edward M. Hartwell, expressed similar sentiments; see Hartwell to Gilman, 11 June 1880, Gilman Papers.

84. "The Johns Hopkins University," *Scribner's Monthly* 19 (1879): 204–6.

85. George H. Boyland, "The Johns Hopkins University and Higher Education: With a Glance at the Hospital Buildings," *Boston Med. Surg. J.* 102 (1880): 98.

86. [George Shrady], "Biological Study at the Johns Hopkins University," *Med. Rec.* 19 (1881): 409.

87. [H. Newell Martin], "Biology: 1876–81," *Johns Hopkins Circ.* (March 1881): 105.

88. H. Newell Martin, "Report to the Trustees containing Suggestions with Reference to the Future of the Biological Department of the Johns Hopkins University," 7 May 1881, J.H.U. Collection, JHUSC.

89. Martin to Gilman, 29 May 1876, Gilman Papers. See also Dennis McCullough, "W. K. Brooks' Role in the History of American Biology," *J. Hist. Biol.* 2 (1969): 411–38, and Benson, "American Morphology in the Late Nineteenth Century."

90. [H. Newell Martin], "Biology: 1876–81," 104. For an assessment of the importance of biology in the medical curriculum at this time by a pupil of Henry Bowditch, see Charles S. Minot, "A Grave Defect in our Medical Education," *Boston Med. Surg. J.* 105 (1881): 565–67.

91. See Thomas H. Huxley, "An Address on the Connection of the Biological Sciences with Medicine," *Brit. Med. J.* 2 (1881): 273–76; James Paget, "President's Address," *Brit. Med. J.* 2 (1881): 195–98; and Rudolf Virchow, "An Address on the Value of Pathological Experiments," *Brit. Med. J.* 2 (1881): 198–203.

92. C. K. Adams, "Science at the University of Michigan," *Pop. Sci. Mon.* 18 (1880): 123–25.

93. "Aid for Original Scientific Research," *American* 3 (1881): 70.

94. "Miscellaneous Items," *Physician and Surgeon* 2 (1880): 430. See also Michael Foster, *A Textbook of Physiology*, 3d ed., rev. (New York: Macmillan Co., 1880); Horace W. Davenport, "Physiology, 1850–1923: The View from Michigan"; and Frederick Novy, "The Laboratories," Bentley.

95. Frederic T. Lewis, "Charles Sedgwick Minot," *Anat. Rec.* 10 (1916): 133–64.

96. Packard to Minot, 23 November 1877, Minot Papers, Countway.

97. See Minot to [James Tyson], 18 September 1879, and Minot to Cadwalader Biddle, 10 November 1879, Pennsylvania Archives.

98. Victor Vaughan, *A Doctor's Memories* (Indianapolis: Bobbs-Merrill, 1926), 209–10. See also University of Michigan Faculty Minutes, 25 June 1881, University Medical School Collection, Bentley.

99. Sewall to Gilman, 8 April 1882, Gilman Papers. See also Sewall to Gilman, July 1881, Gilman Papers.

100. Sewall to "Gentlemen of the Medical Faculty," June 1882, University Medical School Collection, Bentley.

101. *The President's Report to the Board of Regents, for the Year Ending September 30, 1882* (Ann Arbor: University of Michigan, 1882).

102. See Bushrod W. James, *American Resorts: With Notes upon Their Climate* (Philadelphia: F. A. Davis, 1889), and Billy M. Jones, *Health-Seekers in the Southwest, 1817–1900* (Norman: University of Oklahoma Press, 1967).

103. John S. Billings, "An Address on our Medical Literature," *Brit. Med. J.* 2 (1881): 264.

104. *Johns Hopkins Circ.* (Baltimore: Johns Hopkins, July 1882), 223–25.

105. Daniel C. Gilman, "Biology" in *Seventh Annual Report of the Johns Hopkins University* (Baltimore: Johns Hopkins University, 1882), 36. See also "Physiology of the Isolated Mammalian Heart," *Med. News* 40 (1882): 84–85, and W. Bruce Fye, "H. Newell Martin and the Isolated Heart Preparation: The Link between the Frog and Open Heart Surgery," *Circulation* 73 (1986): 857–64.

106. H. Newell Martin, "The Influence upon the Pulse Rate of Variations of Arterial Pressure, of Venous Pressure, and of Temperature" (1882), in *Physiological Papers*. Memoirs from the Biological Laboratory of the Johns Hopkins University, no. 3. (Baltimore: Johns Hopkins Press, 1895), 12.

107. See, for example, Oliver W. Holmes to Henry P. Bowditch, 16 October 1881, Bowditch Papers, and "Book Review. The Human Body . . . by H. Newell Martin," *Pop. Sci. Mon.* 19 (1881): 270–71.

108. B., "Letter from Baltimore, June 1883," *Boston Med. Surg. J.* 109 (1883): 20. See also William A. Kemp, "President's Address," *Trans. Med. Chi.*

Md. (1883): 49–57; Severn Teackle Wallis, "The Johns Hopkins University in Its Relations to Baltimore," *Johns Hopkins Circ.* no. 23, supp. (1883): 107–16; and Abraham Jacobi, *Die Johns Hopkins Universitaet* (New York: E. Steiger & Co., 1881).

109. Gilman to the Johns Hopkins Trustees, 9 June 1881, J.H.U. Collection, JHUSC. See also French, *A History of the University*, 59, for a discussion of the building plans at this time.

110. Ira Remsen, H. Newell Martin, and Henry A. Rowland to George William Brown, 9 January 1882, Remsen Papers, JHUSC.

111. Daniel C. Gilman, *Eighth Report of the President. Johns Hopkins University* (Baltimore, 1883), 20–21. The scientific community learned of the new laboratory in a comprehensive and well-illustrated review. See "The Biological Laboratory of the Johns Hopkins University," *Science* 3 (1884): 350–54.

112. H. Newell Martin, "Modern Physiological Laboratories: What They Are and Why They Are," *Science* 3 (1884): 73–76, 100–103.

113. Alpheus S. Packard, Jr., and Edward D. Cope, "Editors' Table," *Am. Nat.* 18 (1884): 392–93.

114. "The Relation of Laboratories to Medical Science and Medical Education," *Boston Med. Surg. J.* 110 (1884): 233.

115. *Medical Education and the Regulation of the Practice of Medicine in the United States and Canada*, prepared by the Illinois State Board of Health (Chicago: W. T. Keener, 1884).

116. Martin to Gilman, 11 July 1883, Gilman Papers. See also [George Shrady], "Scarcity of Original Workers," *Med. Rec.* 22 (1882): 378–79, and "The Neglect of the Study of Pure Science in America," *Med. Surg. Rep.* 47 (1882): 293–94.

117. Henry A. Rowland, "A Plea for Pure Science," *Pop. Sci. Mon.* 24 (1884): 30–44.

118. Rowland to Gilman, 11 April 1883, Gilman Papers.

119. Martin to Gilman, 15 June 1886, Gilman Papers.

120. Hawkins, *Pioneer*, 131–32.

121. Ludwig to Mall, 19 November 1886, published in Florence Rena Sabin, *Franklin Paine Mall*, 72–73.

122. Eliot to Gilman, 13 April 1887, Gilman Papers.

123. Howell to James B. Angell, 20 July 1889, Angell Papers.

124. Howell to Gilman, 1 January 1893. Gilman Papers. See also Howell to Gilman, 4 January 1893 and 20 January 1893, Gilman Papers.

125. Gilman to Martin 3 November 1892, Gilman Papers.

126. Welch to Mall, 24 April 1893, Mall Papers. See also Fye, "H. Newell Martin" (1985).

127. Benson, "American Morphology in the Late Nineteenth Century."

128. Daniel Gilman, "The Original Faculty," 52.

Chapter 5: The American Physiology Society

1. Alexander Dallas Bache, "Paper Delivered at April 1844 Meeting of the National Institute for the Promotion of Science," Bache Papers, Smithsonian Institution Archives, Washington D.C.

2. *Proc. AAAS* (Philadelphia: John C. Clark, 1849), 144–156. See also Sally Gregory Kohlstedt, *The Formation of the American Scientific Community*.

3. Edward Sharpey-Schafer, *History of the Physiological Society during Its First Fifty Years: 1876–1926*.

4. Ibid., 60–62.

5. "Vivisection," *Brit. Med. J.* 2 (1881): 527. See also Horatio C. Wood, Jr., "The Value of Vivisection," *Scribner's Monthly* (September 1880): 766–70.

6. Benjamin Bryan, ed., *The Vivisectors' Directory: Being a List of Licensed Vivisectors in the United Kingdom, Together with the Leading Physiologists in Foreign Laboratories. Compiled from Authentic Sources* (London: Victoria Street Society for the Protection of Animals from Vivisection, 1884).

7. John G. Curtis, "Report of Committee on Experimental Medicine," *Trans. Med. Soc. N. Y.* (1883): 109.

8. "Antivivisection Agitation," *Med. News* 44 (1884): 339–40.

9. "The Report of the Committee on the Appeal of the American Anti-Vivisection Society. Medical Society of the State of Pennsylvania, 35th Annual Session," *Med. News* 44 (1884): 595.

10. S. Weir Mitchell, *Report of the Special Committee of the Medical Society of the State of Pennsylvania upon an Appeal from the American Antivivisection Society* [Philadelphia, 1884].

11. "Rules Governing Vivisection Adopted by the University Trustees," *Med. News* 46 (1885): 568.

12. H. Newell Martin, "Regulations with Regard to Experiments upon Animals," March 1885, Gilman Papers.

13. D. Hayes Agnew, Joseph Leidy, James Tyson, William Pepper, S. Weir Mitchell, H. C. Wood, William Goodell, Harrison Allen, "Dear Doctor," 30 January 1885. Printed letter. Pennsylvania Archives. Wood, Pepper, and Tyson also served as members of the committee on experimental medicine of the American Medical Association formed in 1884 to combat the growing antivivisection agitation. See "American Medical Association. Thirty-fifth Annual Meeting . . . 1884," *JAMA* 2 (1884): 561–80, esp. 564–65.

14. [George Shrady], "The Anti-vivisection Discussions," *Med. Rec.* 25 (1884): 436.

15. H. Newell Martin, "The Direct Influence of Gradual Variations of Temperature upon the Rate of Beat of the Dog's Heart," *Philosophical Transactions of the Royal Society (London)* 174 (1883): 663–88. Frances Power Cobbe, the indefatigable British antivivisectionist, was active in the founding and early affairs of the *Zoophilist*.

16. H. Newell Martin, *A Correction of Certain Statements Published in the "Zoophilist," also a Castigation and an Appeal* (Baltimore: Isaac Friedenwald, 1885), 4, 10–11.

17. See James B. Herrick, *Memories of Eighty Years* (Chicago: University of Chicago Press, 1949), 35–36.

18. *Illustrations of Vivisections: Or Experiments on Living Animals: From the Works of Physiologists . . . as Reproduced in "Bernard's Martyrs" and*

"Light in Dark Places" by Miss Frances Power Cobbe (Philadelphia: American Society for the Restriction of Vivisection, 1887).

19. *Extracts from an Address from Cannon Wilberforce, for the Society for the Restriction of Vivisection, Made at a Drawing-Room Meeting Held in Germantown, Philadelphia, June 2, 1887,* [1887], 4. Copy in Curtis Papers.

20. John S. Billings, "Medicine in the United States, and Its Relations to Co-operative Investigation," *Brit. Med. J.* 2 (1886): 305.

21. John W. Draper, "Science in America," *Pop. Sci. Mon.* 10 (1876): 313–14.

22. William Osler, "American Association for the Advancement of Science," *Canada Med. Surg. J.* 13 (1878): 63–68.

23. "The Meeting of the American Association for the Advancement of Science," *Med. Rec.* 18 (1880): 325. See also "The Annual Meeting of the American Association for the Advancement of Science," *Med. Rec.* 20 (1881): 295.

24. [William Osler], "British Association for the Advancement of Science, Montreal Meeting, September 1 and 2, 1884," *Med. News* 45 (1884): 360–63.

25. Edwin G. Conklin, "Fifty Years of the American Society of Naturalists," *Am. Nat.* 68 (1934): 385–401.

26. Alpheus S. Packard, Jr., and Edward D. Cope, "Editors' Table," *Am. Nat.* 18 (1884): 160–61. See also "The Society of Naturalists of the Eastern United States," *Science* 1 (1883): 411–12.

27. "Constitution of the American Association for the Advancement of Science," *Proc. AAAS* 33d meeting (Salem, 1885), xxiii.

28. "The International Medical Congress, Washington, 1887," *Med. News* 46 (1885): 390–92, 418–20. For details of the conflict over the International Medical Congress and its consequences see *Med. News* 47 (1885) and *Med. Rec.* 28 (1885) in which several editorials and notes relating to these issues are published, and Fielding H. Garrison, *John Shaw Billings*, 260–63. For a list of individuals who withdrew as well as those who remained on committees of the congress see *Med. News* 47 (1885): 332.

29. "Public Opinion of the Congress Outlook," *Med. News* 47 (1885): 363. The hard feelings that resulted between Austin Flint, Sr., and others as a result of this episode are vividly described in Henry I. Bowditch to Abraham Jacobi, 28 May 1886, Historical Division, National Library of Medicine, Bethesda, Md.

30. John H. Callender, "Introductory Address," *Transactions of the International Medical Congress*, 9th session, 3 vols., ed. John B. Hamilton (Washington, 1887) 3:232–38.

31. I wish to thank Toby Appel, archivist of the American Physiological Society, for pointing out the connection between the formation of the American Physiological Society and the establishment of the Congress of American Physicians and Surgeons.

32. "Historical Introduction," *Transactions of the Congress of American Physicians and Surgeons. First Triennial Session* (New Haven, 1889), xiii–xxii.

33. Henry I. Bowditch, "Address at the Opening of the Annual Meeting of the American Medical Association," *Boston Med. Surg. J.* 96 (1877): 665.

34. Victor C. Vaughan, *A Doctor's Memories* (Indianapolis: Bobbs-Merrill Co., 1926), 444.

35. "Historical Introduction," xx. The original nine specialty societies represented in the Congress of American Physicians and Surgeons were the American Ophthalmological Association, the American Otological Association, the American Gynaecological Association, the American Laryngological Association, the American Dermatological Association, the American Surgical Association, the American Neurological Association, the American Climatological Association, and the Association of American Physicians and Pathologists.

36. "Autobiography of S. Weir Mitchell." Historical Society of Pennsylvania, Philadelphia, Pa., 56. See also William H. Howell, "The American Physiological Society during Its First Twenty-Five Years," esp. 4–6, and William H. Welch, "S. Weir Mitchell, Physician and Man of Science," in S. Weir Mitchell, M.D., LL.D., F.R.S., 1829–1914: Memorial Addresses and Resolutions (Philadelphia, 1914), 97–127, esp. 115.

37. Bowditch to Mitchell, 1 June 1887, Mitchell Papers, Historical Collections, Library of the College of Physicians of Philadelphia, Philadelphia, Pa.

38. Charles Sedgwick Minot, "The Relation of the American Society of Naturalists to Other Scientific Societies," Science n.s. 15 (1902): 242.

39. "The Naturalists' Meeting at Philadelphia," Science 9 (1887): 8.

40. An "American Physiological Society" was established in 1837, inspired by contemporary enthusiasm for hygienic living advocated by William Alcott and Sylvester Graham. The society lasted only a few years, however, and was not concerned with undertaking or encouraging experimentation. See Hebbel E. Hoff and John F. Fulton, "The Centenary of the First American Physiological Society Founded at Boston by William A. Alcott and Sylvester Graham," Bull. Hist. Med. 5 (1937): 687–729.

41. Martin to Bowditch, 4 March 1878, Bowditch Papers.

42. Boston Society of Medical Sciences. Constitution and By-Laws, as Adopted at the Meeting of December 20, 1887. With an Enclosed List of Members (Boston: S. J. Parkhill & Co., 1888), 3.

43. S. Weir Mitchell, "Memoir of John Call Dalton, 1825–1889," Biog. Mem. Nat. Acad. Sci. 3 (1890): 185.

44. The American Physiological Society constitution is published in Howell, "The American Physiological Society," 56–57, and the constitution of the [British] Physiological Society is published in Sharpey-Schafer, "History of the Physiological Society," 8–12.

45. Bowditch (1896), quoted in Howell, "The American Physiological Society," 18.

46. "American Physiological Society Council Minutes," vol. 1, 27 December 1895, APS Archives. Frances Emily White, the unsuccessful candidate, was professor of physiology in the Women's Medical College of Philadelphia. See Gulielma Alsop, History of the Woman's Medical College, Philadelphia, Pennsylvania, 1850–1950 (Philadelphia: J. B. Lippincott Co., 1950), 118–20. The first woman (Ida H. Hyde) was elected to the society in 1902. See Howell, "The American Physiological Society," 71.

47. William H. Howell, "Autobiographical Manuscript," Howell Papers.

48. Ellis to William Howell, 19 May 1937, APS Archives.

49. The characteristics of the original and early members of the American Physiological Society discussed in this chapter were derived from standard biographical sources. See especially Howell, "The American Physiological Society," and J. McKeen Cattell, ed. *American Men of Science*. The attendance data were derived from the "American Physiological Society Minutes," vol. 1, APS Archives.

50. The disproportionate representation of individuals born in the Northeast in the American scientific community in the nineteenth century has been identified by others. See Clark A. Elliott, "The American Scientist, 1800–1863"; Robert V. Bruce, "A Statistical Profile of American Scientists: 1846–1876," in George H. Daniels, ed., *Nineteenth-Century American Science*, 63–64; Donald de Beaver, *The American Scientific Community, 1800–1860: A Statistical-Historical Study* (New York: Arno, 1980), and, for physiologists, see Stephen Sargent Visher, *Scientists Starred, 1903–1943, in "American Men of Science,"* 463–66.

51. Charles R. Bardeen, "Anatomy in America," 189.

52. The laboratories at Harvard, the University of Pennsylvania, and the College of Physicians and Surgeons in the nineteenth century issued volumes of collected papers. See *Physiological Laboratory: Harvard Medical School, Boston, Collected Papers*, vol. 1 (Boston: Harvard Medical School, 1880); *Physiological Laboratory: Harvard Medical School, Boston, Collected Papers*, vol. 2, 1880–1886 (Boston: Harvard Medical School, 1887); N. A. Randolph and Samuel G. Dixon, *Notes from the Physiological Laboratory of the University of Pennsylvania* (Philadelphia: J. B. Lippincott Co., 1885); and *Studies from the Department of Physiology at Columbia University at the College of Physicians and Surgeons of New York, Reprints, 1887–1897* (New York: College of Physicians and Surgeons, 1898). Many of the publications based on research performed in Martin's biology department appeared in *Studies from the Biological Laboratory of the Johns Hopkins University* which appeared irregularly beginning in 1879.

53. Russell H. Chittenden, *The Development of Physiological Chemistry in the United States*, 45.

54. Welch to Gilman, 18 April 1885, Gilman Papers. See also Welch to Gilman, 18 December 1884, Gilman Papers.

55. Welch to Mall, 30 June 1885, Mall Papers.

56. William H. Welch, "Medical Education in the United States," *Harvey Lectures*, ser. 11 (Philadelphia: J. B. Lippincott Co., 1917): 371.

57. Robert E. Kohler, *From Medical Chemistry to Biochemistry*, 110.

58. Curtis to Robert J. Morris, 12 June 1891, Curtis Papers. See also Curtis to Henry P. Bowditch, 11 February 1892, Bowditch Papers, and Russell Chittenden to Curtis, 11 December 1892, Curtis Papers.

59. S. Weir Mitchell, John G. Curtis, William H. Howell, and Henry P. Bowditch, "Dear Sir," 22 November 1895. Printed letter. Copy in Curtis Papers.

60. " 'Vivisection' a Statement in Behalf of Science," *Science* n.s. 3 (1896): 421.

61. Curtis to Mall, 23 March 1891, Mall Papers.

62. Welch to Mall, 1 August 1886, Mall Papers.

63. Ibid., 17 July 1888, Mall Papers.

64. Sewall to the Honorable Board of Regents, 4 July 1888, Angell Papers.

65. Bowditch to Selma Bowditch, 10 April [1889], Bowditch Papers. See also Isaac Ott, *The Actions of Medicines* (Philadelphia: Lindsay & Blakiston, 1878).

66. Porter to Baumgarten, 12 August 1890, Baumgarten Papers. See also W. Bruce Fye, "Acute Coronary Occlusion Always Results in Death: Or Does It? The Observations of William T. Porter," *Circulation* 71 (1985): 4–10.

67. H. Newell Martin, "American Physiological Society," 20 February 1890, Printed Circular, APS Archives. See also Howell, "American Physiological Society," 9.

68. Howell to Angell, 10 July 1889, Angell Papers. See also Howell to Daniel Gilman, 26 May 1887, Gilman Papers, and W. Bruce Fye, "Heparin: The Contributions of William Henry Howell," *Circulation* 69 (1984): 1198–1203.

69. Curtis to James McLane, 19 May 1890, Columbia Archives.

70. John Shrady, ed., *College of Physicians and Surgeons*, 1:238.

71. Edith Finch, *Carey Thomas of Bryn Mawr* (New York: Harper & Brothers, 1947). James Carey Thomas and Francis T. King, trustees of Johns Hopkins, were original trustees of Bryn Mawr College. The first dean of Bryn Mawr was Martha Carey Thomas, James Carey Thomas's daughter. Daniel Gilman delivered an address at the opening of the institution.

72. Wilson also studied under Foster, Huxley, and Ludwig. He briefly held positions at Williams College, where he replaced Samuel Clarke, another of Martin's fellows, when he was on leave, and the Massachusetts Institute of Technology, where he worked under William Sedgwick, one of Martin's earliest fellows.

73. Howell to Bowditch, 5 March 1892, Bowditch Papers.

74. Howell to Bowditch, 28 March 1892, Bowditch Papers.

75. Horace W. Davenport, "Physiology, 1850–1923: The View from Michigan," 50–76.

76. Lombard to Bowditch, 3 April 1885, Bowditch Papers.

77. See Curtis to Mall, 12 November 1886, Mall Papers.

78. Welch to Lombard, 29 August 1888, Lombard Papers, Bentley.

79. Bertha Friedenwald to Harry Friedenwald, [c. 1886], published in Alexandra Lee Levin, *Vision: A Biography of Harry Friedenwald* (Philadelphia: Jewish Publication Society of America, 1964), 86.

80. Davenport, "Physiology, 1850–1923: The View from Michigan," 59–60. See also Dorothy Ross, *G. Stanley Hall: The Psychologist as Prophet* (Chicago: University of Chicago Press, 1972), and Richard J. Storr, *Harper's University, the Beginnings: A History of the University of Chicago*.

81. Porter to Baumgarten, 23 June 1892, Baumgarten Papers.

82. Ibid., 20 August 1892, Baumgarten Papers.

83. The relevant correspondence is ibid., 24 April 1893, 29 May 1893, 15 July 1893, and 22 July 1893, Baumgarten Papers.

84. Ibid., 17 January 1896 [1897], Baumgarten Papers. Content in this letter proves that Porter inadvertently substituted the preceding year.

85. Dana to Bowditch, 25 December 1894, Bowditch Papers. See also Edward Salisbury Dana et al, *A Century of Science in America: With Special Reference to the American Journal of Science, 1818–1918* (New Haven: Yale University Press, 1918). A list of American scientific journals founded between 1867 and 1918 appears on page 55.

86. Welch to Prudden, 30 June 1897, Prudden Papers, Yale University Archives, New Haven, Conn.

87. "American Journal of Physiology," *Boston Med. Surg. J.* 137 (1897): 431.

88. A. Clifford Barger, "The Meteoric Rise and Fall of William Townsend Porter, One of Carl J. Wiggers' 'Old Guard,'" *Physiologist* 25 (1982): 407–13.

89. Henry P. Bowditch, John G. Curtis, Henry H. Donaldson, William H. Howell, Frederic S. Lee, Warren P. Lombard, Graham Lusk, William T. Porter, Edward T. Reichert, Henry Sewall, *An American Text-Book of Physiology*, ed. William H. Howell (Philadelphia: W. B. Saunders Co., 1896).

Chapter 6: A Scientific Prescription for American Medicine

1. See, for example, "The Teaching of Physiology," *Boston Med. Surg. J.* 148 (1903): 240–41.

2. See, for example, Winfield S. Hall, *A Manual of Experimental Physiology for Students of Medicine* (Philadelphia: Lea Brothers & Co., 1904); John C. Hemmeter, *Manual of Practical Physiology, Designed for the Practical Physiology Course in the Curriculum of the American Association of Medical Colleges* (Philadelphia: P. Blakiston's Son & Co., 1912); and Warren P. Lombard, *Laboratory Exercises in Physiology for the Use of Medical Students* (Ann Arbor, Mich.: George Wahr, 1906).

3. Nathan S. Davis, "The Basis of Scientific Medicine and the Proper Methods of Investigation," *JAMA* 16 (1891): 114. See also "The Obligations of Medicine to Physiology, and of Physiology to Medicine," *Boston Med. Surg. J.* 126 (1892): 345–47, and Thomas N. Bonner, "Dr. Nathan Smith Davis and the Growth of Chicago Medicine, 1850–1900," *Bull. Hist. Med.* 26 (1952): 360–74.

4. Quoted in Chesney, *Johns Hopkins Hospital*, 1:88.

5. John S. Billings, "Ideals of Medical Education" (1891), in *Select Papers of John Shaw Billings*, ed. Frank B. Rogers (Chicago: Medical Library Association, 1965), 220.

6. William H. Welch, "The Advancement of Medical Education" (1892), in *Papers and Addresses by William Henry Welch*, 3 vols. (Baltimore: Johns Hopkins Press, 1920), 3:43. See also Owsei Temkin, "The European Background of the Young Doctor Welch," *Bull. Hist. Med.* 24 (1950): 308–18.

7. William H. Welch, "Higher Medical Education and the Need of Its Endowment" (1894), in *Papers and Addresses by William Henry Welch*, 3:53.

8. Franklin P. Mall, "What Is Biology?" *Chautauquan* 18 (1894): 414.

9. Thomas N. Bonner, "German Doctors in America, 1887–1914: Their Views and Impressions of American Life and Medicine," *J. Hist. Med.* 14 (1959): 1. See also Joseph H. Pratt, "The Method of Science in Clinical Training," *Boston Med. Surg. J.* 166 (1912): 835–42.

10. See William Welch to Emeline Welch, 21 April 1878, published in Simon Flexner and James Thomas Flexner, *William Henry Welch and the Heroic Age of American Medicine*, 112–13, and William Osler to August Hoch, [June 1890], published in Harvey Cushing, *Life of Sir William Osler*, 1:331–32.

11. John S. Billings, "Progress of Medicine in the Nineteenth Century," in *Ann. Rep. Smithsonian . . . for the Year ending June 30, 1900* (Washington: Government Printing Office, 1901), 637.

12. Michael Foster, "Recent Progress in Physiology," in *Ann. Rep. Smithsonian . . . to July 1897* (Washington: Government Printing Office, 1898), 440–41.

13. See, for example, John J. Stevenson, "The Debt of the World to Pure Science," *Ann. Rep. Smithsonian . . . to July 1897* (Washington: Government Printing Office, 1898), 325–36.

14. William W. Keen, "The Endowment of Medical Colleges," *Boston Med. Surg. J.* 142 (1900): 584, 585, 586.

15. "The Medical Colleges of the United States," *JAMA* 27 (1896): 624–41.

16. John A. Benson, "The Value to the Medical Student of Physiologic Study," *JAMA* 27 (1896): 621–24.

17. Howell, "The American Physiological Society," 19.

18. See, for example, Nicholas Senn, "Importance and Value of Experimental Research," *Western Medical Reporter* 9 (1887): 55–59, idem, "The Physician as a Scientist," *JAMA* 35 (1900): 1336–38, and idem, "The Final Triumph of Scientific Medicine," *JAMA* 48 (1907): 1824–30.

19. See George Rosen, "Christian Fenger, Medical Immigrant," *Bull. Hist. Med.* 48 (1974): 129–45; Edwin F. Hirsch, *Christian Fenger, M.D., 1840–1902: The Impact of His Scientific Training and His Personality on Medicine in Chicago* (Chicago: Dartnell Press, 1972); and Thomas Neville Bonner, *Medicine in Chicago, 1850–1950: A Chapter in the Social and Scientific Development of a City* (Madison, Wis.: American History Research Center, 1957).

20. *First Annual Conference of the Council on Medical Education of the American Medical Association* (Chicago: American Medical Association, 1905), 11.

21. *Third Annual Conference of the Council on Medical Education of the American Medical Association* (Chicago: American Medical Association, 1907), 10, 11.

22. "Council on Medical Education of the American Medical Association. Fourth Annual Conference," *American Medical Association Bulletin* 3 (1908): 262–63.

23. Abraham Flexner, *The American College: A Criticism* (New York: Century Co., 1908). See also Abraham Flexner, *I Remember: The Autobiography of Abraham Flexner* (New York: Simon & Schuster, 1940).

24. George W. Corner, *A History of the Rockefeller Institute, 1901–1953.*

25. Henry S. Pritchett, "Introduction," in Abraham Flexner, *Medical Education in the United States and Canada,* x.

26. Flexner, *Medical Education in the United States and Canada,* 53–54, 60, 56, 57.

27. John F. Fulton, "A Salute to Abraham Flexner," *J. Hist. Med.* 9 (1956): 439.

28. See Howard S. Berliner, *A System of Scientific Medicine.*

29. "Report of the Sixth Annual Conference of the Council on Medical Education," *American Medical Association Bulletin* 5 (1910): 242–43. See also, William H. Welch, "The Benefits of the Endowment of Medical Research," in *The Rockefeller Institute for Medical Research, Description of the Buildings. Addresses Delivered at the Opening of the Laboratories in New York City* (Lancaster, Pa.: New Era Printing Co., 1907), 26–38.

30. William H. Welch, "Fields of Usefulness of the American Medical Association," (1910), in *Papers and Addresses,* 3:341–43. See also Garfield G. McKinney, "The Part Played by the American Medical Association in the Improvement of Medical Education," 55 (1910): 1396, and Kenneth M. Ludmerer, "Reform of Medical Education at Washington University," *J. Hist. Med.* 35 (1980): 149–73.

31. Howell, "The American Physiological Society," 50.

32. Welch, "Fields of Usefulness of the American Medical Association," 343–44. See also Patricia Peck Gossel, "William Henry Welch and the Antivivisection Legislation in the District of Columbia, 1896–1900," *J. Hist. Med.* 40 (1985): 397–419.

33. These articles were available separately for a nominal fee and were also published in a bound volume entitled *Protection of Medical Research* (Chicago, c. 1911). For an overview of American Medical Association activities in support of research see "Medical Research," in F.J.L. Blasingame, *Digest of Official Actions, 1846–1958, American Medical Association.* (Chicago: American Medical Association, 1959): 608–19.

34. Abraham Flexner, "The History of Full-Time Clinical Teaching." Welch Papers.

35. Mall to Harper, [April 1893], published in Florence Rena Sabin, *Franklin Paine Mall,* 116–17.

36. Lewellys F. Barker, "Medicine and the Universities," *American Medicine* 4 (1902): 146. See also Lewellys F. Barker, *Time and the Physician: The Autobiography of Lewellys F. Barker.* This autobiography was dedicated to William Osler, William Welch, and Franklin Mall.

37. See, for example, John Milton Dodson, "The Research Idea and Methods in Medical Education and Practice," *JAMA* 45 (1905): 81–87. Dodson was dean of the Rush Medical College in Chicago.

38. Charles S. Minot, "Certain Ideals of Medical Education," *JAMA* 53 (1909): 506.

39. See Samuel H. Proger, "Joseph H. Pratt: A Short Biographical Sketch," in *Anniversary Volume: Scientific Contributions in Honor of Joseph*

Hersey Pratt on His Sixty-Fifth Birthday by His Friends (Lancaster, Pa.: Lancaster Press, 1937), xxiii–xxiv, and Joseph H. Pratt, *A Year with Osler, 1896–1897: Notes Taken at His Clinics in the Johns Hopkins Hospital* (Baltimore: Johns Hopkins Press, 1949).

40. Joseph H. Pratt, "The Method of Science in Clinical Training," *Boston Med. Surg. J.* 166 (1912): 835. See also Frederic S. Lee, "The Relation of the Medical Sciences to Clinical Medicine," *JAMA* 63 (1914): 2083–88, and William S. Thayer, "Teaching and Practice," *Science* n.s. 43 (1916): 691–705.

41. A. McGehee Harvey, *Science at the Bedside*, 183.

42. William Henry Howell, "Problems of Physiology of the Present Time," in *Congress of Arts and Sciences, Universal Exposition, St. Louis, 1904*, vol. 5, ed. Howard J. Rogers (Boston: Houghton, Mifflin, 1906).

43. Frederic S. Lee, Walter B. Cannon, and Richard M. Pearce, "Medical Research in Its Relation to Medical Schools," *JAMA* 68 (1917): 1075–79.

44. Richard M. Pearce, William H. Welch, William H. Howell, Franklin P. Mall, Lewellys F. Barker, Charles S. Minot, William B. Cannon, William T. Councilman, Theobold Smith, George N. Stewart, Clarence M. Jackson, Elias P. Lyon, James B. Herrick, John M. Dodson, Charles R. Bardeen, William Ophüls, Samuel J. Meltzer, James Ewing, William W. Keen, Henry H. Donaldson, Christian A. Herter, and Henry P. Bowditch, *Medical Research and Education* ed. J. McKeen Cattell (New York: Science Press, 1913). See also *Richard Mills Pearce, Jr., M.D., 1874–1930: Addresses Delivered at a Memorial Meeting Held April 15, 1930, at the Rockefeller Institute for Medical Research, New York City* (New York, 1930).

45. A valuable study based upon Cattell's diaries and correspondence describes the development of his interest in science: Michael M. Sokal, *An Education in Psychology: James McKeen Cattell's Journal and Letters from Germany and England, 1880–1888* (Cambridge: MIT Press, 1981), see esp. 194–99. By the time his volume on medical research and education appeared, Cattell was quite successful. He held a chair at Columbia University and had established the Science Press, a company that published *Science, Popular Science Monthly*, and *American Men of Science*, a biographical directory that Cattell edited.

46. Cattell to Selma Bowditch, 19 July 1913, Bowditch Papers.

47. Richard M. Pearce, "Research in Medicine," in *Medical Research and Education*, 68–69, 87, 86. See also Charles W. Eliot, "The Qualities of the Scientific Investigator," in *The Rockefeller Institute for Medical Research: Description of the Buildings: Addresses Delivered at the Opening of the Laboratories in New York City* (Lancaster, Pa.: New Era Printing Co., 1907), 42–50.

48. William H. Howell, "Biographical Memoir of Samuel James Meltzer, 1851–1923." *Biog. Mem. Nat. Acad. Sci.* 21 (1923): 11.

49. Samuel J. Meltzer, "The Science of Clinical Medicine: What It Ought to Be and the Men to Uphold It," in *Medical Research and Education*, ed. J. McKeen Cattell, 437.

50. William H. Welch, "The Place of Dr. Meltzer in American Medicine," in *Memorial Number for Samuel James Meltzer, M.D., Founder and First Pres-*

ident of the Society for Experimental Biology and Medicine (New York, 1921): 40–41.

51. Abraham Flexner, "Report on the Johns Hopkins Medical School," in Alan M. Chesney, *The Johns Hopkins Hospital*, 3:289, 301.

52. Joseph Ben-David, "Scientific Productivity and Academic Organization in Nineteenth-Century Medicine," in *The Sociology of Science*, ed. Bernard Barber and Walter Hirsch (New York: Free Press of Glencoe, 1962), 308–9.

53. [Fielding Garrison], "Texts Illustrating the History of Medicine in the Library of the Surgeon-General's Office," in *Index-Catalogue of the Library of the Surgeon General's Office, United States Army*, 2d ser. (Washington: Government Printing Office, 1912), 17:89–178. See also Leslie T. Morton, *A Medical Bibliography (Garrison and Morton), an Annotated Check-list of Texts Illustrating the History of Medicine*, 4th ed. (Hampshire, England: Gower Publishing Co., 1983).

54. Henry Chapman, *On Medical Education* (Philadelphia: Collins, 1876).

55. Carrel to Anne-Marie Ricard Carrel, [1905], excerpts published in W. Sterling Edwards and Peter D. Edwards, *Alexis Carrel, Visionary Surgeon* (Springfield, Ill.: Charles C Thomas, 1974): 34–35.

56. Alexis Carrel, "Suture of Blood-Vessels and Transplantation of Organs," in *Nobel Lectures Including Presentation Speeches and Laureate's Biographies, Physiology or Medicine, 1901–1921* (Amsterdam: Elsevier Publishing Co., 1967), 464. Carrel's transplantation experiments became the target of antivivisectionists. See *Experiments on Cats Performed in Rockefeller Institute (Transplantation of Kidneys)* (New York: New York Anti-vivisection Society, [1908]).

57. Charles W. Greene, "History of the American Physiological Society during Its Second Quarter Century," in *History of the American Physiological Society Semicentennial, 1887–1937*, 90.

Bibliography

Manuscript Collections

ANGELL PAPERS. James B. Angell Papers, Michigan Historical Collections, Bentley Historical Library, University of Michigan, Ann Arbor, Mich.

APS ARCHIVES. Archives, The American Physiological Society, Bethesda, Md.

BAUMGARTEN PAPERS. Baumgarten Family Papers, Washington University School of Medicine Archives, St. Louis, Mo.

BENTLEY. Michigan Historical Collections, Bentley Historical Library, University of Michigan, Ann Arbor, Mich.

BILLINGS PAPERS. John Shaw Billings Papers, Rare Books and Manuscripts Division, New York Public Library, Astor, Lenox, and Tilden Foundations, New York, N.Y.

BOWDITCH PAPERS. Bowditch Papers, Rare Books and Manuscripts Division, Francis A. Countway Library of Medicine, Boston, Mass.

CHESNEY ARCHIVES. Alan Mason Chesney Medical Archives, Johns Hopkins Medical Institutions, Baltimore, Md.

COLUMBIA ARCHIVES. Special Collections Section, Augustus C. Long Health Sciences Library, Columbia University, New York, N.Y.

COUNTWAY. Rare Books and Manuscripts Division, Francis A. Countway Library of Medicine, Boston, Mass.

CURTIS PAPERS. Curtis Papers, Augustus C. Long Health Sciences Library, Columbia University, New York, N.Y.

ELIOT PAPERS. Eliot Papers, Harvard University Archives, Harvard University Library, Cambridge, Mass.

GILMAN PAPERS. Daniel Coit Gilman Papers, Special Collections, Milton S. Eisenhower Library, Johns Hopkins University, Baltimore, Md.

HAMBURGER ARCHIVES. Milton S. Eisenhower Library, Johns Hopkins University, Baltimore, Md.

HAROLD BOWDITCH NOTES. [Harold Bowditch], "Henry Pickering Bowditch, M.D.," Bowditch Papers, Rare Books and Manuscripts Division, Francis A. Countway Library of Medicine, Boston, Mass.

HENRY PAPERS. Joseph Henry Papers, Smithsonian Institution Archives, Washington, D.C.

HOWELL PAPERS. William H. Howell Papers, Alan Mason Chesney Medical Archives, Johns Hopkins Medical Institutions, Baltimore, Md.

JEFFERSON ARCHIVES. Archives, Scott Memorial Library, Thomas Jefferson University, Philadelphia, Pa.

JHUSC. Special Collections, Milton S. Eisenhower Library, Johns Hopkins University, Baltimore, Md.

LEIDY PAPERS. Joseph Leidy Collection, Library, Academy of Natural Sciences of Philadelphia, Philadelphia, Pa.

MALL PAPERS. Franklin Paine Mall Papers, Alan Mason Chesney Medical Archives, Johns Hopkins Medical Institutions, Baltimore, Md.

PENNSYLVANIA ARCHIVES. University of Pennsylvania Archives, Philadelphia, Pa.

PEPPER COLLECTION. William Pepper Collection, Special Collections, Charles Patterson Van Pelt Library, University of Pennsylvania, Philadelphia, Pa.

PUTNAM PAPERS. James J. Putnam Collection, Rare Books and Manuscripts Division, Francis A. Countway Library of Medicine, Boston, Mass.

REYNOLDS COLLECTION. Reynolds Historical Library, University of Alabama in Birmingham, Birmingham, Ala.

SHARPEY-SCHAFER COLLECTION. Sharpey-Schafer Collection, Contemporary Medical Archives, Wellcome Institute for the History of Medicine, London, England.

TRENT COLLECTION. Trent Collection, Duke University Medical Center Library, Durham, N.C.

WELCH PAPERS. William H. Welch Papers, Alan Mason Chesney Medical Archives, Johns Hopkins Medical Institutions, Baltimore, Md.

WYMAN PAPERS. Wyman Papers, Rare Books and Manuscripts Division, Francis A. Countway Library of Medicine, Boston, Mass.

Secondary Sources

Abrahams, Harold J. *Extinct Medical Schools of Nineteenth-Century Philadelphia.* Philadelphia: University of Pennsylvania Press, 1966.

Ackerknecht, Erwin H. *Medicine at the Paris Hospital, 1794–1848.* Baltimore: Johns Hopkins Press, 1967.

Allen, Garland E. "Naturalists and Experimentalists: The Genotype and the Phenotype." *Studies in History of Biology* 3 (1979): 179–209.

———. *Thomas Hunt Morgan: The Man and His Science.* Princeton: Princeton University Press, 1978.

Allen, Gay Wilson. *William James: A Biography.* New York: Viking Press, 1967.

Atkinson, William B., ed. *A Biographical Dictionary of Contemporary American Physicians and Surgeons.* 2d ed., enl. and rev. Philadelphia: D. G. Brinton, 1880.

Atwater, Edward C. "'Squeezing Mother Nature': Experimental Physiology in the United States before 1870." *Bull. Hist. Med.* 52 (1978): 313–35.

Bardeen, Charles Russell. "Anatomy in America." *Bulletin of the University of Wisconsin no. 115.* Science Series, Vol. 3, no. 4, 85–208. Madison: University of Wisconsin, 1905.

Barker, Lewellys F. *Time and the Physician: The Autobiography of Lewellys F. Barker.* New York: G. P. Putnam's Sons, 1942.

Barnes, Sherman. "The Entry of Science and History in the College Curriculum." *History of Education Quarterly* 4 (1964): 44–58.

Basalla, George; William Coleman; and Robert H. Kargon, eds. *Victorian Science: A Self-portrait from the Presidential Addresses of the British Association for the Advancement of Science.* Garden City, N.Y.: Doubleday & Co., 1970.

Bates, Ralph S. *Scientific Societies in the United States.* 3d ed. Cambridge: MIT Press, 1965.

Bauer, Edward Louis. *Doctors Made in America.* Philadelphia: J. B. Lippincott Co., 1963.

Beach, Mark B. *A Bibliographic Guide to American Colleges and Universities from Colonial Times to the Present.* Westport, Conn.: Greenwood Press, 1975.

———. "Professors, Presidents, and Trustees: A Study of University Governance, 1825–1918." Ph.D. diss., University of Wisconsin, 1966.

Beardsley, Edward H. *The Rise of the American Chemistry Profession, 1850–1900.* University of Florida Monographs, Social Sciences, no. 23. Gainsville: University of Florida Press, 1964.

Beaver, Donald deB. *The American Scientific Community, 1800–1860: A Statistical-Historical Study.* New York: Arno Press, 1980.

Becker, Howard S., and James Carper. "The Elements of Identification with an Occupation." *American Sociological Review* 21 (1956): 341–48.

Beecher, Henry K., and Mark D. Altschule. *Medicine at Harvard: The First Three Hundred Years.* Hanover, N.H.: University Press of New England, 1977.

Bell, Whitfield, J., Jr. "The Medical Institution of Yale College, 1810–1885." *Yale J. Biol. Med.* 33 (1960): 169–83.

Bellot, H. Hale. *University College London, 1826–1926.* London: University of London Press, 1929.

Ben-David, Joseph. *Centers of Learning: Britain, France, Germany, United States.* New York: McGraw–Hill, 1977.

———. *The Scientist's Role in Society: A Comparative Study.* Englewood Cliffs, N.J.: Prentice-Hall, 1971.

———, and Avraham Zloczower. "Universities and Academic Systems in Modern Societies." *European Journal of Sociology* 3 (1972): 45–84.

Benison, Saul. "In Defense of Medical Research." *Harvard Medical Alumni Bulletin* 44 (1970): 16–23.

Benson, Keith R. "American Morphology in the Late Nineteenth Century: The Biology Department at Johns Hopkins University." *J. Hist. Biol.* 18 (1985): 163–205.

————. "Problems of Individual Development: Descriptive Embryological Morphology in America at the Turn of the Century." *J. Hist. Biol.* 14 (1981): 115–28.

Berliner, Howard, S. *A System of Scientific Medicine: Philanthropic Foundations in the Flexner Era.* New York: Tavistock Publications, 1985.

Bernard, Claude. *An Introduction to the Study of Experimental Medicine.* Translated by Henry Copley Greene. New York: Macmillan Co., 1927.

Bibby, Cyril. *T. H. Huxley: Scientist, Humanist, and Educator.* New York: Horizon Press, 1960.

Billroth, Theodor. *The Medical Sciences in the German Universities: A Study in the History of Civilization.* New York: Macmillan Co., 1924.

Bledstein, Burton. *The Culture of Professionalism: The Middle Class and the Development of Higher Education in America.* New York: W. W. Norton, 1976.

Bonner, Thomas Neville. *American Doctors and German Universities: A Chapter in International Intellectual Relations, 1870–1914.* Lincoln: University of Nebraska Press, 1963.

Bordley, James, III, and A. McGehee Harvey. *Two Centuries of American Medicine, 1776–1976.* Philadelphia: W. B. Saunders Co., 1976.

Bowditch, Henry Pickering. *The Life and Writings of Henry Pickering Bowditch.* 2 vols. New York: Arno Press, 1980.

Bowditch, Manfred. "Henry Pickering Bowditch: An Intimate Memoir." *Physiologist* 1 (1958): 7–11.

Bowditch, Vincent Y. *Life and Correspondence of Henry Ingersoll Bowditch.* 2 vols. Boston: Houghton Mifflin, 1902.

Bowers, John Z. "The Influence of Charles W. Eliot on Medical Education." *Pharos* 35 (1972): 156–59.

Bracegirdle, Brian. "The History of Histology: A Brief Survey of Sources." *Hist. Sci.* 15 (1977): 77–101.

Brooks, Chandler McC. "The Development of Physiology in the Last Fifty Years." *Bull. Hist. Med.* 33 (1959): 249–62.

————, and Paul F. Cranefield, eds., *The Historical Development of Physiological Thought.* New York: Hafner Publishing Co., 1959.

Brown, E. Richard. *Rockefeller Medicine Men: Medicine and Capitalism in America.* Berkeley and Los Angeles: University of California Press, 1979.

Brown, W. Norman. *Johns Hopkins Half-Century Directory: A Catalogue of the Trustees, Faculty, Holders of Honorary Degrees, and Students, Graduates and Non-Graduates, 1876–1926.* Baltimore: Johns Hopkins Press, 1926.

Browning, William. "The Relation of Physicians to Early American Geology." *Ann. Med. Hist.* n.s. 3 (1931): 547–67.

Burdon-Sanderson, John. "Ludwig and Modern Physiology." *Science Progress* 5 (1896): 1–21.

Burket, Walter C., ed. *Papers and Addresses by William Henry Welch.* 3 vols. Baltimore: Johns Hopkins Press, 1920.

Burr, Anna Robeson. *Weir Mitchell: His Life and Letters.* New York: Duffield & Co., 1929.

Calhoun, Daniel H. *Professional Lives in America: Structure and Aspiration, 1750–1850.* Cambridge: Harvard University Press, 1975.

Calvert, Monte A. *The Mechanical Engineer in America, 1830–1910: Professional Cultures and Conflict.* Baltimore: Johns Hopkins Press, 1967.

Campbell, Edward D. *History of the Chemical Laboratory of the University of Michigan, 1856–1916.* Ann Arbor: University of Michigan, 1916.

Cannon, Walter B. "President Eliot's Relations to Medicine." *New England Journal of Medicine* 210 (1934): 730–38.

Carson, Gerald. *Men, Beasts, and Gods: A History of Cruelty and Kindness to Animals.* New York: Charles Scribner's Sons, 1972.

Cattell, J. McKeen, ed. *American Men of Science: A Biographical Directory.* New York: Science Press, 1906.

Caullery, Maurice. *Universities and Scientific Life in the United States.* Translated by James Houghton Woods and Emmet Russell. Cambridge: Harvard University Press, 1922.

Chasis, Herbert. "History of Collaboration by Department of Physiology at New York University School of Medicine." *Physiologist* 26 (1983): 64–70.

Chesney, Alan M. *The Johns Hopkins Hospital and the Johns Hopkins University School of Medicine: A Chronicle. Vol. 1. Early Years, 1867–1893.* Baltimore: Johns Hopkins Press, 1943.

————. *The Johns Hopkins Hospital and the Johns Hopkins University School of Medicine: A Chronicle. Vol. 2, 1893–1905.* Baltimore: Johns Hopkins Press, 1958

————. *The Johns Hopkins Hospital and the Johns Hopkins University School of Medicine: A Chronicle. Vol. 3, 1905–1914.* Baltimore: Johns Hopkins Press, 1963.

Chittenden, Russell H. *The Development of Physiological Chemistry in the United States.* New York: Chemical Catalog Co., 1930.

————. *History of the Sheffield Scientific School of Yale University, 1846–1922.* 2 vols. New Haven: Yale University Press, 1928.

Chubin, Daryl E. "The Conceptualization of Scientific Specialties." *Sociological Quarterly* 17 (1976): 448–76.

Cohen, Saul, ed. *Education in the United States: A Documentary History.* 5 vols. New York: Random House, 1974.

Coleman, Sydney, H. *Humane Society Leaders in America: With a Sketch of the Early History of the Humane Movement in England.* Albany: American Humane Association, 1924.

Coleman, William. *Biology in the Nineteenth Century: Problems of Form, Function, and Transformation.* New York: John Wiley & Sons, 1971.

————. "The Cognitive Basis of the Discipline: Claude Bernard on Physiology." *Isis* 76 (1985): 49–70.

————, ed. *Physiological Programmatics of the Nineteenth Century.* New York: Arno Press, 1981.

Conklin, Edwin G. "Fifty Years of the American Society of Naturalists." *Am. Nat.* 68 (1934): 385–401.

Cordasco, Franceso. *The Shaping of American Graduate Education: Daniel Coit Gilman and the Protean Ph.D.* Totowa, N.J.: Rowman & Littlefield, 1973.

———, and David N. Alloway. *Medical Education in the United States: A Guide to Information Sources.* Education Information Guide Series, vol. 8. Detroit: Gale Research Co., 1980.

———, and William W. Brickman. *A Bibliography of American Educational History.* New York: A.M.S. Press, 1975.

Cordell, Eugene Fauntleroy. *The Medical Annals of Maryland, 1799–1899.* Baltimore: Medical & Chirurgical Faculty of Maryland, 1903.

Corner, George W. *A History of the Rockefeller Institute, 1901–1953: Origins and Growth.* New York: Rockefeller Institute Press, 1964.

———. *Two Centuries of Medicine: A History of the School of Medicine, University of Pennsylvania.* Philadelphia: J. B. Lippincott Co., 1965.

Coulson, Thomas. *Joseph Henry: His Life and Work.* Princeton: Princeton University Press, 1950.

Cranefield, Paul F. "The Organic Physics of 1847 and the Biophysics of Today." *J. Hist. Med.* 12 (1957): 407–23.

———. "The Philosophical and Cultural Interests of the Biophysics Movement of 1847." *J. Hist. Med.* 21 (1966): 1–7.

———, English translation ed. *Two Great Scientists of the Nineteenth Century: Correspondence of Emil Du Bois-Reymond and Carl Ludwig.* Edited by Paul Diepgen, translated by Sabine Lichtner-Ayed. Baltimore: Johns Hopkins University Press, 1982.

Cravens, Hamilton. "American Science Comes of Age: An Institutional Perspective, 1850–1930." *American Studies* 17 (1976): 49–70.

———. "The Role of Universities in the Rise of Experimental Biology." *Science Teacher* 44 (1977): 33–37.

Crosland, Maurice P., ed. *The Emergence of Science in Western Europe.* New York: Science History Publications, 1976.

"Curricula of Professional Schools, Medicine." *Report of the Commissioner of Education for the Year 1889–1890,* 875–913. Washington: Government Printing Office, 1893.

Curti, Merle, and Roderick Nash. *Philanthropy in the Shaping of American Higher Education.* New Brunswick: Rutgers University Press, 1965.

Cushing, Harvey. *The Life of Sir William Osler.* 2 vols. Oxford and New York: Oxford University Press, 1925.

Dalton, John C., Jr. *The Experimental Method in Medical Science.* New York: G. P. Putnam's Sons, 1882.

———. *History of the College of Physicians and Surgeons in the City of New York; Medical Department of Columbia College.* New York: College of Physicians and Surgeons, 1888.

Daniels, George H. "Finalism and Positivism in Nineteenth Century American Physiological Thought." *Bull. Hist. Med.* 38 (1964): 343–63.

———. "The Process of Professionalization in American Science: The Emergent Period, 1820–1860." *Isis* 58 (1967): 151–66.

————. *Science in American Society: A Social History*. New York: Alfred A. Knopf, 1971.

————, ed. *Nineteenth-Century American Science: A Reappraisal*. Evanston: Northwestern University Press, 1972.

Davenport, Horace W. "Physiology, 1850–1923: The View from Michigan." *Physiologist* 24, supp. no. 1 (1982): 1–96.

Diehl, Carl. *Americans and German Scholarship, 1770–1870*. New Haven: Yale University Press, 1978.

di Gregorio, Mario A. *T. H. Huxley's Place in Natural Science*. New Haven: Yale University Press, 1984.

Dolby, R.G.A. "The Transmission of Two New Scientific Disciplines from Europe to North America in the Late Nineteenth Century." *Annals of Science* 34 (1977): 287–310.

Dupree, A. Hunter. *Science in the Federal Government: A History of Policies and Activities*. 1957. Reprint. Baltimore: Johns Hopkins University Press, 1986.

Durbin, Paul T., ed. *A Guide to the Culture of Science, Technology, and Medicine*. New York: Free Press, a division of Macmillan Co., 1980.

Eggerth, Arnold H. *The History of the Hoagland Laboratory*. Brooklyn, N.Y., 1960.

Eliot, Charles W. *Educational Reform: Essays and Addresses*. New York: Century Co., 1901.

Elliot, Clark A. "The American Scientist, 1800–1863: His Origins, Career, and Interests." Ph.D. diss., Case Western Reserve University, 1970.

Ellis, Frederick W. "Henry Pickering Bowditch and the Development of the Harvard Laboratory of Physiology." *New England Journal of Medicine* 219 (1938): 819–28.

Eulner, Hans-Heinz. *Die Entwicklung der medizinischen Specialfächer an den Universitäten des Deutschen Sprachgebietes*. Stuttgart: Ferdinand Enke, 1970.

Faber, Knud. *Nosography: The Evolution of Clinical Medicine in Modern Times*. 2d ed. New York: Paul B. Hoeber, 1930.

Farber, Paul L. "The Transformation of Natural History in the Nineteenth Century." *J. Hist. Biol.* 15 (1982): 145–52.

Fearing, Franklin. *Reflex Action: A Study in the History of Physiological Psychology*. Baltimore: Williams & Wilkins Co., 1930.

Fishbein, Morris. *A History of the American Medical Association, 1847–1947*. Philadelphia: W. B. Saunders Co., 1947.

Fleming, Donald. *William H. Welch and the Rise of Medicine*. Boston: Little, Brown & Co., 1954. Reprint. Baltimore: Johns Hopkins University Press, 1987.

Flexner, Abraham. *Daniel Coit Gilman: Creator of the American Type of University*. New York: Harcourt, Brace & Co., 1946.

————. *Medical Education: A Comparative Study*. New York: Macmillan Co., 1925.

————. *Medical Education in Europe: A Report to the Carnegie Foundation for the Advancement of Teaching.* Bull. no. 6. New York: Carnegie Foundation for the Advancement of Teaching, 1912.

———. *Medical Education in the United States and Canada: A Report to the Carnegie Foundation for the Advancement of Teaching.* Bull. no. 4. New York: Carnegie Foundation for the Advancement of Teaching, 1910.

Flexner, Simon, and James Thomas Flexner. *William Henry Welch and the Heroic Age of American Medicine.* New York: Viking Press, 1941.

Foster, Michael. *Claude Bernard.* London: T. Fisher Unwin, 1899.

———. "Progress of Physiology during the Last Thirteen Years." *Brit. Med. J.* 2 (1897): 445–50.

———. "Reminiscences of a Physiologist." *Colorado Medical Journal* 6 (1900): 419–29.

Franklin, Fabian. *The Life of Daniel Coit Gilman.* New York: Dodd, Mead & Co., 1910.

Franklin, Kenneth J. "A Short History of the International Congresses of Physiologists." *Annals of Science* 3 (1938): 241–335.

French, John C. *A History of the University Founded by Johns Hopkins.* Baltimore: Johns Hopkins Press, 1946.

French, Richard D. *Antivivisection and Medical Science in Victorian Society.* Princeton: Princeton University Press, 1975.

———. "Some Problems and Sources in the Foundations of Modern Physiology in Great Britain." *Hist. Sci.* 10 (1971): 28–55.

Fulton, John F. "A Note on the Origin of the Term 'Physiology,'" *Yale J. Biol. Med.* 3 (1930): 59–61.

———. *Physiology.* New York: Paul B. Hoeber, 1931.

Funkenstein, Daniel. *Medical Students, Medical Schools and Society during Five Eras: Factors Affecting the Career Choices of Physicians, 1958–1976.* Cambridge, Mass.: Ballinger, 1978.

Galdston, Iago. "Research in the United States." *CIBA Symposia* 8 (1946): 362–72.

Garrison, Fielding H. *John Shaw Billings: A Memoir.* New York: G. P. Putnam's Sons, 1915.

———. "Sir Michael Foster and the Cambridge School of Physiologists." *Maryland Medical Journal* 58 (1915): 106–18.

Geison, Gerald. "Divided We Stand: Physiologists and Clinicians in the American Context." In *The Therapeutic Revolution: Essays in the Social History of Medicine,* edited by Morris J. Vogel and Charles E. Rosenberg, 67–90. Philadelphia: University of Pennsylvania Press, 1979.

———. *Michael Foster and the Cambridge School of Physiology: The Scientific Enterprise in Late Victorian Society.* Princeton: Princeton University Press, 1978.

———. "Scientific Change, Emerging Specialties, and Research Schools." *Hist. Sci.* 19 (1981): 20–40.

Gerard, Ralph W. *Mirror to Physiology: A Self-Survey of Physiological Science.* Washington: American Physiological Society, 1958.

Gifford, George E., Jr. "Medicine and Natural History: Crosscurrents in Philadelphia in the Nineteenth Century." *Trans. Coll. Phys. Phila.* 4th ser., 45 (1978), 139–49.

Gilman, Daniel Coit. *The Launching of a University and Other Papers: A Sheaf of Remembrances*. New York: Dodd, Mead & Co., 1906.

———. *University Problems in the United States*. New York: Century Co., 1898.

Goodfield, G. J. *The Growth of Scientific Physiology: Physiological Method and the Mechanist-Vitalist Controversy, Illustrated by the Problems of Respiration and Animal Heat*. 1960. Reprint. New York: Arno Press, 1975.

Gougher, Ronald L. "Comparison of English and American Views of the German University, 1840–1865: A Bibliography." *History of Education Quarterly* 4 (1969): 477–91.

Gould, George L., ed. *The Jefferson Medical College of Philadelphia, Benefactors, Alumni, Hospitals, Etc., Its Founders, Officers, Instructors, 1826–1904: A History*. 2 vols. New York: Lewis Publishing Co., 1904.

Gregg, Alan. The Furtherance of Medical Research. New Haven: Yale University Press, 1944.

Gregory, Frederick. *Scientific Materialism in Nineteenth Century Germany*. Studies in the History of Modern Science. Vol. 1. Boston: D. Reidel Publishing Co., 1977.

Gross, Michael. "The Lessened Locus of Feelings: A Transformation in French Physiology in the Early Nineteenth Century." *J. Hist. Biol.* 12 (1979): 231–71.

Guralnick, Stanley M. "The American Scientist in Higher Education, 1820–1910." In *The Sciences in the American Context: New Perspectives*, edited by Nathan Reingold, 99–141. Washington: Smithsonian Institution Press, 1979.

Haines, George, IV. *Essays on German Influence upon English Education and Science, 1850–1919*. Connecticut College Monograph, no. 9. Hamden, Conn.: Shoe String Press, 1969.

Hall, Thomas S. *Ideas of Life and Matter: Studies in the History of General Physiology, 600 B.C.–1900 A.D.* 2 vols. Chicago: University of Chicago Press, 1969.

Haller, John S., Jr. *American Medicine in Transition, 1840–1910*. Urbana: University of Illinois Press, 1981.

Harrington, Thomas Francis. *The Harvard Medical School: A History, Narrative, and Documentary*. Edited by James Gregory Mumford. 3 vols. New York: Lewis Publishing Co., 1905.

The Harvard Medical School, 1782–1906. Boston: Harvard Medical School, 1906.

Harvey, A. McGehee. *Adventures in Medical Research: A Century of Discovery at Johns Hopkins*. Baltimore: Johns Hopkins University Press, 1976.

———. *Research and Discovery in Medicine: Contributions from Johns Hopkins*. Baltimore: Johns Hopkins University Press, 1981.

———. *Science at the Bedside: Clinical Research in American Medicine, 1905–1945*. Baltimore: Johns Hopkins University Press, 1981.

Haskell, Thomas L. *The Emergence of Professional Social Science: The American Social Science Association and the Nineteenth-Century Crisis of Authority.* Urbana: University of Illinois Press, 1977.

Hawkins, Hugh. *Between Harvard and America: The Educational Leadership of Charles Eliot.* New York: Oxford University Press, 1972.

————. *Pioneer: A History of the Johns Hopkins University, 1874–1889.* Ithaca: Cornell University Press, 1960.

————. "University Identity: The Teaching and Research Functions." In *The Organization of Knowledge in Modern America, 1860–1920*, edited by Alexandra Oleson and John Voss, 285–312. Baltimore: Johns Hopkins University Press, 1979.

Hemmeter, John C. "Tendencies of Modern Physiological Discipline in Medical Schools." *N.Y. Med. J.* 96 (1912): 1153–59.

Henry, Frederick P. *Founders' Week Memorial Volume, Containing an Account of the Two Hundred and Twenty-Fifth Anniversary of the Founding of the City of Philadelphia, and Histories of Its Principal Scientific Institutions, Medical Colleges, Hospitals, etc.* Philadelphia, 1909.

Hering, Ewald. "Das Physiologische Institut." In *Festschrift zur Feier des 500 Jährigen Bestehens der Universität Leipzig Herausgegeben von Rektor und Senat.* 3 vols. Leipzig: S. Hirzel, 1909, 3:21–38.

History of the American Physiological Society Semicentennial, 1887–1937. Baltimore, 1938.

Hoff, Hebbel. "Medical Progress a Century Ago: The Physiological Laboratory Comes to America." *Connecticut Medicine* 36 (1972): 57–60, 109–13.

Hollis, Ernest Victor. *Philanthropic Foundations and Higher Education.* New York: Columbia University Press, 1938.

Honan, James Henry. *Honan's Handbook to Medical Europe: A Ready Reference Book to the Universities, Hospitals, Clinics, Laboratories and General Medical Work of the Principal Cities of Europe.* Philadelphia: P. Blakiston's Son & Co., 1912.

Howell, William H. "The American Physiological Society during Its First Twenty-Five Years." In *History of the American Physiological Society Semicentennial, 1887–1937*, 1–89. Baltimore, 1938.

Hudson, Robert P. "Abraham Flexner in Perspective: American Medical Education, 1865–1910." *Bull. Hist. Med.* 46 (1972): 545–61.

Hughes, Arthur F. W. *The American Biologist through Four Centuries.* Springfield, Ill.: Charles C Thomas, 1982.

Hun, Henry. *A Guide to American Medical Students in Europe.* New York: William Wood & Co., 1883.

Huxley, Leonard. *Life and Letters of Thomas Henry Huxley.* 2 vols. New York: D. Appleton & Co., 1901.

Huxley, Thomas H. *Science and Education: Essays* [1893]. New York: D. Appleton & Co., 1910.

James, Henry. *Charles W. Eliot, President of Harvard University, 1869–1909.* 2 vols. Boston: Houghton Mifflin, 1930.

Jones, Russell M. "American Doctors in Paris, 1820–1861: A Statistical Profile." *J. Hist. Med.* 25 (1970): 143–57.

Kaufman, Martin. *American Medical Education: The Formative Years, 1765–1910.* Westport, Conn.: Greenwood Press, 1976.

Kelly, Howard A., and Walter A. Burrage, eds. *Dictionary of American Medical Biography: Lives of Eminent Physicians of the United States and Canada, from the Earliest Times.* New York: D. Appleton & Co., 1928.

Kett, Joseph F. *The Formation of the American Medical Profession: The Role of Institutions, 1780–1860.* New Haven: Yale University Press, 1968.

King, Lester S. *American Medicine Comes of Age, 1840–1920: Essays to Commemorate the Founding of "The Journal of the American Medical Association," July 14, 1883.* Chicago: American Medical Association, 1984.

Kohler, Robert E. *From Medical Chemistry to Biochemistry: The Making of a Biomedical Discipline.* New York: Cambridge University Press, 1982.

Kohlstedt, Sally Gregory. *The Formation of the American Scientific Community: The American Association for the Advancement of Science, 1848–60.* Urbana: University of Illinois Press, 1976.

———. "The Nineteenth-Century Amateur Tradition: The Case of the Boston Society of Natural History." In *Science and Its Public: The Changing Relationship,* edited by Gerald Holton and William A. Blanpied. Boston Studies in the Philosophy of Science. Vol. 33, 173–90. Boston: D. Reidel Publishing Co., 1976.

Kuritz, Hyman. "The Popularization of Science in Nineteenth-Century America." *History of Education Quarterly* 21 (1981): 259–74.

Lankford, John. "Amateurs and Astrophysics: A Neglected Aspect in the Development of a Scientific Specialty." *Social Studies of Science* 11 (1981): 275–303.

Larson, Magla Sarfatti. *The Rise of Professionalism: A Sociological Analysis.* Berkeley and Los Angeles: University of California Press, 1977.

Leavitt, Emily S. *Animals and Their Legal Rights. Animal Welfare Institute. A Survey of American Laws from 1641 to 1978.* 3d ed. Washington: Animal Welfare Institute, 1978.

Leikind, Morris. "The Evolution of Medical Research in the United States." *International Record of Medicine* 171 (1958): 455–68.

Lemaine, Gerard; Roy Macleod; Michael Mulkay; and Peter Weingart, eds. *Perspectives on the Emergence of Scientific Disciplines.* Maison des Sciences de l'Homme, Paris Publications no. 4. Chicago: Aldine, 1977.

Lenoir, Timothy. "Teleology without Regrets: The Transformation of Physiology in Germany, 1790–1847." *Studies in the History and Philosophy of Science* 12 (1981): 293–354.

Lepore, Michael J. *Death of the Clinician: Requiem or Reveille?* Springfield, Ill.: Charles C Thomas, 1982.

Lesch, John E. *Science and Medicine in France: The Emergence of Experimental Physiology, 1790–1855.* Cambridge: Harvard University Press, 1984.

Lesky, Erna. *The Vienna Medical School of the Nineteenth Century.* Baltimore: Johns Hopkins University Press, 1976.

Lombard, Warren P. "The Life and Work of Carl Ludwig." *Science* n.s. 4 (1916): 363–75.

Long, Esmond R. *A History of American Pathology*. Springfield, Ill.: Charles C
Thomas, 1962.

Ludmerer, Kenneth M. *Learning to Heal: The Development of American Medical Education*. New York: Basic Books, 1985.

———. "Reform at Harvard Medical School, 1869–1909." *Bull. Hist. Med.* 55
(1981): 343–70.

Lurie, Edward. *Louis Agassiz: A Life in Science*. Chicago, University of Chicago Press, 1960.

McCaughey, Robert A. "The Transformation of American Academic Life: Harvard University, 1821–1892." *Perspectives in American History* 8 (1974):
239–332.

MacLeod, Roy M. "Resources of Science in Victorian England: The Endowment of Science Movement, 1868–1900." In *Science and Society, 1600–
1900*, edited by Peter Mathias, 110–66. Cambridge and New York: Cambridge University Press, 1972.

Magel, Charles R. *A Bibliography on Animal Rights and Related Matters*.
Washington: University Press of America, 1981.

Markowitz, Gerald E., and David K. Rosner. "Doctors in Crisis: A Study of the
Use of Medical Education Reform to Establish Modern Professional Elitism
in Medicine." *American Quarterly* 25 (1973): 83–107.

Meek, Walter J. "The Beginnings of American Physiology." *Ann. Med. Hist.* 10
(1928): 111–25.

A Memoir of Henry Jacob Bigelow. Boston: Little, Brown & Co., 1900.

"A Memorial of George Brown Goode, Together with a Selection of His Papers
on Museums and on the History of Science in America." *Annual Report of
the Board of Regents of the Smithsonian Institution. Report of the U.S.
National Museum*. Part 2. Washington: Government Printing Office,
1901.

Mendelsohn, Everett. "The Biological Sciences in the Nineteenth Century:
Some Problems and Sources," *Hist. Sci.* 3 (1964): 39–59.

———. "The Emergence of Science as a Profession in Nineteenth-Century Europe." In *The Management of Scientists*, edited by Karl Hill, 3–48. Boston:
Beacon Press, 1964.

Merz, John Theodore. *History of European Scientific Thought in the Nineteenth Century*. 1904–1912. Reprint. 4 vols. Gloucester, Mass.: Peter
Smith, 1976.

Miller, Howard S. *Dollars for Research: Science and Its Patrons in Nineteenth-
Century America*. Seattle: University of Washington Press, 1970.

Morison, Samuel Eliot. *The Development of Harvard University Since the Inauguration of President Eliot, 1869–1929*. Cambridge: Harvard University
Press, 1930.

Mosley, Russell. "From Avocation to Job: The Changing Nature of Scientific
Practice." *Social Studies of Science* 9 (1979): 511–22.

Newman, Charles. *The Evolution of Medical Education in the Nineteenth Century*. New York and London: Oxford University Press, 1957.

Norwood, William Frederick. *Medical Education in the United States before
the Civil War*. Philadelphia: University of Pennsylvania Press, 1944.

Numbers, Ronald L. "Together But Not Equal: Amateurs and Professionals in Early American Scientific Societies." *Reviews in American History* 4 (1976): 497–503.

————, ed. *The Education of American Physicians: Historical Essays*. Berkeley and Los Angeles: University of California Press, 1980.

————, and John Harley Warner. "The Maturation of American Medical Science." In *Sickness and Health in America: Readings in the History of Medicine and Public Health*. 2d ed. Edited by Judith Walzer Leavitt and Ronald L. Numbers, 113–25. Madison: University of Wisconsin Press, 1985.

Ober, William B. "American Pathology in the Nineteenth Century: Notes for the Definition of a Specialty." *Bull. N. Y. Acad. Med.* 52 (1976): 326–47.

O'Hara, Leo James. "An Emerging Profession: Philadelphia Medicine, 1860–1900." Ph.D. diss., University of Pennsylvania, 1976.

Oleson, Alexandra, and Sanborn C. Brown, eds. *The Pursuit of Knowledge in the Early American Republic: American Scientific and Learned Societies from Colonial Times to the Civil War*. Baltimore: Johns Hopkins University Press, 1976.

————, and John Voss, eds. *The Organization of Knowledge in Modern America, 1860–1920*. Baltimore: Johns Hopkins University Press, 1979.

Olmsted, James M.D. *Charles-Edouard Brown-Séquard: A Nineteenth-Century Neurologist and Endocrinologist*. Baltimore: Johns Hopkins Press, 1946.

————. *François Magendie: Pioneer in Experimental Physiology and Scientific Medicine in Nineteenth-Century France*. New York: Schuman's, 1944.

————. "Physiology as an Independent Science." In *Science in the University by Members of the Faculties of the University of California*, 293–303. Berkeley and Los Angeles: University of California Press, 1944.

————, and E. Harris Olmsted. *Claude Bernard and the Experimental Method in Medicine*. New York: Henry Schuman, 1952.

O'Malley, Charles D., ed. *The History of Medical Education*. UCLA Forum in Medical Sciences, no. 12. Berkeley and Los Angeles: University of California Press, 1970.

Parascandola, John, and Elizabeth Keeney. *Sources in the History of American Pharmacology*. Madison, Wis.: American Institute of the History of Pharmacy, 1983.

Paul, Harry W. *The Sorcerer's Apprentice: The French Scientist's Image of German Science, 1840–1919*. University of Florida Social Sciences Monograph, no. 44. Gainesville: University of Florida Press, 1972.

Paul, Robert. "German Academic Science and the Mandarin Ethos, 1850–1880." *British Journal of the History of Science* 17 (1984): 1–29.

Paulsen, Frederich. *The German Universities and University Study*. Translated by Frank Thilly and William L. Elwang. New York: Charles Scribner's Sons, 1906.

Pauly, Philip J. "The Appearance of Academic Biology in Late Nineteenth-Century America." *J. Hist. Biol.* 17 (1984): 369–97.

Price, Derek J. De Solla. *Little Science, Big Science.* New York: Columbia University Press, 1963.

Prudden, Lillian E., ed. *Biographical Sketches and Letters of T. Mitchell Prudden, M.D.* New Haven: Yale University Press, 1927.

Radbill, Samuel X. "The Autobiographical Ana of Robley Dunglison, M.D." *Trans. Am. Philo. Soc.* 53, part 8 (1963): 1–212.

Rather, Lelland J. *Disease, Life, and Man: Selected Essays by Rudolf Virchow.* Stanford: Stanford University Press, 1958.

Rattner, Sidney. "Evolution and the Rise of the Scientific Spirit in America." *Philosophy of Science* 3 (1936): 104–22.

Reingold, Nathan. "Definitions and Speculations: The Professionalization of Science in America in the Nineteenth-Century." In *The Pursuit of Knowledge in the Early American Republic: American Scientific and Learned Societies from Colonial Times to the Civil War*, edited by Alexandra Oleson and Sanborn C. Brown, 33–69. Baltimore: Johns Hopkins University Press, 1976.

———. *Science in Nineteenth-Century America: A Documentary History.* London: Macmillan Co., 1966.

———, ed. *Science in America Since 1820.* New York: Science History Publications, 1976.

Reiser, Stanley Joel. *Medicine and the Reign of Technology.* New York and Cambridge: Cambridge University Press, 1978.

Richards, Stewart. "Drawing the Life-Blood of Physiology: Vivisection and the Physiologists' Dilemma, 1870–1900." *Annals of Science* 43 (1986): 27–56.

Richmond, Phyllis A. "The Nineteenth-Century American Physician as a Research Scientist." In *History of American Medicine: A Symposium*, edited by Felix Marti-Ibanez, 142–55. New York: MD Publications, 1959.

Robinson, G. Canby. *Adventures in Medical Education: A Personal Narrative of the Great Advance of American Medicine.* Cambridge: Harvard University Press, 1957.

Roderick, Gordon W., and Michael D. Stephens. *Scientific and Technical Education in Nineteenth-Century England.* New York: Barnes & Noble, 1973.

Rosen, George. "Carl Ludwig and His American Students." *Bull. Hist. Med.* 4 (1936): 609–50.

———. "Changing Attitudes of the Medical Profession to Specialization." *Bull. Hist. Med.* 12 (1942): 342–54.

———. "Special Medical Societies in the United States after 1860." *CIBA Symposia* 9 (1947): 785–92.

———. *The Specialization of Medicine with Particular Reference to Ophthalmology.* New York: Froben Press, 1944.

———. *The Structure of American Medical Practice, 1875–1941.* Edited by Charles E. Rosenberg. Philadelphia: University of Pennsylvania Press, 1983.

Rosenberg, Charles E. *No Other Gods: On Science and American Social Thought.* Baltimore: Johns Hopkins University Press, 1976.

———. "Science and Social Values in Nineteenth-Century America: A Case

Study in the Growth of Scientific Institutions." In *Science and Values: Patterns of Tradition and Change*, edited by Arnold Thackray and Everett Mendelsohn, 21–42. New York: Humanities Press, 1975.

Ross, Sydney. "*Scientist:* The Story of a Word." *Annals of Science* 18 (1962): 65–85.

Rossiter, Margaret W. *The Emergence of Agricultural Science: Justus Liebig and the Americans, 1840–1880.* New Haven: Yale University Press, 1975.

Rothschuh, Karl E. *Entwicklungsgeschichte Physiologischer Probleme in Tabellenform.* Munich: Urban & Schwarzenberg, 1952.

———. *History of Physiology.* Translated and edited by Guenter B. Risse. Huntington, N.Y.: Robert E. Krieger Publishing Co., 1973.

Rothstein, William G. *American Physicians in the Nineteenth Century: From Sects to Science.* Baltimore: Johns Hopkins University Press, 1972.

———. "Pathology, the Evolution of a Specialty in American Medicine." *Medical Care* 17 (1979): 975–88.

Russell, Colin A. *Science and Social Change in Britain and Europe, 1700–1900.* New York: St. Martin's Press, 1983.

Ryan, W. Carson. *Studies in Early Graduate Education: The Johns Hopkins, Clark University, the University of Chicago.* Bull. no. 30. New York: Carnegie Foundation for the Advancement of Teaching, 1930.

Sabin, Florence Rene. *Franklin Paine Mall: The Story of a Mind.* Baltimore: Johns Hopkins Press, 1934.

Schiller, Joseph. "Claude Bernard and Brown-Séquard: The Chair of General Physiology and the Experimental Method." *J. Hist. Med.* 21 (1966): 260–70.

———. "The Genesis and Structure of Claude Bernard's Experimental Method." In *Foundations of Scientific Method: The Nineteenth Century*, edited by Ronald N. Giere and Richard S. Westfall, 133–60. Bloomington: Indiana University Press, 1973.

———. "The Influence of Physiology on Medicine." *Episteme* 6 (1972): 116–27.

———. "Physiology's Struggle for Independence in the First Half of the Nineteenth Century." *Hist. Sci.* 7 (1968): 64–89.

Schröer, Heinz. *Carl Ludwig: Begründer der Messenden Experimentalphysiologie, 1816–1895.* Grosse Naturforscher. Vol. 33. Stuttgart: Wissenschaftlische Verlagsgessellschaft M. B. H., 1967.

Sewall, Henry. "The Beginnings of Physiological Research in America." *Science* n.s. 58 (1923): 187–95.

Sharpey-Schafer, Edward. *History of the Physiological Society during Its First Fifty Years, 1876–1926.* Supplement to *Journal of Physiology.* London: Cambridge University Press, 1927.

Shortt, Samuel E. D. "Physicians, Science, and Status: Issues in the Professionalization of Anglo-American Medicine in the Nineteenth Century." *Med. Hist.* 27 (1983): 51–68.

Shrady, John, ed. *The College of Physicians and Surgeons, New York, and Its Founders, Officers, Instructors, Benefactors and Alumni: A History.* 2 vols. New York: Lewis Publishing Co., c. 1903.

Shryock, Richard H. "The Advent of Modern Medicine in Philadelphia, 1800–1850." *Yale J. Biol. Med.* 13 (1941): 715–38.

―――. *American Medical Research, Past and Present.* New York: Commonwealth Fund, 1947.

―――. "The History of Quantification in Medical Science." *Isis* 52 (1961): 215–37.

―――. "The Interplay of Social and Internal Factors in Modern Medicine: An Historical Analysis." *Centaurus* 3 (1953): 107–25.

―――. *The Unique Influence of the Johns Hopkins University on American Medicine.* Copenhagen: Ejnar Munksgaard, 1953.

Shultz, William J. *The Humane Movement in the United States, 1910–1922.* New York: Columbia University Press, 1924.

Starr, Paul. *The Social Transformation of American Medicine.* New York: Basic Books, 1982.

Stevens, Rosemary. *American Medicine and the Public Interest.* New Haven: Yale University Press, 1971.

Stevenson, Lloyd G. "Physiology, General Education and the Anti-Vivisection Movement." *Clio Medica* 12 (1977): 17–31.

Stirling, William. "Carl Ludwig, Professor of Physiology in the University of Leipzig." *Science Progress* 4 (1895): 11–64.

Storr, Richard J. *The Beginnings of Graduate Education in America.* Chicago: University of Chicago Press, 1953.

―――. *Harper's University, the Beginnings: A History of the University of Chicago.* Chicago: University of Chicago Press, 1966.

Swanson, Carl P. "A History of Biology at the Johns Hopkins University." *Bios* 22 (1951): 223–62.

Taylor, D. W. "The Life and Teaching of William Sharpey (1802–1880): 'Father of Modern Physiology' in Britain." *Medical History* 15 (1971): 126–53, 241–59.

Temkin, Owsei. "Materialism in French and German Physiology of the Early Nineteenth Century." *Bull. Hist. Med.* 20 (1946): 322–27.

―――. "The Philosophical Background of Magendie's Physiology." *Bull. Hist. Med.* 20 (1946): 10–35.

Thwing, Charles Franklin. *The American and the German University: One Hundred Years of History.* New York: Macmillan Co., 1928.

Tobey, Ronald C. *The American Ideology of National Science, 1919–1930.* Pittsburgh: University of Pittsburgh Press, 1971.

Turner, G. L'E, ed. *The Patronage of Science in the Nineteenth Century.* Leiden: Noordhoff International Publishing, 1976.

Turner, James. *Animals, Pain, and Humanity in the Victorian Mind: Reckoning with the Beast.* Baltimore: Johns Hopkins University Press, 1980.

Turner, Steven; Edward Kerwin; and David Woolwine. "Careers and Creativity in Nineteenth-Century Physiology: Zloczower *Redux,*" *Isis* 75 (1984): 523–29.

Veysey, Lawrence R. *The Emergence of the American University.* Chicago: University of Chicago Press, 1965.

SECONDARY SOURCES   295

Visher, Stephen Sargent. *Scientists Starred, 1903–1943, in "American Men of Science": A Study of Collegiate and Doctoral Training, Birthplace, Distribution, Backgrounds, and Developmental Influences.* Baltimore: Johns Hopkins Press, 1947.

Vivisection. Hearing before the Senate Committee on the District of Columbia, February 21, 1900, on the Bill (S. 34) for the Further Prevention of Cruelty to Animals in the District of Columbia. Washington, D.C.: Government Printing Office, 1900.

Vivisection: The Royal Society for the Prevention of Cruelty to Animals and the Royal Commission. London: Smith Elder & Co., 1876.

Vogel, Morris J., and Charles E. Rosenberg, eds. *The Therapeutic Revolution: Essays in the Social History of American Medicine.* Philadelphia: University of Pennsylvania Press, 1979.

Warner, John Harley. "Science in Medicine." *Osiris* 2d ser., 1 (1985): 37–58.

Wartman, William B. *Medical Teaching in Western Civilization: A History Prepared from the Writings of Ancient & Modern Authors.* Chicago: Yearbook Medical Publishers, 1961.

Webb, Gerald B., and Desmond Powell. *Henry Sewall: Physiologist and Physician.* Baltimore: Johns Hopkins Press, 1946.

Westacott, E. *A Century of Vivisection and Anti-Vivisection: A Study of Their Effect upon Science, Medicine and Human Life during the Past Hundred Years.* Ashingdon, England: C. W. Daniel Co., 1949.

Wiebe, Robert H. *The Search for Order, 1877–1920.* New York: Hill & Wang, 1967.

Wiggers, Carl J. "The Evolution of Experimental Physiology at the University of Michigan and Western Reserve University." *Bulletin of the Cleveland Medical Library* 10 (1963): 5–18.

Wilson, Leonard G., ed. *Benjamin Silliman and His Circle: Studies on the Influence of Benjamin Silliman on Science in America.* New York: Science History Publications, 1979.

Index

Abel, John Jacob, 190, 198, 207
Academy of Natural Sciences of Philadelphia, 31, 55, 60, 63, 69, 82
Agassiz, Louis, 2, 64, 68, 93, 98, 140, 154, 171; and Mitchell, 64, 68–69
Allen, Harrison, 63, 86, 87, 132
Alumni. *See* Medical education, alumni
American Academy of Arts and Sciences, 31
American Association for the Advancement of Science, 96, 170, 176–77, 178
American Chemical Society, 176
American Institute for the Cultivation of Science, 170
American Journal of Physiology, 201–3, 227
American Medical Association (AMA), 121, 211; and antivivisection movement, 46, 219–20; Committee on Experimental Medicine, 46; Committee on International Congress of 1887, 178–80; Committee on Medical Literature, 31–32; Committee on Medical Research, 223–24; Council on Defense of Medical Research, 219; Council on Medical Education, 26, 212–13, 217, 218; and reformers, 211–12, 219, 220; on specialization, 98; Welch as president of, 218
American Philosophical Society, 55, 62

American Physiological Society (APS)
—and career opportunities, 192, 195, 200–201, 207
—conception of, 168–69
—formalizes networks of scientists, 13, 181, 195
—founding members of, 171, 231–32; characteristics of, 186–87; institutional affiliations of, 76, 184, 185, 186, 187, 188, 190, 233
—founding of, 6, 168–70, 180–83; meeting for (1887), 168, 181, 184–85
—meetings of: agenda, 184; patterns of attendance, 189–90, 234; timing of, 189
—members' contributions to other fields, 228–30
—membership: of amateurs vs. professionals, 169, 181–82, 183, 193; benefits of, 169–70, 183–84, 225; eligibility criteria, 185, 186; growth of, 190; institutional affiliation of, 233
—prizes for research, 194
—role of, in vivisection debate, 170, 175–76, 183, 190–92, 219
American Society for the Prevention of Cruelty to Animals (ASPCA), 35
American Society for the Restriction of Vivisection, 175
American Society of Naturalists, 178
American Surgical Association, 180